Magnetic Resonance Imaging in Stroke

Magnetic resonance imaging (MRI) provides non-invasive information about the brain's blood flow, water movement and biochemical abnormalities following stroke, and advances in MRI are transforming the investigation and treatment of cerebrovascular disease. Echoplanar techniques with diffusion- and perfusion-weighted imaging, together with developments in magnetic resonance spectroscopy and angiography, are replacing CT scanning as the diagnostic modality of choice. In this profusely illustrated book, world leaders in these technologies review the scientific basis and clinical applications of MRI in stroke. It will appeal to a broad readership including stroke physicians, neurologists, neurosurgeons, rehabilitation specialists, and others with a clinical or research interest in cerebrovascular disease.

Stephen Davis is Professor of Neurology at the University of Melbourne. He heads the Stroke Research Group and is Co-Director of the Brain Imaging Laboratory at the Royal Melbourne Hospital, where he is Director of Neurology.

Marc Fisher is Professor of Neurology at the University of Massachusetts, and a leading authority on the use of MRI in the evaluation of stroke therapies.

Steven Warach is Chief of the Section on Stroke Diagnostics and Therapeutics in the Stroke Branch at NINDS, National Institutes of Health, Bethesda, Maryland. He pioneered the use of diffusion and perfusion MRI in the evaluation of stroke and in clinical trials.

Magnetic Resonance Imaging in Stroke

Edited by

Stephen Davis
University of Australia, Melbourne

Marc Fisher
University of Massachusetts Memorial Medical Care, USA

Steven Warach
National Institutes of Health, Bethesda, MD, USA

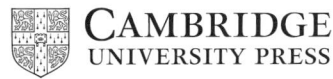

PUBLISHED BY THE PRESS SYNDICATE OF THE UNIVERSITY OF CAMBRIDGE
The Pitt Building, Trumpington Street, Cambridge, United Kingdom

CAMBRIDGE UNIVERSITY PRESS
The Edinburgh Building, Cambridge CB2 2RU, UK
40 West 20th Street, New York, NY 10011–4211, USA
477 Williamstown Road, Port Melbourne, VIC 3207, Australia
Ruiz de Alarcón 13, 28014 Madrid, Spain
Dock House, The Waterfront, Cape Town 8001, South Africa

http://www.cambridge.org

© Cambridge University Press 2003

This book is in copyright. Subject to statutory exception
and to the provisions of relevant collective licensing agreements,
no reproduction of any part may take place without
the written permission of Cambridge University Press.

First published 2003

Printed in the United Kingdom at the University Press, Cambridge

Typeface Utopia 9.5/14pt   System QuarkXPress® [SE]

A catalogue record for this book is available from the British Library

Library of Congress Cataloguing in Publication data
Magnetic resonance imaging in stroke / edited by Stephen Davis,
Marc Fisher, Stephen Warach.
     p.   cm.
  Includes bibliographical references and index.
  ISBN 0 521 80683 6
  1. Cerebrovascular disease – Magnetic resonance imaging. I. Davis,
Stephen M. II. Fisher, Marc. III. Warach, Steven.

RC388.5 .M246 2002
616.8′1–dc21   2002023435

ISBN 0 521 80683 6 hardback

Every effort has been made in preparing this book to provide accurate and
up-to-date information which is in accord with accepted standards and
practice at the time of publication. Nevertheless, the authors, editors and
publisher can make no warranties that the information contained herein is
totally free from error, not least because clinical standards are constantly
changing through research and regulation. The authors, editors and
publisher therefore disclaim all liability for direct or consequential
damages resulting from the use of material contained in this book. Readers
are strongly advised to pay careful attention to information provided by
the manufacturer of any drugs or equipment that they plan to use.

Contents

List of contributors	*page* vii
Preface	xiii

1 The importance of specific diagnosis in stroke patient management — 1
John N. Fink and Louis R. Caplan

2 Limitations of current brain imaging modalities in stroke — 15
P. Alan Barber and Stephen M. Davis

3 Clinical efficacy of CT in acute cerebral ischemia — 31
Rüdiger von Kummer

4 Computerized tomographic-based evaluation of cerebral blood flow — 47
Lawrence R. Wechsler, Steven Goldstein and Howard Yonas

5 Technical introduction to MRI — 55
Rohit Sood and Michael Moseley

6 Clinical use of standard MRI — 69
Brian M. Tress

7 MR angiography of the head and neck: basic principles and clinical applications — 85
Robert R. Edelman and Joel Meyer

8 Stroke MRI in intracranial hemorrhage — 103
Peter D. Schellinger, Olav Jansen and Werner Hacke

9 Using diffusion-perfusion MRI in animal models for drug development — 113
Marc Fisher

10 **Localization of stroke syndromes using diffusion-weighted MR imaging (DWI)** 121
Max Wintermark, Marc Reichhart, Reto Meuli and Julien Bogousslavsky

11 **MRI in transient ischemic attacks: clinical utility and insights into pathophysiology** 135
Jeffrey L. Saver and Chelsea Kidwell

12 **Perfusion-weighted MRI in stroke** 147
William A. Copen and A. Gregory Sorensen

13 **Perfusion imaging with arterial spin labelling** 161
David C. Alsop and John A. Detre

14 **Clinical role of echoplanar MRI in stroke** 175
Stephen Davis and Mark Parsons

15 **The ischemic penumbra: the evolution of a concept** 191
Geoffrey A. Donnan, Peter M. Wright, Romesh Markus, Thanh Phan and David C. Reutens

16 **New MR techniques to select patients for thrombolysis in acute stroke** 207
Vincent N. Thijs and Gregory W. Albers

17 **MRI as a tool in stroke drug development** 223
Steven Warach

18 **Magnetic resonance spectroscopy in stroke** 233
Dawn E. Saunders and Martin M. Brown

19 **Functional MRI and stroke** 251
Amy Brodtmann, Leeanne Carey and David G. Darby

Index 263
Colour figures between pp. 120 and 121.

Contributors

Stephen M. Davis,
Department of Neurology,
Royal Melbourne Hospital,
Parkville,
Victoria 3050,
Australia

Marc Fisher,
Department of Neurology,
UMACS,
Memorial Health Care,
119 Belmont Street,
Worcester,
MA 01605,
USA

Steven Warach,
National Institutes of Health,
NINDS,
10 Center Drive,
MSC 1063, Room B1D733,
Bethesda,
MD 29892-1063,
USA

Gregory W. Albers,
Stanford Stroke Center,
Stanford University Medical Center,
Palo Alto,
CA 94394,
USA

David C. Alsop,
Department of Radiology,
Beth Israel Deaconess Medical Center and Harvard Medical School,
USA

P.A. Barber,
Department of Neurology,
Royal Melbourne Hospital,
University of Melbourne,
Parkville,
Victoria 3050,
Australia

Julien Bogousslavsky,
Department of Neurology,
University Hospital (CHUV) BH07,
1011 Lausanne,
Switzerland

Amy Brodtmann,
Department of Neurology,
Royal Melbourne Hospital,
Parkville,
Victoria 3050,
Australia

Martin M. Brown,
Stroke Medicine,
Institute of Neurology,
University College London,
The National Hospital for Neurology and Neurosurgery,
Queen Square,
London,
UK

Louis R. Caplan,
Department of Neurology,
Beth Israel Deaconess Medical Center,
Boston,
MA,
USA

Leeanne Carey,
Department of Neurology,
Royal Melbourne Hospital,
Parkville,
Victoria,
Australia

William A. Copen,
Department of Radiology,
Massachusetts General Hospital,
PO Box 9657,
55 Fruit Street,
Boston,
MA 02114,
USA

David G. Darby,
Department of Neurology,
Royal Melbourne Hospital,
Parkville,
Victoria 3050,
Australia

Stephen M. Davis,
Department of Neurology,
Royal Melbourne Hospital,
University of Melbourne,
Parkville,
Victoria 3050,
Australia

John A. Detre,
Departments of Neurology and Radiology,
University of Pennsylvania Medical Center,
3 W Gates,
3400 Spruce Street,
Philadelphia,
PA 19104–4283,
USA

Geoffrey A. Donnan,
National Stroke Research Institute,
Heidelberg,
Victoria,
Australia

List of contributors

Robert R. Edelman,
Department of Radiology, Room 5106
Evanston Hospital,
2650 Ridge Avenue,
Evanston,
IL 60201,
USA

John N. Fink,
Department of Neurology,
Christchurch School of Medicine,
New Zealand

Marc Fisher,
Department of Neurology,
UMACS,
Memorial Health Care,
119 Belmont Street,
Worcester,
MA 01605,
USA

S. Goldstein,
University of Pittsburgh Health System,
Stroke Institute,
Departments of Neurology and Neurosurgery,
200 Lothrop Street,
PA 15213,
USA

Werner Hacke,
Department of Neurology,
University of Heidelberg,
Germany

Olav Jansen,
Department of Neuroradiology,
University of Kiel,
Germany

Chelsea Kidwell,
UCLA Stroke Center,
710 Westwood Plaza,
Los Angeles,
CA 90095,
USA

Rüdiger von Kummer,
Department of Neuroradiology,
University of Technology,
Fetscherstr. 74,
Dresden,
Saxonia D-01307,
Germany

Romesh Markus,
National Stroke Research Institute,
Heidelberg,
Victoria,
Australia

Reto Meuli,
Department of Diagnostic and Interventional
 Radiology,
University Hospital (CHUV) BH07,
1011 Lausanne,
Switzerland

Joel Meyer,
Department of Radiology,
Evanston Northwestern Healthcare,
Northwestern University School of Medicine,
2650 Ridge Avenue,
Evanston,
IL 60201
USA

Michael Moseley,
Department of Radiology,
1201 Welch Road,
Stanford University,
CA 94305-5488,
USA

Mark Parsons,
Department of Neurology,
Royal Melbourne Hospital,
University of Melbourne,
Parkville,
Victoria 3050,
Australia

Thanh Phan,
National Stroke Research Institute,
Heidelberg,
Victoria,
Australia

Marc Reichhart,
Department of Neurology,
University Hospital (CHUV) BH07,
1011 Lausanne,
Switzerland

David C. Reutens,
National Stroke Research Institute,
Heidelberg,
Victoria,
Australia

Dawn E. Saunders,
Department of Neuroradiology,
The National Hospital of Neurology and Neurosurgery,
Queen Square,
London,
UK

Jeffrey L. Saver,
UCLA Stroke Center,
710 Westwood Plaza,
Los Angeles,
CA 90095,
USA

Peter D. Schellinger,
Department of Neurology,
University of Heidelberg,
Im Neuenheimer Feld 400,
D69120 Heidelberg,
Germany

Rohit Sood,
Department of Radiology,
Stanford University,
CA 94305-5488,
USA

A. Gregory Sorensen,
Massachusetts General Hospital,
NMR Center,
149 13th Street,
Charlestown,
MA 02129,
USA

Vincent N. Thijs,
Department of Neurology,
U2 Gasthuisberg,
Herestraat 49,
3000 Leuven,
Belgium

Brian M. Tress,
The University of Melbourne Department of Radiology,
c/o Post Office,
Parkville,
Victoria 3050,
Australia

Steven Warach
National Institutes of Health,
NINDS,
10 Center Drive,
MSC 1063, Room B1D 733
Bethesda
MD 29892–1063,
USA

Lawrence R. Wechler,
University of Pittsburgh Health System,
Stroke Institute,
Departments of Neurology and Neurosurgery,
200 Lothrop Street,
PA 15213,
USA

Max Wintermark,
Department of Diagnostic and Interventional Radiology,
University Hospital (CHUV) BH07,
1011 Lausanne,
Switzerland

Peter M. Wright,
National Stroke Research Institute,
Heidelberg,
Victoria,
Australia

H. Yonas,
University of Pittsburgh Health System,
Stroke Institute,
Departments of Neurology and Neurosurgery,
200 Lothrop Street,
PA 15213,
USA

Preface

Stroke is a leading cause of death in Western countries, with a mortality rate higher than most forms of cancer and now the commonest cause of long-term adult disability. Stroke diagnosis and management were revolutionized by the widespread introduction of computed tomographic (CT) scanning in the 1970s. CT scanning sensitively excludes cerebral hemorrhage, but early ischemic changes can be subtle. In the first few hours after stroke onset, when acute therapies such as thrombolysis are being considered, CT is often normal, although acute ischemic changes have become better recognized in recent years. Conventional magnetic resonance imaging (MRI) became widely available in most countries a decade after the advent of CT scanning, but has had a limited role in stroke diagnosis and management. Although MRI provides far better imaging of posterior fossa structures and facilitated non-invasive angiography (MRA), its sensitivity in acute stroke is not much better than CT. Other functional imaging techniques such as single photon emission computed tomography (SPECT) and positron emission tomography (PET) have been valuable research tools, but have not been of routine clinical use in the management of stroke.

Since the 1990s, the increasingly widespread availability of echoplanar MRI technology facilitated the introduction of diffusion-weighted imaging (DWI), perfusion imaging (PWI) and magnetic resonance spectroscopy (MRS). Diffusion-weighted imaging allows the hyperacute evaluation of the ischemic core within minutes of stroke onset and the distinction between acute and chronic ischemic lesions. It represents an extraordinary advance in stroke imaging, specifically in the region of ischemic tissue that is usually destined for infarction. PWI provides a measure of the hypoperfused tissue at risk, particularly in the ischemic penumbra, where acute therapies are targeted. Currently, PWI is dependent on contrast injection, but arterial spin labelling may well supersede this technique. These new MRI methods also permit topographic analysis of acute infarcts and some insights into stroke pathophysiology and prognosis. Concurrent MRA allows analysis of acute arterial occlusion and monitors recanalization. Magnetic resonance spectroscopy provides insights into metabolically deranged cerebral tissues and provides information that is complementary to DWI and PWI. These new techniques are transforming the diagnosis and management of acute stroke. We believe that CT is likely to be widely replaced by these new MR techniques within the next few years. This has already occurred in many expert stroke centres.

In this book we have aimed to provide a comprehensive and up-to-date summary of the dramatic developments that have occurred in this field in the last few years and have also tried to predict likely advances. The scope of the text includes background on the importance of precise stroke diagnosis, the current uses of CT including perfusion imaging and an introduction to standard and echoplanar MRI techniques. Recent advances in MRI permit exclusion of intracerebral hemorrhage and this is currently being tested in randomized trials. A series of chapters details the diagnostic advances facilitated by MRA, DWI, PWI and MRS. Following a review of the pathophysiology and clinical importance of the ischemic penumbra, our contributors illustrate the role of MRI in drug development and selection of acute therapies. Recent studies provide insights into the use of MRI in individualization of the time window, providing a 'tissue clock' for therapeutic interventions such as thrombolysis. Currently, MR-based studies are testing the hypothesis that perfusion–diffusion mismatch, the postulated MR signature of the ischemic penumbra, can suggest the benefit of thrombolysis beyond the clinically established 3-hour time window. Finally, functional brain imaging using brain activation studies and MRI are leading to a better understanding of brain processing and brain recovery after stroke.

In this book, we have targeted neurologists, other stroke physicians, neuroradiologists and other clinicians involved in stroke diagnosis, imaging and management. We have aimed to encapsulate the development, current and emerging clinical role of MRI in stroke. We are grateful for the contributions of our chapter authors, all leaders in the field of MRI and stroke. A few years ago, experts debated whether MRI, in acute stroke diagnosis, was ready for 'prime time'. After reading this book, we suspect you will agree that it is.

Stephen Davis, Marc Fisher and Steven Warach, 2002

The importance of specific diagnosis in stroke patient management

John N. Fink[1] and Louis R. Caplan[2]

[1]Department of Neurology, Christchurch School of Medicine, New Zealand
[2]Department of Neurology Beth Israel Deaconess Medical Center, Boston, MA, USA

Introduction: A stroke is not a 'stroke'

Stroke cannot be considered a diagnosis in itself. Stroke refers to any damage to the brain or spinal cord caused by a vascular abnormality, the term generally being reserved for when symptoms begin abruptly. Stroke is anything but a homogeneous entity, encompassing disorders as different as rupture of a large blood vessel that causes flooding of the subarachnoid space with blood, the occlusion of a tiny artery supplying a small but strategic brain site and thrombosis of a venous conduit obstructing outflow of blood from the brain. Each stroke subtype carries with it different implications for acute treatment, prognosis and secondary prevention. Each stroke patient has additional variables that influence management, including the time from onset to presentation, the severity of the lesion, and associated comorbidities as well as social and psychological factors. The availability of non-invasive imaging techniques has revolutionized the diagnostic process, enabling a much greater understanding of the relevant pathophysiological processes active in the individual patient. This chapter provides an overview of how the specific diagnostic information available from non-invasive investigations can be applied to the management of individual patients.

'Lumping' vs. 'splitting'

The goal of every clinician is to provide the best care for his or her patients. Where possible, physicians should manage patients according to methods that have been tested by well-designed randomized controlled trials. Unfortunately, few therapies for patients with stroke have been tested with randomized trials, and even fewer have been thoroughly investigated for patients with specific stroke subtypes.

Randomized trials have limitations, including the issue of numbers v. specificity, or 'lumping' v. 'splitting'. To provide statistically valid results, randomized trials must contain large numbers of patients with enough end points to analyse within a relatively short period; therefore 'lumping' must predominate over 'splitting'. But, if the results are to be useful for clinical practice, the data must be specifically applicable to individual patients. Too often, there are significant obstacles to doing this. Investigators have continued to design trials as if they expect a single treatment to be effective for all ischemic stroke patients, resulting in inevitable disappointment. Even when treatments have been found effective, there is still a great deal of room for improvement. For example, aspirin has been proven to be effective for early secondary prevention of 'stroke' generally, but only prevents 25% of recurrent strokes within 14 days.[1,2] Cost containment and the need to involve a large number of centres with varying expertise and resources in trials results in a minimum of patient investigation. As a result, accurate subgroup comparisons in trials become impossible, even when these are reported in a *post hoc* analysis. Patients who are too ill, old, young, or of child-bearing age are often excluded from trials. Those unable to give informed consent or who have too complex, or multiple, illnesses are also frequently left out. The type of patients that are excluded from these trials are those that doctors are called on to care for every day.

The term 'evidence-based' must be used cautiously when applied to a particular circumstance if that circumstance has not been specifically studied. Information from trials must be weighed according to the context of specific treatment decisions for individual patients. George Thibault said it well:[3]

> We then need to decide which approach in our large therapeutic armamentarium will be most appropriate in a particular patient, with a particular stage of diseases and particular coexisting conditions, and at a particular age. Even when randomized clinical trials have been performed (which is true for only a small minority of clinical problems), they will often not answer this question specifically for the patient sitting in front of us in the office or lying in the hospital bed.

The complexity of managing stroke patients is increasing. Improvements in diagnostic accuracy have raised new questions about the correct application of existing treatments. There have been many new developments in stroke therapeutics, including intravenous and intra-arterial thrombolysis, catheter-based interventions such as angioplasty and stenting for both extracranial and intracranial stenoses, the development of new antiplatelet agents with potentially complimentary mechanisms of action, and hypothermic treatment, to name a few. The exact place for all of these therapies is not established, yet it is extremely likely that many of the new treatments that are currently 'unproven' will be able to deliver improved outcomes for carefully selected patients. Ignoring these new diagnostic and therapeutic developments is not an option, although a conservative approach must be taken when potentially hazardous therapies have not been rigorously tested. A specific diagnosis is required to optimize treatment selection.

Advances in imaging and stroke diagnosis

Advances in imaging have led to dramatic changes in our understanding of stroke pathophysiology

Table 1.1. Stroke classification

(a) Clinical stroke classification systems
   'Traditional'
      Transient ischemic attack (TIA)
      Minor stroke
      Reversible ischemic neurologic deficit (RIND)
      Stroke in progress
      Completed stroke
   Oxfordshire Community Stroke Project[6]
      Total anterior cerebral infarction syndrome (TACI)
      Partial anterior cerebral infarction syndrome (PACI)
      Lacunar infarction syndrome (LACI)
      Posterior cerebral infarction syndrome (POCI)
(b) Etiologic classification systems
   TOAST[7]
      Large artery
      Cardioembolism
      Small vessel
      Other determined etiology
      Undetermined etiology
   Baltimore-Washington[8]
      Atherosclerotic vasculopathy
      Non-atherosclerotic vasculopathy
      Vasculopathy of uncertain cause (lacunar infarct)
      Cardiac/transcardiac embolism
      Hematological/other
      Migrainous stroke
      Oral contraceptive or exogenous estrogen use
      Other drug related
      Indeterminate

and how we diagnose stroke. Early stroke classifications relied on clinical information. Terms such as 'transient ischemic attack (TIA)', 'minor stroke', 'reversible ischemic neurologic deficit (RIND)', 'stroke in progress' and 'completed stroke' were used to distinguish stroke subtypes.[4] These simplistic distinctions now have little clinical usefulness. Even the term 'TIA' is becoming obsolete as smaller infarctions have become detectable with magnetic resonance imaging (MRI).[5]

Subsequent classifications have increasingly focused on stroke etiology, because of its importance in determining treatment strategies for secondary prevention of stroke (Table 1.1). This has required an increasing emphasis on the results of imaging investigations, rather than clinical features. The authors of the Trial of Org 10172 in Acute

Stroke Treatment (TOAST) classified strokes as being due to large artery atherosclerosis, cardioembolism, small vessel occlusion, other determined etiology or undetermined etiology.[7] This system of stroke classification represents an important advance, but still has shortcomings that limit its application to the diagnosis and management of individual patients. One major limitation is the oversimplified 'large artery' classification. This category 'lumps' embolic strokes from sources in the aorta, large vessel origins in the thorax, cervical arterial lesions, and intracranial arterial stenoses with strokes due to thrombotic occlusion of cervical or intracranial vessels of either anterior or posterior circulations.

Stroke subtype classifications used today, such as the TOAST system, reflect the type of stroke imaging techniques that were generally available a decade ago, namely non-contrast computed tomography (CT) head scan and ultrasound examinations of the cervical carotid arteries and of the heart. A diagnostic strategy that continues to rely solely on these modalities will not achieve a more accurate diagnosis. Not only are important parts of the vascular system overlooked entirely by such an approach, but the accuracy of even these simple classifications is often poor.[9] A lacunar stroke cannot be reliably diagnosed on the basis of clinical and acute CT findings.[10] Some patients with a lacunar syndrome have multiple acute lesions on diffusion-weighted MRI, consistent with an embolic etiology.[11] Moreover, diagnosis using the traditional approach is not made in real time, but retrospectively. A subacute CT scan is required if the diagnosis of lacunar infarction is to be confirmed and a cortical lesion excluded. Ultrasound tests may be obtained days after the initial presentation. This is a critical limitation that prevents a specific diagnosis prior to consideration of acute stroke therapies that can only be overcome if other protocols for acute imaging and assessment are used.[9]

Newer imaging techniques that allow rapid, non-invasive assessment of a much greater extent of the vascular system are now widely available. MRI, as this book demonstrates, is an extremely powerful technique for imaging the brain and cerebrovascular system. Brain MRI examinations for stroke should routinely include magnetic resonance angiography (MRA) of the intracranial vasculature. Magnetic resonance venography (MRV) and MRA of the cervical carotid and vertebral arteries can easily be performed at the same sitting as brain imaging, without the need for contrast. Assessment of the aortic arch and proximal vessels is possible with gadolinium-enhanced MRA. Diffusion-weighted MR imaging (DWI) and perfusion imaging (PI) enable determination in real time of the presence and severity of an ischemic deficit and the response of the brain to the insult. These new techniques enable the concept of stroke diagnosis to go beyond that of simple stroke etiology to establish a comprehensive and dynamic model of stroke pathophysiology for individual patients.

Initial stroke diagnosis

Stroke or stroke-mimic

The initial diagnostic step should be to determine if the event is due to stroke or a non-vascular stroke mimic. Clinical information remains very important in distinguishing disorders such as migraine, seizure, and factitious and psychogenic disorders from stroke. Sometimes the diagnosis is relatively clear, but when this is not the case, imaging results are critical. A typical appearance on a CT scan will often confirm the diagnosis of stroke; however, false-negative CT findings are common in the acute phase, particularly if image quality is poor, readers are inexperienced or if the patient presents with lacunar or brainstem stroke.[10,12–14] Diffusion-weighted MRI is extremely sensitive to acute brain ischemia and false-negatives are very rare, with the exception of small brainstem lacunes.[12,15] DWI is therefore the diagnostic modality of choice when the diagnosis of stroke is uncertain and positive evidence of a stroke is required. The importance of an accurate diagnosis even at this level should not be underestimated; as many as 20% of initial stroke diagnoses are erroneous,[16] and some patients with stroke mimic have been treated with thrombolysis as a result.[17]

Arterial occlusion, arterial rupture, or venous thrombosis

The next level of stroke diagnosis is primarily to distinguish hemorrhagic from ischemic stroke. However, conceptualizing the mechanism and its vascular pathology ensures that stroke due to venous thrombosis is not overlooked. The majority of the remainder of the chapter considers diagnosis of ischemic stroke; cerebral venous thrombosis and hemorrhagic stroke are considered briefly below.

Cerebral venous thrombosis

Although cerebral venous thrombosis (CVT) is rare in comparison with other stroke types, it is treatable and the diagnosis is frequently missed on CT scan. MRI is very sensitive in the detection of CVT;[18] however, the diagnosis can be overlooked if it is not considered in the differential diagnosis, or if susceptibility-weighted (T_2^*) imaging or MR venography is not specifically requested. Patients presenting with what appear to be lobar hemorrhages on CT (young patients with temporal lobe hemorrhage especially) are particularly at risk of being misdiagnosed and mismanaged before the correct diagnosis is made.[19]

Hemorrhagic Stroke

CT scanning has generally been considered the investigation of choice for identification of intracranial blood; however MRI protocols including T_2^* imaging are now able to reliably detect acute cerebral hemorrhage, and are far superior to CT in the detection of subacute and chronic hemorrhage.[20–23] The sensitivity of T_2^* and FLAIR MRI for the detection of acute subarachnoid hemorrhage is comparable with CT.[24]

Clinicians are already familiar with the need to make a specific diagnosis of the cause of hemorrhage, when it is detected. The development of catheter-based interventions for treatment of aneurysms and arterio-venous malformations (AVM) has meant that an even more detailed characterization of the size, morphology and anatomic location of these lesions is required to determine the appropriate therapeutic approach. Digital subtraction angiography (DSA) is generally required before final management decisions are made. MRI is very sensitive for the initial detection of AVM and other vascular abnormalities in the brain, including cavernous angiomata, which are often undetectable with DSA. MRA has a role in follow-up of any untreated lesions and screening of high-risk families.[25–27]

Specific diagnosis and management of ischemic stroke

Acute stroke

The NINDS trial[28] established the effectiveness of intravenous tissue plasminogen activator (tPA) for acute ischemic 'stroke' within 3 hours of symptom onset. While this is a major advance in stroke treatment, the advancement must not stop there. Thrombolysis according to the NINDS protocol adds one favourable outcome for every 13 patients treated, while causing harm to one in 17.[28] The NINDS trial and other negative multi-centre trials of intravenous thrombolysis[29–33] relied on a CT scan and a clock to characterize their patients before treatment decisions were made. This was appropriate at the time as other rapid methods of more detailed assessment were not generally available, but inevitably resulted in some patients being exposed to the risk of treatment without hope of benefit, such as patients whose vessels have spontaneously recanalized,[34] or those with little salvageable brain tissue within the hypoperfused region. At the same time, some patients who might benefit beyond 3 hours were denied treatment on the basis of time alone, not individual pathophysiological features.[35] The PROACT trials have subsequently demonstrated the potential of intra-arterial thrombolytic agents.[36,37] Occlusions of the internal carotid artery and proximal middle cerebral artery do not respond as well as more distal occlusions to intravenous thrombolysis, and may be better treated via the intra-arterial route.[37–39] Determining the appropriate applications for these potentially hazardous therapies requires a specific diagnosis.

More advanced, rapid, non-invasive imaging

techniques for assessment of acute ischemia are increasingly available. Multimodal stroke MRI protocols that include diffusion-weighted imaging, perfusion imaging, MRA and susceptibility-weighted imaging can be performed rapidly, exclude brain hemorrhage, define areas of hypoperfusion and tissue damage and identify occluded arteries, enabling decisions about thrombolysis to be made according to individual pathophysiological criteria.[34,35] DWI and MRA can enable an unequivocal diagnosis of acute stroke to allow stroke patients who might be excluded from thrombolysis on CT-based criteria to be treated, such as patients presenting with seizure at stroke onset, hypoglycemia or hyperglycemia. Definition of the 'ischemic penumbra' with diffusion and perfusion MRI may allow expansion of the therapeutic window beyond the current 3-hour guideline for selected patients.[35] Parameters are being established to identify those with an unacceptably high risk of hemorrhage due to the severity of the ischemic damage present at the infarct core.[40] Continued refinements in MR perfusion imaging techniques promise to allow more accurate predictions of the volume of brain tissue that is at risk of infarction if reperfusion does not occur, based on perfusion thresholds.[41]

In addition to enabling more specific application of thrombolytic therapies, physicians can use detailed knowledge of their patients' pathophysiology to select candidates for other acute stroke therapies. In particular, patients who are not candidates for t-PA but who have a persistent vascular occlusion and a significant volume of brain at risk of infarction due to tenuous collateral supply may benefit from hypertensive therapy to improve collateral circulation.[42]

Practical application of acute stroke MRI

Multimodal stroke MRI has been in use for several years in institutions in many countries, including our own hospital. The hardware and software required are increasingly available. Stroke fellows can be trained to perform the studies enabling 24-hour coverage independent of technician rosters. Acute hemorrhagic stroke can be accurately identified using an MRI protocol that includes susceptibility images, and additional CT scanning is not required before administering acute treatments.[20–22] Patients with multifocal small chronic hemorrhagic lesions due to presumed amyloid angiopathy can also be identified, who may be at increased risk of hemorrhage if thrombolytic agents are given.[23,43] The scanning time of an acute imaging protocol is less than 15 minutes. In the last 4 years at our institution, we have performed perfusion studies in over 300 acute stroke patients and have treated 29 acute stroke patients with t-PA on the basis of MRI results alone.

Stroke etiology and secondary prevention

A detailed diagnosis of stroke etiology is required to plan management strategies for secondary stroke prevention. This requires identification of the location and nature of the vascular lesions responsible, identification of systemic stroke risk factors and consideration of the likely pathophysiological mechanism of stroke. The elements of specific diagnosis of ischemic stroke are summarized in Table 1.2.

Diagnosis of vascular lesions

All levels of the vascular supply to the brain should be considered when determining stroke etiology, that is: the heart, aorta, proximal carotid or vertebral arteries in the thoracic cavity, cervical carotid and vertebral arteries and intracranial vessels. Not only must the anatomical location of vascular lesions be determined, but knowledge of the nature and severity of lesions is required, also. MRA can provide a comprehensive assessment of the vascular tree to determine the location and severity of vascular lesions. MRI with MRA is the non-invasive investigation of choice for the diagnosis and follow-up of carotid and vertebral artery dissection.[44] Duplex ultrasound remains more established than MRA for assessment of cervical internal carotid artery lesions, but promising results are being shown with contrast-enhanced MRA,[45] and vertebral artery assessment is superior with MRA. MRA has great promise in the evaluation of aortic lesions;[46] it is possible that in the future, MRI of the heart and great vessels will reduce the need for the

Table 1.2. Approach to ischemic stroke diagnosis

1. Initial ischemic stroke diagnosis:
   (a) stroke vs. non-vascular stroke mimic
   (b) ischemic stroke vs. hemorrhagic stroke vs. venous thrombosis
2. Acute stroke pathophysiology
   (a) severity and extent of ischemic brain injury
   (b) persistence and severity of cerebral hypoperfusion
   (c) identification of vascular occlusive lesion
3. Stroke etiology: vascular lesion
   (a) location of vascular lesion(s)
       e.g. cardiac, aorta, vascular origins, cervical vessels, intracranial vessels
   (b) nature of vascular lesion(s)
       e.g. cardiac: thrombus, AF, valvular, PFO, akinesis, endocarditis, other
       vascular: atherosclerosis – severity, ulceration, other high risk features
       other lesions – dissection, vasospasm, fibromuscular dysplasia, arteritis, drug-associated vasculopathy
4. Systemic stroke risk factors
   (a) traditional risk factor identification: hypertension, smoking, diabetes, hyperlipidemia.
   (b) thrombophilia
       acquired: antiphospholipid syndrome, polycythemia, thrombocytosis, hyperfibrinogenemia, other
       inherited: protein C, S, ATIII deficiency, prothrombin mutation
   (c) other, e.g. hyperhomocysteinemia
5. Stroke mechanism
   (a) embolic stroke
   (b) *in situ* thrombosis
   (c) lacunar infarction
   (d) hemodynamic / 'watershed' stroke
   (e) vasospasm
6. Stroke severity
   (a) clinical features, e.g. NIH Stroke Scale Score
   (b) lesion volume / location
7. Patient factors
   (a) premorbid functioning, age
   (b) comorbidities
   (c) psychological, social and economic factors

more invasive procedure of transesophageal echocardiography. Transcranial Doppler Ultrasonography is a useful method of assessing the major intracranial vessels but MRA or CTA offer the convenience of being performed at the same time as brain imaging. Digital subtraction angiography is still required when intravascular interventions are contemplated, on occasion to distinguish between critical stenosis and occlusion of the internal carotid artery, and to confirm the diagnosis of certain non-atherosclerotic vasculopathies, such as fibromuscular dysplasia, inflammatory and infectious arteritides, drug abuse-associated vasculopathy, and radiation-induced stenosis.

Specific vascular diagnosis and management

Cardiac-origin embolism

A full discussion of the diagnosis and management of cardiac-origin embolism is beyond the scope of this chapter and is available elsewhere.[47] Secondary prevention strategies can include anticoagulants, antiplatelet agents or their combination, antibiotics, antiarrhythmics and cardioversion, pacemaker, surgery, or catheter-based interventions. Therapeutic decisions depend on a specific diagnosis of the structural lesions involved and the likely composition of the embolic particle itself.[47,48]

Lesions of the aorta and great vessels

That the aorta is an important source of brain embolism is now well established.[49,50] The embolic risk is greatest for thick, complex and mobile plaques.[51,52] Gadolinium-enhanced MRA can establish this diagnosis quickly and accurately.[46] The best treatment to prevent embolism from aortic lesions is not yet known. Cases have been reported where aortic thrombotic masses have disappeared after anticoagulant therapy.[53,54] Intravenous thrombolytic treatment[55] and surgical removal of protruding atheromas[56] have also been reported to be successful in treating patients with aortic atheromas.

Atheromatous disease of the origins of the vertebral arteries is a common, yet often overlooked source of posterior circulation TIA and stroke.[57] Antiplatelet agents or anticoagulants are generally the first line of treatment, but angioplasty and stenting of such lesions may sometimes be appropriate.[58]

Cervical vascular lesions
Carotid endarterectomy is well-established for the treatment of symptomatic severe (70–99%) internal carotid artery (ICA) stenosis.[59,60] The benefit of endarterectomy for symptomatic moderate (50–69%) stenosis is more modest and decisions about treatment must take individual and surgeon characteristics into account.[60,61] The benefit–risk ratio for carotid endarterectomy for unselected patients with asymptomatic ICA lesions is even lower[62] and treatment decisions must be individualized.[63,64] A significant increase in severity of stenosis increases stroke risk and favours surgery.[65] Identification of individual patients with higher stroke risk who would benefit most from surgical treatment may be possible using TCD microembolus detection,[66] or possibly platelet scintigraphy[67] or indicators of cerebral perfusion or vascular 'reserve'[68,69] including MRI perfusion techniques;[70] however, more studies are still required.[71]

Certain cervical carotid artery lesions may be better treated with intravascular interventions than traditional endarterectomy. Careful patient selection is required; indications might include high cervical lesions with difficult surgical access, radiation-induced stenosis, postsurgical restenosis, fibromuscular dysplasia and patients with high surgical risk due to severe medical comorbidity. A randomized controlled trial of carotid stenting and endarterectomy is planned.[72]

Dissection of the internal carotid artery generally does not require surgical intervention, even when aneurysms are associated;[73] however, patients may benefit from a period of anticoagulation.

Intracranial stenoses
The identification of intracranial stenoses can have important prognostic implications.[74,75] Whether anticoagulation is more appropriate treatment than aspirin for patients with intracranial disease is currently the subject of a multicentre randomized controlled trial.[76] Intracranial angioplasty and stenting, in the hands of experienced operators, may be beneficial for carefully selected patients with poor untreated prognosis refractory to medical therapy.[77]

Pathophysiological stroke diagnosis
Vascular imaging studies define the structural lesions important in stroke etiology, but may not show whether the stroke was due to thrombotic, embolic or hemodynamic mechanism, and do not inform about the nature of the embolic material itself. Some stroke subtypes, such as migrainous stroke, may not be associated with a structural vascular lesion. Clinical information must be combined with imaging data to achieve a specific diagnosis and tailor management for the individual patient.

Thrombosis and embolism
Our understanding of stroke pathophysiology has changed dramatically during recent years, emphasizing the importance of embolism in stroke pathogenesis.[47,48] The majority of non-lacunar ischemic strokes are likely to be embolic in origin. Secondary prevention strategy depends on identification of the donor source, risk factors, and consideration of the likely nature of the embolic particle itself.[47,48]

Thrombosis is likely when complete ICA occlusion is found, although even then embolism from the distal ICA thrombus may be the final stroke mechanism, and embolism from the heart may have caused the ICA occlusion.[78–80] Thrombosis may be an important mechanism when intracranial vascular stenoses are present. It may be difficult to know in some cases whether intracranial stenoses detected in the subacute period represent chronic lesions or partial recanalization of an embolus. Repeat imaging at a chronic time point with MRA, CTA or TCD may be required.

Hemodynamic stroke
The importance of hemodynamic factors as sole mechanism in stroke etiology has also been overemphasized in the past. Many strokes that may previously have been considered 'hemodynamic', particularly 'posterior borderzone' infarctions are likely to be caused by embolism.[81–84] However, impaired regional blood flow due to severe vascular stenosis or occlusion is likely to contribute to the

pathogenesis of embolic stroke. A small embolic vascular occlusion is more likely to result in infarction when insufficient collateral circulation is present, and low flow may impair clearance of emboli, or 'washout'.[85] Possibly the most reliable marker for hemodynamic infarction is the topographic pattern of infarction seen on acute multimodal MRI, including DWI, MRA and perfusion imaging, along with the appropriate clinical setting. Multiple small acute lesions are seen in widespread distribution within the internal borderzone region, in the absence of a vascular occlusion.[86] Evidence of a hemodynamic cause for stroke warrants consideration of reduction of antihypertensive medications or other measures to raise blood pressure, as well as consideration of revascularization procedures. Magnetic resonance perfusion and other methods of brain perfusion imaging such as SPECT, or TCD assessment of 'vascular reserve' may provide helpful information in the management of these patients in the future.[70,71]

Migraine and vasoconstriction
The diagnosis of migrainous stroke remains primarily clinical. Infarction can be caused by prolonged intense vasoconstriction[87,88] either directly as a result of impeded blood flow or due to secondary thrombosis.[88,89] Treatment for secondary prevention of migrainous infarction should include a migraine prophylactic agent as well as antiplatelet therapy. We have most often used verapamil in this setting.

Systemic stroke risk factors
Modifiable systemic stroke risk factors must be incorporated into the patient's diagnosis. Management must be individualized. Risk factors are not simply present or absent, but there is a continuum of increasing stroke risk with higher blood pressure and cholesterol levels.[90–93] The actual stroke risk may differ between individuals with the same blood pressure recordings, depending on how accurately recordings in the office reflect true daily levels, the duration of hypertension and the presence of additional risk factors. Evidence of significant end-organ damage such as extensive cerebral white-matter disease on CT or MRI scanning in a patient with apparently 'well-controlled' blood-pressure should prompt consideration of intensification of treatment. Ambulatory blood pressure recording may be very helpful to optimize the management in individual patients. The role of intensive lipid-lowering therapy in secondary stroke prevention is currently the subject of a large randomized trial.

Young patients and those without major vascular risk factors for stroke should also be tested for hereditary and acquired thrombophilic states (Table 1.2), the discovery of which can lead to modification of treatments prescribed, such as the use of higher intensity anticoagulation for patients with the antiphospholipid antibody syndrome,[94] or the introduction of additional treatments such as venesection for polycythemia, folate supplementation for hyperhomocysteinemia and use of agents such as eicosapentanoic acid (fish-oil) to reduce fibrinogen levels in hyperfibrinogenemia.[95,96]

Multiple possible causes of stroke
Some individuals presenting with stroke may have more than one potential cause identified. The major risk factors that predispose to atherosclerosis, such as hypertension, cigarette smoking, diabetes and hypertension promote plaque formation and occlusive disease in the coronary arteries, aorta and peripheral vasculature, as well as the craniocervical arteries.[97] Hypertension also predisposes the penetrating arteries of the brain to lipohyalinosis and atheromatous branch disease. The true frequency of multiple potential causes for stroke in the stroke population is not known. Variation in reported frequencies in the literature have been due to definitions used, such as the degree of carotid artery stenosis required before it is considered an etiological candidate, and how thoroughly the patients in each series were investigated. Improvements in diagnostic techniques will inevitably result in more such patients being identified.

Understanding of the activity of all of these processes in the individual patient is important. Data from the Lausanne Stroke Registry indicated that 46 (38%) out of 121 recurrent strokes had a different etiology than the initial index stroke.[98] In asymptomatic carotid stenosis, 40% of strokes observed ipsilateral to severe carotid lesions were attributable to cardioembolic or lacunar etiologies.[99] In addition, the coexistence of coronary artery disease in patients presenting with stroke should not be overlooked. Patients who survive ischemic stroke face a similar risk of death from future myocardial infarction to that from recurrent ischemic stroke.[100]

Stroke severity

Stroke severity is an important diagnostic consideration in determining stroke prognosis, which in turn influences management decisions. Clinical features, which can be quantified using clinical scales such as the NIH Stroke Scale generally provide the most important prognostic information.[101] Early ischemic lesion volume detected with DWI is also an independent predictor of stroke outcome.[102] Imaging studies can be particularly important for prognosis in specific cases. The use of diffusion and perfusion MR imaging techniques and MRA in determining the prognosis of patients presenting with acute stroke has already been discussed. Detection of a large infarction involving the entire middle cerebral artery territory in a younger stroke patient is associated with a high risk of 'malignant' cerebral edema.[103] Large infarctions or hemorrhages in the posterior fossa may also be associated with the development of raised intracranial pressure.[104] Recognition of these patterns allows early discussion of treatment options that may include hematoma excision, hypothermia[105] and hemicraniectomy.[106]

Patient variables

Individualized stroke management requires consideration of the whole individual. Even once a specific pathophysiological diagnosis of stroke is achieved, other variables peculiar to that individual patient must also be considered before planning management. Pre-existent or coexistent illness may limit or affect treatment. The patient's premorbid function is also an important consideration. Age is never an absolute contraindication to stroke therapy, however elderly patients do not tolerate medical and surgical treatments as well as younger patients, nor do they rehabilitate as well from the effects of a stroke. Secondary prevention studies have demonstrated that the absolute benefit of treatments such as antihypertensive medication and carotid endarterectomy may be greater for elderly patients.[60,107] Socioeconomic and psychological factors may influence treatment decisions for some patients and their families.

Specific diagnosis and stroke patient management

The implications of the enormous heterogeneity of stroke and stroke patients for patient management should be obvious. Patients should be regarded as individuals and modern non-invasive imaging techniques should be used to obtain a specific diagnosis of stroke pathophysiology for each, in order to ensure optimal management. Acute stroke therapy should be offered when possible, preferably on the basis of pathophysiological, rather than arbitrary, criteria. All patients deserve assessment of potential risk factors, such as hypertension, diabetes, smoking, lifestyle, etc, and appropriate modifications should be instituted. The mechanism of stroke must be considered. Patients with atherosclerosis who have had evidence of cerebral ischemia should have an evaluation of their heart, coronary arteries, aorta and extracranial and intracranial arteries. When atherosclerosis is not the cause, a careful search for a specific alternative diagnosis must be made. Therapeutic strategies should then be instituted for each of the potential risks found and clinicians should carefully weigh the risk–benefit ratio of each strategy based on the totality of their knowledge of that individual patient. Some treatments such as antiplatelet medications or standard anticoagulants might be effective against more than one of the lesions found, while other treatments such as carotid endarterectomy or intracranial angioplasty are effective only for the lesions treated. Some treatments that should benefit one lesion (e.g. coronary artery bypass grafting) might pose a risk for patients with other lesions such as severe extracranial and intracranial occlusive disease.

Treatment decisions should be based on information gained about the individual patient, not on assumptions or arbitrary criteria. The availability of powerful non-invasive imaging technology makes thorough evaluation of each patient a realistic expectation. The increasing use of these techniques in randomized controlled trials will provide answers to important unresolved questions in stroke therapeutics and continue to improve outcomes for our patients.

REFERENCES

1 International Stroke Trial Collaborative Group. The International Stroke Trial (IST): a randomised trial of aspirin, subcutaneous heparin, both, or neither among 19435 patients with acute ischaemic stroke. *Lancet* 1997; 349: 1569–1581.

2 CAST (Chinese Acute Stroke Trial) Collaborative Group. CAST: randomized placebo-controlled trial of early aspirin use in 20 000 patients with acute ischaemic stroke. *Lancet* 1997; 349: 1641–1649.

3 Thibault GE. Clinical problem solving: too old for what? *N Engl J Med* 1993; 328: 946–950.

4 Caplan LR. Are terms such as *completed stroke* or *RIND* of continued usefulness? *Stroke* 1983; 14: 431–433.

5 Kidwell CS, Alger JR, Di Salle F et al. Diffusion MRI in patients with transient ischemic attacks. *Stroke* 1999; 30: 1174–1180.

6 Bamford J, Sandercock P, Dennis M, Burn J, Warlow C. Classification and natural history of clinically identifiable subtypes of cerebral infarction. *Lancet* 1991; 337: 1521–1526.

7 Adams HP, Bendixen BH, Kappelle LJ et al. Classification of subtype of acute ischemic stroke. Definitions for use in a multicenter clinical trial. TOAST. Trial of Org 10172 in Acute Ischemic Stroke. *Stroke* 1993; 24: 35–41.

8 Johnson CJ, Kittner SJ, McCarter RJ et al. Interrater reliability of an etiologic classification of ischemic stroke. *Stroke* 1995; 26: 46–51.

9 Lee LJ, Kidwell CS, Alger J, Starkman S, Saver JL. Impact on stroke subtype diagnosis of early diffusion-weighted magnetic resonance imaging and magnetic resonance angiography. *Stroke* 2000; 31: 1081–1089.

10 Toni D, Iweins F, von Kummer R et al. Identification of lacunar infarcts before thrombolysis in the ECASS I study. *Neurology* 2000; 54: 684–688.

11 Ay H, Oliveira-Filho J, Buonanno FS et al. Diffusion-weighted imaging identifies a subset of lacunar infarction associated with embolic source. *Stroke* 1999; 30: 2644–50.

12 Lansberg MG, Albers GW, Beaulieu C, Marks MP. Comparison of diffusion-weighted MRI and CT in acute stroke. *Neurology* 2000; 54: 1557–1561.

13 Schriger DL, Kalafut M, Starkman S, Krueger M, Saver JL. Cranial computed tomography interpretation in acute stroke: physician accuracy in determining eligibility for thrombolytic therapy. *J Am Med Assoc* 1998; 279: 1293–1297.

14 Beauchamp NJ, Barker PB, Wang PY, vanZijl PC. Imaging of acute cerebral ischemia. *Radiology* 1999; 212: 307–324.

15 Ay H, Buonanno FS, Rordorf G et al. Normal diffusion-weighted MRI during stroke-like deficits. *Neurology* 1999; 52: 1784–1792.

16 Libman RB, Wirkowski E, Alvir J, Rao TH. Conditions that mimic stroke in the emergency department: implications for acute stroke treatment trials. *Arch Neurol* 1995; 52: 1119–1122.

17 Katzan IL, Furlan AJ, Lloyd LE et al. Use of tissue-type plasminogen activator for acute ischemic stroke: the Cleveland area experience. *J Am Med Assoc* 2000; 283: 1151–1158.

18 Dormont D, Anxionnat R, Evrard S, Louaille C, Chiras J, Marsault C. MRI in cerebral venous thrombosis. *Am J Neuroradiol* 1994; 21: 81–99.

19 Fink JN, McAuley DL. Cerebral venous sinus thrombosis – a diagnostic challenge. *Intern Med J* 2001; 31: 384–90.

20 Linfante I, Llinas RH, Caplan LR, Warach S. MRI features of intracerebral hemorrhage within 2 hours from symptom onset. *Stroke* 1999; 30: 2263–2267.

21 Patel MR, Edelman RR, Warach S. Detection of hyperacute primary intraparenchymal hemorrhage by magnetic resonance imaging. *Stroke* 1996; 27: 2321–2324.

22 Schellinger PD, Jansen O, Fiebach JB, Hacke W, Sartor K. A standardized MRI stroke protocol: comparison with CT in hyperacute intracerebral hemorrhage. *Stroke* 1999; 30: 765–768.

23 Roob G, Schmidt R, Kapeller P, Lechner A, Hartung HP, Fazekas F. MRI evidence of past cerebral microbleeds in a healthy elderly population. *Neurology* 1999; 52: 991–994.

24 Mitchell P, Wilkinson ID, Hoggard N et al. Detection of subarachnoid haemorrhage with magnetic resonance imaging. *J Neurol Neurosurg Psychiatry* 2001; 70: 205–211.

25 Ross JS, Masaryk TJ, Modic MT, Ruggieri PM, Haacke EM, Selman WR. Intracranial aneurysms: evaluation by MR angiography. *Am J Neuroradiol* 1990; 11: 449–455.

26 Ronkainen A, Hernesniemi J, Puranen M et al. Familial intracranial aneurysms. *Lancet* 1997; 349: 380–384.

27 Crawley F, Clifton A, Brown MM. Should we screen for familial intracranial aneurysm? *Stroke* 1999; 30: 312–316.

28 The National Institute of Neurological Disorders and Stroke rt-PA Stroke Study Group. Tissue plasminogen activator for acute ischemic stroke. *N Engl J Med* 1995; 333: 1581–1587.

29 The Multicentre Acute Stroke Trial – Italy (MAST-I) Group. Randomised controlled trial of streptokinase, aspirin, and combination of both in treatment of acute ischemic stroke. *Lancet* 1995; 346: 1509–1514.

30 Clark WM, Wissman S, Albers GW, Jhamandas JH, Madden KP, Hamilton S. Recombinant tissue-type plasminogen activator (Alteplase) for ischemic stroke 3 to 5 hours after symptom onset. The ATLANTIS Study: a randomized controlled trial. *J Am Med Assoc* 1999; 282: 2019–2026.

31 Hacke W, Kaste M, Fieschi C et al. for the ECASS Study Group. Intravenous thrombolysis with recombinant tissue plasminogen activator for acute hemispheric stroke. The European Cooperative Acute Stroke Study (ECASS). *J Am Med Assoc* 1995; 274: 1017–1025.

32 Hacke W, Kaste M, Fieschi C et al. for the Second European-Australasian Acute Stroke Study Investigators. Randomised double-blind placebo-controlled trial of thrombolytic therapy with intravenous alteplase in acute ischaemic stroke (ECASS II). *Lancet* 1998; 352: 1245–1251.

33 The Multicentre Acute Stroke Trial – Europe Study Group. Thrombolytic therapy with streptokinase in acute ischemic stroke. *N Engl J Med* 1996; 335: 145–150.

34 Caplan LR, Mohr JP, Kistler JP, Koroshetz W. Should thrombolytic therapy be the first-line therapy for acute ischemic stroke? Thrombolysis: not a panacea for ischemic stroke. *N Engl J Med* 1997; 337: 1309–1313.

35 Albers GW. Expanding the window for thrombolytic therapy in acute stroke: the potential role of acute MRI for patient selection. *Stroke* 1999; 30: 2230–2237.

36 del Zoppo GJ, Higashida RT, Furlan AJ, Pessin MS, Rowley HA, Gent M. PROACT: a phase II randomized trial of recombinant pro-urokinase by direct arterial delivery in acute middle cerebral artery stroke. *Stroke* 1998; 29: 4–11.

37 Furlan A, Higashida R, Wechsler L et al. for the PROACT Investigators. Intra-arterial prourokinase for acute ischemic stroke. The PROACT II study: a randomized controlled trial. *J Am Med Assoc* 1999; 282: 2003–2011.

38 Pessin MS, del Zoppo GJ, Furlan AJ. Thrombolytic treatment in acute stroke: review and update of selective topics. In: Moskowitz MA, Caplan LR, eds. *Cerebrovascular Diseases: Nineteenth Princeton Stroke Conference*. Boston: Butterworth-Heinemann, 1995: 409–418.

39 Linfante I, Llinas RH, Chaves C, Caplan LR, Schlaug G. Reperfusion rates and clinical outcome of MCA versus ICA occlusion: MRI/CT before and after t-PA within 3 hours of symptom onset [Abstract]. American Academy of Neurology, 53rd Annual Meeting, 2001.

40 Kidwell CS, Saver JL, Mattiello J et al. A diffusion-perfusion MRI signature predicting hemorrhagic transformation following intra-arterial thrombolysis [Abstract]. *Stroke* 32: 318.

41 Schlaug G, Benfield A, Baird AE et al. The ischemic penumbra: operationally defined by diffusion and perfusion MRI. *Neurology* 1999; 53: 1528–1537.

42 Hillis AE, Barker PB, Beauchamp NJ, Winters BD, Mirski M, Wityk RJ. Restoring blood pressure reperfused Wernicke's area and improved language. *Neurology* 2001; 56: 670–672.

43 Wijdicks EF, Jack CR Jr. Intracerebral hemorrhage after fibrinolytic therapy for acute myocardial infarction. *Stroke* 1993; 24: 554–557.

44 Kasner SE, Hankins LL, Bratina P, Morganstern LB. Magnetic resonance angiography demonstrates vascular healing of carotid and vertebral artery dissections. *Stroke* 1997; 28: 1993–1997.

45 Nederkoorn PJ, Kappelle LJ, van der Graaf Y, Hunink MG, Eikelboom BC, Mali WP. Duplex ultrasound, MR angiography and conventional angiography in carotid artery disease: interpretation of separate test results and their combinations [Abstract]. *Stroke* 2001; 32: 335.

46 Fayad ZA, Nahar T, Fallon JT et al. In vivo magnetic resonance evaluation of atherosclerotic plaques in the human thoracic aorta: a comparison with trans-esophageal echocardiography. *Circulation* 2000; 101: 2503–2509.

47 Caplan LR. Brain embolism. In: Caplan LR, Hurst JW, Chimowitz MI, eds. *Clinical Neurocardiology*. New York: Marcel Dekker; 1999: 35–185.

48 Caplan LR. Brain embolism, revisited. *Neurology* 1993; 43: 1281–1287.
49 Amarenco P, Duyckaerts C, Tzourio C, Hennin D, Bousser MG, Hauw JJ. The prevalence of ulcerated plaques in the aortic arch in patients with stroke. *N Engl J Med* 1992; 326: 221–225.
50 Amarenco P, Cohen A, Baudrimont M, Bousser M-G. Transesophageal echocardiographic detection of aortic arch disease in patients with cerebral infarction. *Stroke* 1992; 23: 1005–1009.
51 The French Study of Aortic Plaques in Stroke Group. Atherosclerotic disease of the aortic arch as a risk factor for recurrent ischemic stroke. *N Engl J Med* 1996; 334: 1216–1221.
52 Mitusch R, Doherty C, Wucherpfennig H et al. Vascular events during follow-up in patients with aortic arch atherosclerosis. *Stroke* 1997; 28: 36–39.
53 Blackshear JL, Jahangir A, Oldenberg WA, Safford RE. Digital embolization from plaque-related thrombus in the thoracic aorta: identification with transesophageal echocardiography and resolution with warfarin therapy. *Mayo Clin Proc* 1993; 68: 268–272.
54 Freedberg RS, Tunick PA, Culliford AT, Tatelbaum RJ, Kronzon I. Disappearance of a large intraaortic mass in a patient with prior systemic embolization. *Am Heart J* 1993; 125: 1445–1447.
55 Hausmann D, Gulba D, Bargheer K, Niedermeyer J, Comess KA, Daniel WG. Successful thrombolysis of an aortic-arch thrombus in a patient after mesenteric embolism. *N Engl J Med* 1992; 327: 500–501.
56 Belden JR, Caplan LR, Bojar RM, Payne DD, Blachman P. Treatment of multiple cerebral emboli from an ulcerated, thrombogenic ascending aorta with aortectomy and graft replacement. *Neurology* 1997; 49: 621–622.
57 Caplan LR. *Posterior Circulation Disease. Clinical Findings, Diagnosis and Management.* Boston: Blackwell, 1996.
58 Spelle PM, Martin JB, Weill A et al. Percutaneous transluminal angioplasty and stenting of the proximal vertebral artery from symptomatic stenosis. *Am J Neuroradiol* 2000; 21: 727–731.
59 NASCET Collaborators. Beneficial effect of carotid endarterectomy in symptomatic patients with high-grade carotid stenosis. *N Engl J Med* 1991; 325: 445–453.
60 European Carotid Surgery Trialists Collaborative Group. Randomised trial of endarterectomy for recently symptomatic carotid stenosis: final results of the MRC European Carotid Surgery Trial (ECST). *Lancet* 1998; 351: 1379–1387.
61 Barnett HJM, Taylor DW, Eliasziw M et al. for the North American Symptomatic Carotid Endarterectomy Trial Collaborators. Benefit of carotid endarterectomy in patients with symptomatic moderate or severe stenosis. North American Symptomatic Carotid Endarterectomy Trial Collaborators. *N Engl J Med* 1998; 339: 1415–1425.
62 Executive Committee for the Asymptomatic Carotid Atherosclerosis Study (ACAS). Endarterectomy for asymptomatic carotid artery stenosis. *J Am Med Assoc* 1995; 273: 1421–1428.
63 Caplan LR. A 79 year-old musician with asymptomatic carotid artery disease. *J Am Med Assoc* 1995; 274: 1383–1389.
64 Caplan LR. *Caplan's Stroke: a Clinical Approach.* 3rd edn. Boston: Butterworth-Heinemann; 2000: 175–176.
65 Chambers BR, Norris JW. Outcome in patients with asymptomatic neck bruits. *N Engl J Med* 1986; 315: 860–865.
66 Seibler M, Nachtman A, Sitzer M et al. Cerebral microembolism and the risk of ischemia in asymptomatic high-grade internal carotid artery stenosis. *Stroke* 1995; 26: 2184–2186.
67 Manca G, Parenti G, Bellina R et al. [111]In platelet scintigraphy for the noninvasive detection of carotid plaque thrombosis. *Stroke* 2001; 32: 719.
68 Markus H, Cullinane M. Severely impaired cerebrovascular reactivity predicts stroke and TIA risk in patients with carotid artery stenosis and occlusion. *Brain* 2001; 124: 457–467.
69 Gur AY, Bova I, Bornstein NM. Is impaired cerebral vasomotor reactivity a predictive factor of stroke asymptomatic patients? *Stroke* 1996; 27: 2188–2190.
70 Kim JH, Lee SJ, Shin T et al. Correlative assessment of hemodynamic parameters obtained with T2*-weighted perfusion MR imaging and SPECT in symptomatic carotid artery occlusion. *Am J Neuroradiol* 2000; 21: 1450–1456.
71 Derdeyn CP, Grubb RL Jr, Powers WJ. Cerebral hemodynamic impairment: methods of measurement and association with stroke risk. *Neurology* 1999; 53: 251–259.
72 Hobson RW. Carotid angioplasty-stent: clinical experience and role for clinical trials. *J Vasc Surg* 2001; 33 (Suppl): S117–123.
73 Guillon B, Brunereau L, Biousse V, Djouhri H, Levy C, Bousser MG. Long-term follow-up of aneurysms developed during extracranial internal carotid artery dissection. *Neurology* 1999; 53: 117–122.
74 The Warfarin-Aspirin Symptomatic Intracranial Disease (WASID) Study Group. Prognosis of patients

with symptomatic vertebral or basilar artery stenosis. *Stroke* 1998; 29: 1389–1392.
75 Bogousslavsky J, Barnett HJM, Fox AJ, Hachinski VC, Taylor W, EC/IC Bypass Study Group. Atherosclerotic disease of the middle cerebral artery. *Stroke* 1986; 17: 1112–1120.
76 Benesch CG, Chimowitz MI. Best treatment for intracranial arterial stenosis? 50 years of uncertainty. *Neurology* 2000; 55: 465–466.
77 Gomez CR, Misra VK, Liu MW et al. Elective stenting of symptomatic basilar artery stenosis. *Stroke* 2000; 31: 95–99.
78 Jorgenson L, Tovrik A. Ischemic cerebrovascular diseases in an autopsy series. Part 2: prevalence, location, pathogenesis and clinical course of cerebral infarcts. *J Neurol Sci* 1969; 9: 285–320.
79 Castaigne P, L'hermitte F, Gautier JC, Escourolle R, Derouesne C. Internal carotid artery occlusion. A study of 61 instances in 50 patients with postmortem data. *Brain* 1970; 93: 231–258.
80 Blackwood W, Hallpike JF, Kocen RS, Mair WG. Atheromatous disease of the carotid arterial system and embolism from the heart in cerebral infarction: a morbid anatomical study. *Brain* 1969; 92: 897–910.
81 Chaves CJ, Silver B, Schlaug G, Dashe J, Caplan LR, Warach S. Diffusion- and perfusion-weighted MRI patterns in borderzone infarcts. *Stroke* 2000; 31: 1090–1096.
82 Belden JR, Caplan LR, Pessin MS, Kwan E. Mechanisms and clinical features of posterior border-zone infarct. *Neurology* 1999; 53: 1312–1318.
83 Angeloni U, Bozzao L, Fantozzi L, Bastianello S, Kushner M, Fieschi C. Internal borderzone infarction following acute middle cerebral artery occlusion. *Neurology* 1990; 40: 1196–1198.
84 Baird AE, Donnan GA, Saling M. Mechanisms and clinical features of internal watershed infarction. *Clin Exp Neurol* 1991; 28: 50–55.
85 Caplan LR, Hennerici M. Impaired clearance of emboli (washout) is an important link between hypoperfusion, embolism, and ischemic stroke. *Arch Neurol* 1998; 55: 1475–1482.
86 Darby DG, Barber PA, Gerraty RP et al. Pathophysiological topography of acute ischemia by combined diffusion-weighted and perfusion MRI. *Stroke* 1999; 30: 2043–2052.
87 Solomon S, Lipton RB, Harris PY. Arterial stenosis in migraine: spasm or arteriopathy? *Headache* 1990; 30: 52–61.
88 Caplan LR. Migraine and posterior circulation stroke. In: ed. Caplan LR, ed. *Posterior Circulation Disease: Clinical Findings, Diagnosis, and Management.* Boston: Blackwell; 1996: 544–568.
89 Caplan LR. Migraine and vertebrobasilar ischemia. *Neurology* 1991; 41: 55–61.
90 Voko Z, Bots ML, Hofman A, Koudstaal PJ, Witteman JC, Breteler MM. J-shaped relation between blood pressure and stroke in treated hypertensives. *Hypertension* 1999; 34: 1181–1185.
91 Hansson L, Zanchetti A, Carruthers SG et al. for the HOT Study Group. Effects of intensive blood-pressure lowering and low-dose aspirin in patients with hypertension: principal results of the Hypertension Optimal Treatment (HOT) randomised trial. *Lancet* 1998; 351: 1755–62.
92 Tell GS, Crouse JR, Furberg CD. Relation between blood lipids, lipoproteins, and cerebrovascular atherosclerosis. A review. *Stroke* 1988; 19: 423–430.
93 Iso H, Jacobs DR, Wentworth D, Neaton JD, Cohen JD. Serum cholesterol and six-year mortality from stroke in 350,977 men screened for the multiple risk factor intervention trial. *N Engl J Med* 1989; 320: 904–910.
94 Khamashta MA, Cuadrado MJ, Mujic F, Taub NA, Hunt BJ, Hughes GR. The management of thrombosis in the antiphospholipid-antibody syndrome. *N Engl J Med* 1995; 332: 993–997.
95 Radack K, Deck C, Huster G. Dietary supplementation with low-dose fish oils lowers fibrinogen levels: a randomized double-blind controlled study. *Ann Intern Med* 1989; 111: 757–758.
96 Kobayashi S, Hirai A, Terano T, Hamazaki T, Tamura Y, Kumagai A. Reduction in blood viscosity by eicosopentanoic acid. *Lancet* 1981; 2: 197.
97 Caplan LR. Lice, fleas and strokes. *Arch Neurol* 2000; 57: 1113–1114.
98 Yamamoto H, Bogousslavsky J. Mechanism of second and further strokes. *J Neurol Neurosurg Psychiatry* 1998; 64: 771–776.
99 Barnett HJM, Meldrum HE. Carotid endarterectomy: a neurotherapeutic advance. *Arch Neurol* 2000; 57: 40–45.
100 CAPRIE Steering Committee. A randomised, blinded, trial of clopidogrel versus aspirin in patients at risk of ischemic events (CAPRIE) *Lancet* 1996; 348: 1329–1339.
101 Adams HP Jr, Davis PH, Leira EC et al. Baseline NIH Stroke Scale score strongly predicts outcome after stroke: a report of the Trial of Org 10172 in Acute Stroke Treatment (TOAST). *Neurology* 1999; 53: 126–131.
102 Thijs VN, Lansberg MG, Beaulieu C, Marks MP, Moseley

ME, Albers GW. Is early ischemic lesion volume on diffusion-weighted imaging an independent predictor of stroke outcome? A multivariable analysis. *Stroke* 2000; 31: 2597–2602.

103 Hacke E, Schwab S, Horn M, Spranger M, De Georgia M, von Klummer R. 'Malignant' middle cerebral artery territory infarction: clinical course and prognostic signs. *Arch Neurol* 1996; 53: 309–315.

104 Koh MG, Phan TG, Atkinson JLD, Wijdicks EFM. Neuroimaging in deteriorating patients with cerebellar infarcts and mass effect. *Stroke* 2000; 31: 2062–2067.

105 Schwab S, Schwarz S, Spranger M, Keller E, Bertram M, Hacke W. Moderate hypothermia in the treatment of patients with severe middle cerebral artery infarction. *Stroke* 1998; 29: 2461–2466.

106 Schwab S, Steiner T, Schwarz S, Steiner HH, Jansen O, Hacke W. Early hemicraniectomy in patients with complete middle cerebral artery infarction. *Stroke* 1998; 29: 1888–1893.

107 Staessen JA, Gasowski J, Wang JG et al. Risks of untreated and treated isolated systolic hypertension in the elderly: meta-analysis of outcome trials. *Lancet* 2000; 355: 865–872.

Limitations of current brain imaging modalities in stroke

P. Alan Barber and Stephen M. Davis

Department of Neurology, Royal Melbourne Hospital, University of Melbourne, Parkville, Victoria, Australia

Introduction

The successful management of stroke patients requires the ability to confirm the diagnosis, identify the site, extent and age of the lesion, and determine underlying pathophysiology. Several studies have made it clear that this cannot be done on the basis of clinical findings alone.[1-3] At the most basic level, clinicians are unable to accurately differentiate between cerebral infarction and primary intracerebral hemorrhage.[4] Cerebral imaging is therefore a prerequisite in the management of almost all stroke patients.

Techniques such as computed tomography (CT), magnetic resonance imaging (MRI), positron emission tomography (PET) and single photon emission computed tomography (SPECT) have provided a window onto the structural and functional changes that occur during stroke can be examined and have revolutionized our understanding of the pathophysiology of ischemia. The advent of thrombolytic therapy has exposed a need for imaging techniques that enable the more rational selection of patients for potentially hazardous treatments. Each of these currently used brain imaging techniques has limitations in such a role and these will form the focus of this chapter.

Patient factors

There are a number of logistic and technical problems related to the performance of all imaging studies in stroke patients. These difficulties relate to a patient's emotional and physical state in the immediate hours after symptom onset. Fear, confusion, language disturbance, and physical deficits may all affect the ability to comprehend or follow commands. Patients are often restless, and frequently become more so with prolonged scanning protocols. Many become claustrophobic within the confined spaces of scanners. Head movement is a considerable problem and can result in image quality degradation. While this may be minimized by moulded head holders or masks, ill-fitting devices may be uncomfortable and increase patient agitation and movement. The use of sedatives to reduce patient movement may mask neurological deterioration, and is therefore relatively contraindicated in the acute stroke setting.

Computed tomography

Computed tomography is more widely available and is less expensive than other tomographic imaging modalities and has been the investigation of choice in stroke. CT images can be obtained rapidly and non-invasively in unwell and frequently uncooperative patients. CT identifies cerebral hemorrhage and is the investigation of choice for subarachnoid hemorrhage. In contrast to MRI, CT can be performed in patients with ferromagnetic metallic foreign bodies. CT is less affected by patient motion than conventional MRI and also allows full access to a patient during scanning, making it of use in restless or critically ill patients. Bony anatomy is also well delineated. This is an advantage when bony injury is suspected, but a

Table 2.1. Advantages and limitations of cerebral computed tomography (CT) in acute stroke

Advantages of CT in stroke	Limitations of CT in stroke
Widely available and relatively inexpensive	Exposure to radiation
Non-invasive	Low sensitivity for infarction at the hyperacute stage
Sensitive to hemorrhage, investigation of choice for subarachnoid hemorrhage	Difficulties distinguishing acute from chronic infarction
Good visualization of bony anatomy	Poor imaging of posterior fossa structures
Good access to patients during scanning procedure	Low interobserver agreement on the degree of ischemic change
Rapid image acquisition, useful in restless patients	Inability to stratify patients in acute stroke trials
CT angiography and CT perfusion imaging can be added to conventional protocols	Inability to delineate hypoperfused but viable cerebral tissue

limitation in the posterior cranial fossa where 'beam hardening' artefacts are produced by bone at the base of the skull. A summary of the advantages and limitations of CT in stroke can be found in Table 2.1 and a full discussion of the role of CT in stroke can be found in Chapter 3.

The principle behind CT is similar to conventional X-ray imaging. Radiation passes through tissue from multiple directions; detectors measure the degree of attenuation of the exiting radiation, and images are reconstructed in cross-section.[5] Thus, CT scanning requires exposure to radiation, with the average dose equivalent to the background radiation received in 1 year.[6] Repeated studies should therefore be avoided unless absolutely necessary. Pregnancy is also a relative contraindication to CT, although the risks to the fetus must be weighed against the potential benefits of the information provided.

Sequence of changes that are seen on CT following a stroke

The early CT changes of ischemia include parenchymal hypodensity and cerebral swelling. Parenchymal hypodensity corresponds to an increase in the intracellular water components of affected brain tissue and is best seen as a loss of grey–white matter differentiation in the cerebral cortex, insular ribbon or basal ganglia (Figs. 2.1 and 2.2). Cerebral swelling is the result of the accumulation of extracellular water and can be seen as a flattening of cortical sulci, an asymmetry between the sylvian fissures and compression of the ventricles.[7–11]

These early ischemic changes are frequently subtle and CT is often normal in the therapeutically critical first hours after stroke onset. Furthermore, these changes mean that it can be particularly difficult to visualize small strokes on acute CT studies. This is a result of the small volume of hypodense ischemic tissue and the minimal compressive effects on surrounding brain. Thus, CT is not particularly effective in identifying small subcortical or brainstem lacunar strokes.[12–14]

Over the first days following stroke onset, infarcted tissue becomes more hypodense and clearly demarcated.[15] Cerebral swelling also increases reaching a maximum between one and five days. During the second week, some patients may develop a progressive increase in the density of the infarct, which may result in 'fogging' of the infarct. This phenomenon may persist for up to a fortnight and as a result strokes may become more difficult to identify and smaller strokes may be overlooked completely. The density of an infarct then decreases leaving a hypodense and atrophic lesion.[16,17]

Despite this temporal sequence of changes, it is often difficult to differentiate between an acute or subacute, and chronic infarction on CT. This is a particular problem with small subcortical lesions that occur on a background of periventricular white matter disease. The presence of such a lesion does

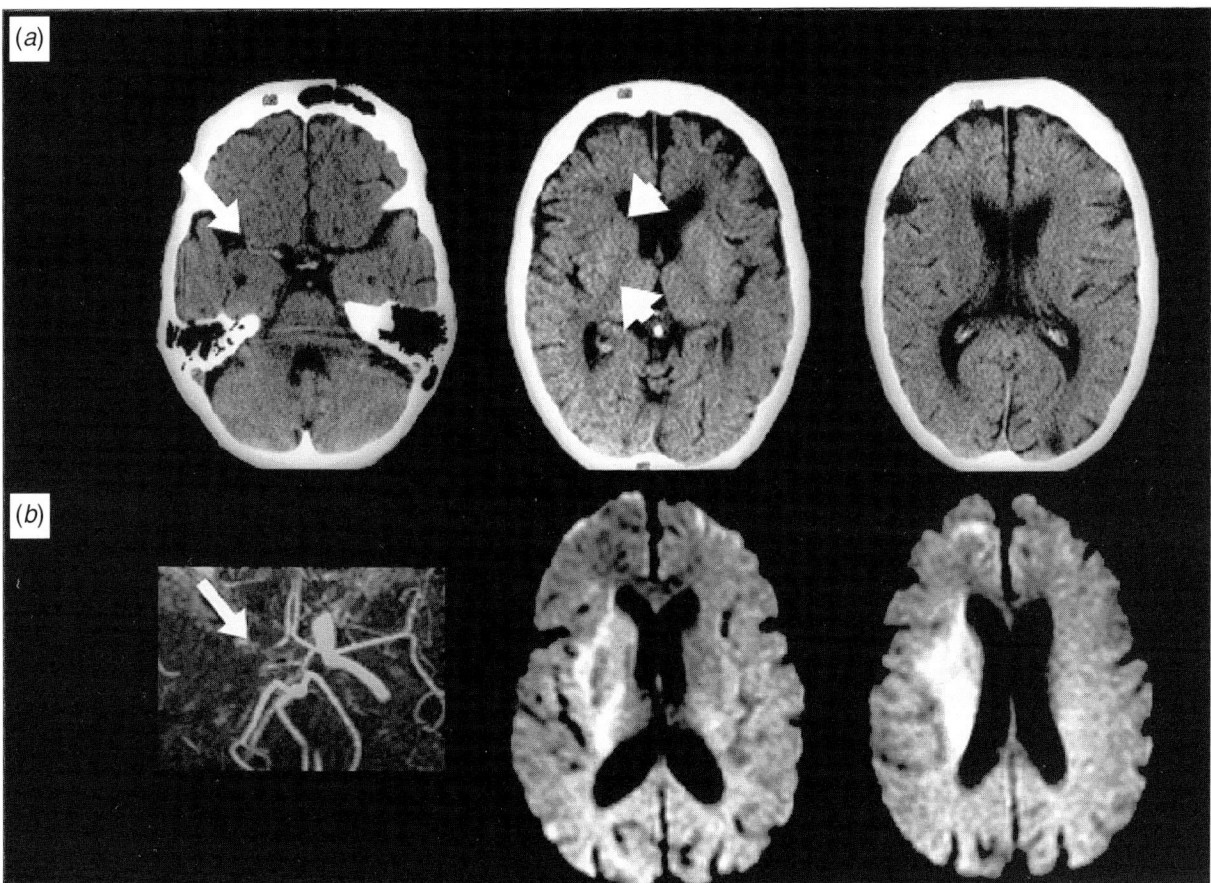

Fig. 2.1. Early ischemic changes on computed tomography (CT) may be subtle. (*a*) CT obtained at 2 hours 45 minutes in a patient who presented with left hemineglect and hemiparesis, show a hyperdense right middle cerebral artery (MCA) sign (arrow), with a subtle loss of distinction between the basal ganglia and surrounding white matter (arrowheads). (*b*) Magnetic resonance angiography and diffusion-weighted imaging in the same patient at 2 hours 15 minutes show an occluded right MCA and a hyperintense region of ischemia in the right subcortical and basal ganglia regions.

not necessarily mean that the lesion is relevant to a patient's clinical presentation.

The subtlety of the early changes of ischemia results in a low sensitivity for cerebral infarction at the hyperacute stage. Indeed the sensitivity of CT for stroke in patients imaged within 5 hours has been reported to be as low as 58%.[18] The difficulty identifying hyperacute ischemia on CT also results in a substantial interobserver variability in the detection of acute infarction.[19,20] Furthermore, the reliability and reproducibility of CT in the estimation of the degree of ischemic change is modest.[11,21] This is of importance, as some guidelines recommend that tissue plasminogen activator (t-PA) be avoided in patients with CT evidence of major ischemia on a screening CT scan.[22,23] As these patients may have a greater risk of hemorrhagic transformation and worse outcome following t-PA.[11,21,24]

In practical terms, these limitations mean that the presence, location and size of an infarct cannot be reliably determined in the first hours after stroke onset. As a consequence, many patients are treated with thrombolytic therapy without definite pre-therapy cerebral CT confirmation of diagnosis of stroke. The major role for hyperacute CT is to exclude primary intracerebral hemorrhage and other non stroke pathology. CT

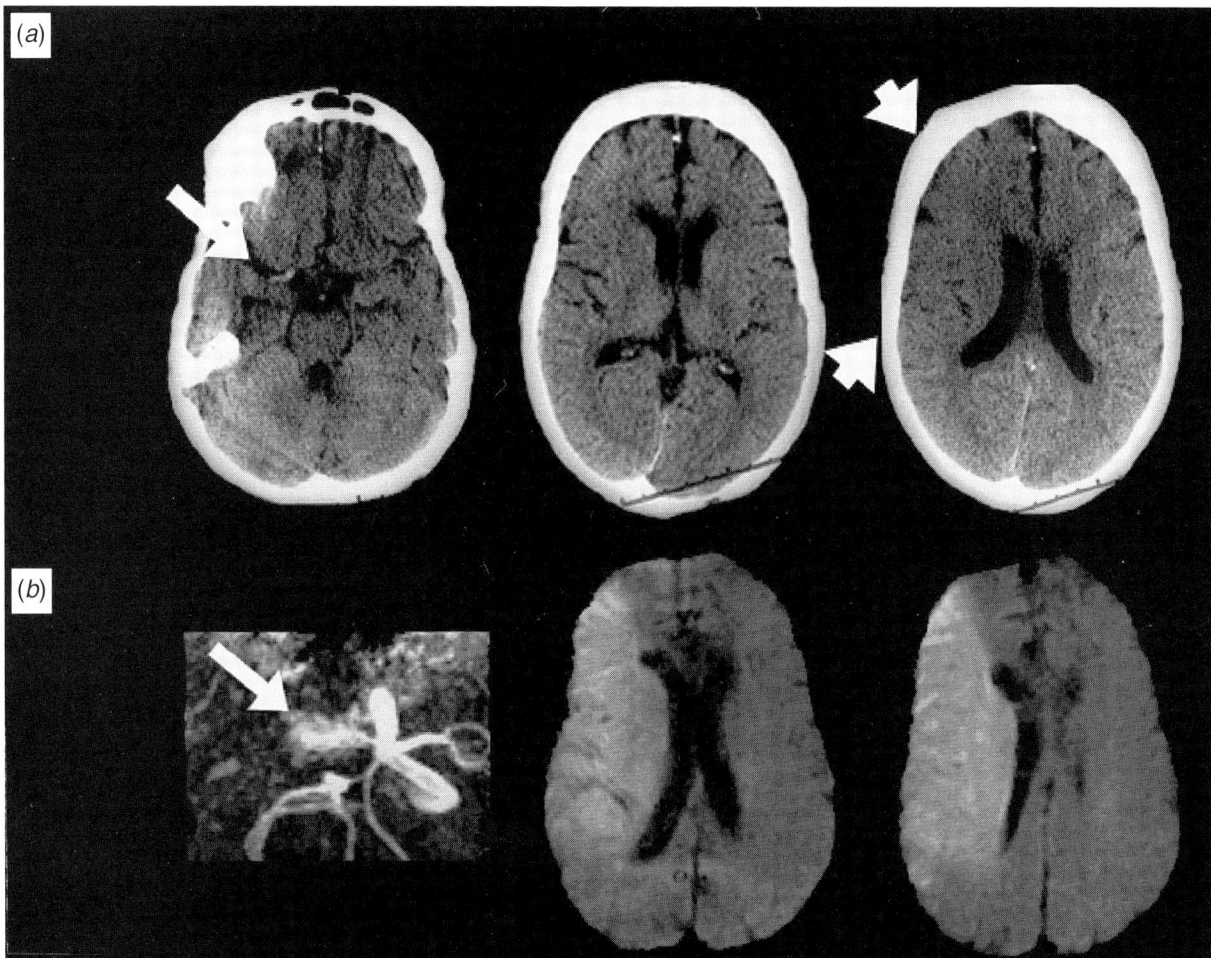

Fig. 2.2. Early ischemic changes on computed tomography (CT) may be subtle. (*a*) CT obtained at 2 hours in a patient who presented with left hemineglect and hemiparesis, shows a hyperdense right middle cerebral artery (MCA) sign (arrow) and subtle loss of distinction between cortical grey and white matter in the right middle cerebral artery territory (arrowheads). (*b*) Magnetic resonance angiography and diffusion-weighted imaging in the same patient at 4 hours shows an occluded right MCA with a hyperintense region of ischemia involving the whole of the right MCA territory.

may also lead to an underestimation of the volume of ischemic change so that patients are exposed to the risks of thrombolytic therapy, despite guidelines to the contrary. Conversely, excessive concern about the degree of ischemic change on CT can lead to treatment being inappropriately withheld.[25] In acute stroke trials, CT cannot be used to reliably stratify participants according to infarct location or size before therapy is commenced. Patients with similar strokes can only be compared retrospectively after treatment has been given.

Computed tomographic angiography and perfusion imaging

Computed tomographic angiography (CTA) is a rapid, reliable and safe method for imaging the intracranial vasculature. Data is acquired following the administration of an intravenous contrast agent. Reconstruction of this data produces angiographic images that can be displayed in three dimensions. CTA is able to delineate the site of vessel occlusion and length of occluded segment in acute stroke patients, and

Table 2.2. Advantages and limitations of conventional magnetic resonance imaging (MRI) in acute stroke

Advantages of MRI in stroke	Limitations of MRI in stroke
Widely available	Expensive
Rapid and non-invasive	Contraindicated in patients with metal fragments, pacemakers and other electrically or magnetically active implanted devices
High soft tissue resolution	Low sensitivity for infarction in the hyperacute stage
Sensitive to brainstem ischemia	Difficulties estimating the degree of ischemic change
Can 'weight' images to augment tissue contrast	Unable to delineate hypoperfused but viable cerebral tissue
Multiple sequences can be obtained providing more information than from any one sequence alone	Unable to stratify patients in acute stroke trials

compares well with other vascular imaging techniques.[26–29]

CT can also be used to produce maps of cerebral perfusion by following the change in Hounsfield number that occurs with the passage of an intravenous contrast agent through the cerebral vascular bed. This change in density is proportional to the concentration of the contrast agent, and can therefore be used to determine flow information. CT perfusion-imaging techniques have been used to calculate maps of tracer transit time and, more recently, perfused cerebral blood volume.[30,31] A further CT perfusion imaging technique used in stroke is xenon enhanced CT (XeCT).[32–34] However, xenon is a mild short acting anesthetic and the use of XeCT is not widespread.

While the clinical role of CTA and CT perfusion imaging is still yet to be defined, these techniques have enormous potential in acute stroke. As almost all patients have CT scans, clinically useful vascular and blood flow information can be obtained with little added time or expense. In addition, CTA is less invasive than conventional angiography and both CTA and perfusion CT can be performed in patients who are critically ill or claustrophobic, or who have metallic foreign bodies such as pacemakers. Multimodal CT may therefore directly compete with the MR imaging techniques discussed in later chapters. However, CT is unable to delineate hypoperfused but potentially salvageable tissue of the ischemic penumbra.

Magnetic resonance imaging

Magnetic resonance imaging is the imaging modality of choice for most neurologic conditions. MR images can be obtained rapidly, non-invasively and with no exposure to ionizing radiation. Images can be generated in any orientation. MRI has high soft tissue resolution and sensitivity to tissue edema. MRI has a higher sensitivity than CT to brainstem and cerebellar ischemia, making it of particular use in the posterior fossa. MR images can be 'weighted' to augment contrast between tissue types. Furthermore, specialized pulse sequences have been developed to highlight specific tissue properties. A number of different sequences can be obtained at the same imaging session, providing more information than from any single sequence alone. For example, information provided by T_1- and T_2-weighted imaging can be augmented by that provided by susceptibility-weighted sequences (sensitive to hemorrhage), diffusion-weighted imaging (tissue destined to infarct without prompt intervention), MR angiography (vascular anatomy), MR perfusion imaging (cerebral perfusion), and MR spectroscopy (concentration of specific cerebral metabolites). The technical aspects and role of MRI in stroke will be discussed in later chapters.

However, MRI has a number of limitations in stroke (Table 2.2). First, MRI is approximately twice as expensive as CT. Claustrophobic patients may have difficulties tolerating the studies. MRI is contraindicated in patients with fragments of metal, for example within the eyes, and in patients with intracranial aneurysm clips, cardiac pacemakers or any other electrically or magnetically active implanted devices that could interact with the magnetic field.

Early ischemic changes are subtle

Ischemic changes may be seen in conventional MR studies within 1 to 2 hours of stroke onset. The earliest findings include loss of the normal flow void within major intracranial vessels and the presence of arterial enhancement if contrast has been used.[35,36] The first morphological changes are due to the development of parenchymal swelling with effacement of cortical sulci and distortion of the ventricular system. These changes are first seen in T_1-weighted sequences and may be present in up to half of patients within 6 hours.[36] This early swelling occurs without signal change and is most likely related to the onset of cytotoxic edema, which can develop within minutes in experimental ischemia.[37] Signal changes only appear with the development of vasogenic edema and are not usually found before eight hours on T_2-weighted sequences or 16 hours on T_1-weighted sequences.

As a consequence, the overall sensitivity of MRI for ischemia is low in the first few hours following the onset of symptoms.[36,38,39] Conventional MRI is also subject to the same limitations as cerebral CT when it comes to delineating acute from chronic infarction, and stratifying patients according to infarct presence, location and size prior to therapy or randomization in acute stroke trials (Fig. 2.3).

MRI in intracerebral hemorrhage

There has been a widespread belief that conventional MRI is less sensitive than CT in the detection of intracerebral hemorrhage. Much of this pessimism is based on a number of early trials using MR scanners with low field strengths. However, there is increasing evidence that echoplanar gradient-echo T_2^*-weighted imaging, also termed susceptibility weighted imaging, is reliable in the detection of acute intraparenchymal hemorrhage.[40–44] In addition, fluid-attenuated inversion recovery (FLAIR)

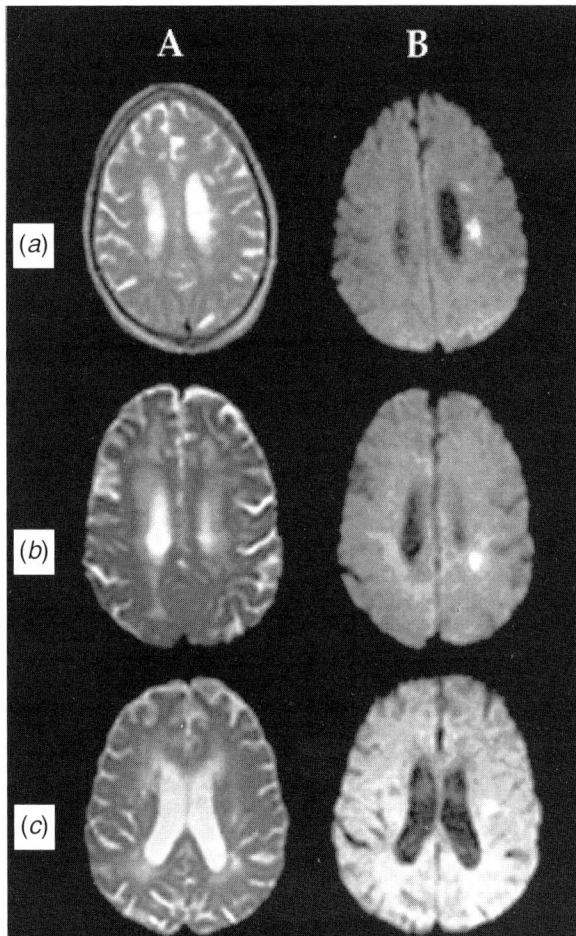

Fig. 2.3. Conventional magnetic resonance imaging sequences may not differentiate acute from chronic infarction. Conventional T_2-weighted imaging (T_2-WI) (A) and diffusion-weighted imaging (DWI) (B) in three patients with subcortical infarction imaged at 11 hours (a), 10 hours (b) and 10.5 hours (c) after the onset of symptoms. Ischemic changes are seen in the periventricular and subcortical white matter on T_2-WI but there is no way of distinguishing acute from chronic infarction. Hyperintense regions of acute infarction are clearly seen on DWI.

imaging may detect subarachnoid hemorrhage.[45] However, until large randomized controlled trials confirm the ability of MRI to detect intraparenchymal and subarachnoid hemorrhage, a screening CT must be considered in all stroke patients. The expense of any screening CT must be added to the cost of performing MRI.

Table 2.3. Advantages and limitations of single photon emission computed tomography (SPECT) in stroke

Advantages of SPECT in stroke	Limitations of SPECT in stroke
Generally well tolerated	Technically and logistically complex
Images cerebral perfusion	Exposure to ionizing radiation
Can demonstrate collateral flow or remote phenomena such as diaschisis	Still require CT or MRI imaging
Can demonstrate ischemic tissue while CT and conventional MRI are normal	No standardized image acquisition or analysis protocols
With ^{99}Tc-HMPAO, images reflect perfusion at the time of injection, so that scanning can be delayed	Unable to delineate the ischemic penumbra
	SPECT has no established clinical role in stroke

Echoplanar magnetic resonance imaging

Echoplanar MRI (EPI) offers advantages over conventional MRI or CT. Echoplanar images can be obtained after a single measurement or *shot*, so that all data may be collected after a single excitation.[46–48] This is in contrast to conventional MR spin- and gradient-echo sequences in which only a small portion of the data required to construct an image is collected after each excitation. As a result, EPI enables whole brain imaging in seconds. This in turn has facilitated the development of functional brain imaging. EPI may be sensitized to flow and diffusion in the same way as conventional spin-echo or gradient-echo imaging sequences.[47] However, because of EPI's very rapid imaging capabilities, whole brain perfusion-weighted imaging (PWI) and diffusion-weighted imaging (DWI) can be obtained within minutes. This rapid imaging capability renders EPI relatively insensitive to movement artefact.

EPI has several limitations in stroke patients. Firstly, it is as expensive and subject to the same contraindications as conventional MRI. EPI is sensitive to chemical shift artefacts that require the use of fat suppression corrections. Susceptibility artefacts, which result in image distortions, are a particular problem in the posterior fossa and around the paranasal sinuses. EPI also has the potential to generate electric currents, which is related to the rate of switching of the magnetic field when rapidly alternating radiofrequency pulses are applied. A change in magnetic field causes a change in electric field and results in the generation of electric currents within the body. This raises concerns about the generation of cardiac dysrhythmias or tetanic muscle contractions and some patients have reported mild twitching or pain. However, the current frequencies for switched gradient fields are usually well below the threshold for neuromuscular stimulation.[48–50]

Single photon emission computed tomography

Single photon emission computed tomography (SPECT) is a rapid, relatively non-invasive perfusion imaging modality that has been used since the late 1970s to study cerebral blood flow changes. SPECT is particularly well suited to the investigation of stroke patients (Table 2.3). SPECT can provide assessments of the degree and extent of ischemia, give an indication of likely underlying pathogenesis, and demonstrate the presence of collateral flow and remote physiological phenomena such as diaschisis (Fig. 2.4, see colour plate section). However, SPECT is technically and logistically complex, and at present has no established clinical role in stroke. A full discussion of the limitations of SPECT in stroke requires some understanding of its underlying principles. These will be summarized in the following section.

Acquisition of SPECT studies

Perfusion SPECT acquires three-dimensional data that represent regional perfusion by localizing gamma ray-emitting radiotracers. These radiotracers are distributed in the brain according to the rate of CBF. The emitted photons are then detected using gamma cameras or one of several different ring-type gamma-ray detector systems. These may be rotating gamma detector arrays, fixed detector systems, or single or multihead camera systems. Image acquisition time depends on the desired quality of the image, as well as the imaging system and radiotracer used. In general, high-resolution images can be obtained within 20–30 minutes.[51]

After data acquisition, individual count rates at each location are calculated and filtered to avoid excessive amplification of noise. Computer generated reconstruction then enables data to be presented three-dimensionally or as a series of two-dimensional slices in the axial, coronal or sagittal planes. An image consists of a matrix of pixels, each reflecting the number of 'counts' emitted by the gamma rays.[52] In areas of reduced perfusion, less radiotracer is emitted and consequently the region appears less bright.

Radiolabelled tracers

The most commonly used tracer for cerebral perfusion SPECT is ^{99m}-Technetium hexamethylpropyleneamine oxime (^{99}Tc-HMPAO, exametazime, Ceretec, Amersham International). ^{99}Tc-HMPAO is a commercially available, low molecular weight, lipophilic macrocyclic amine. It is less expensive and offers better spatial resolution than earlier radiotracers. ^{99}Tc-HMPAO is unstable in vitro and needs to be injected soon after preparation, which assuming technicians are available, takes approximately 30 minutes. ^{99}Tc-HMPAO has an in vivo half-life of approximately 6 hours so that imaging may proceed immediately or be delayed for several hours with images reflecting the state of cerebral perfusion at the time of the injection.[53–56] The in vivo retention of ^{99}Tc-HMPAO prevents early repeat imaging and results in a greater exposure to radiation than other tracers.[57,58] ^{99}Tc-ethyl cysteinate dimer (ECD, Neurolite) is also used in perfusion SPECT and has the advantage over ^{99}Tc-HMPAO of being stable in vitro for approximately 6 hours.[51] Other perfusion SPECT radiotracers such as ^{123}I N-isopropyl-p-iodoamphetamine (IMP, Spectamine) and the inert gas ^{133}xenon have been largely superseded by the newer radiotracers.

SPECT analysis

SPECT studies can provide both semiquantitative and qualitative assessments of cerebral perfusion. This is in contrast to PET in which absolute measures of blood flow can be determined. Semiquantitative SPECT analysis takes into account the number of radioactive 'counts' within a region of interest, expressed as a fraction of the total counts within the brain or with respect to some unaffected region such as the contralateral hemisphere or cerebellum.[59] This requires high-resolution whole brain imaging, so that image acquisition and analysis may take 30 minutes or more. Simpler qualitative acquisition protocols have been developed that require fewer slices with lower resolution. These protocols can be combined with visual analysis so that perfusion may be reported as simply being normal, low, absent or high.[60] This results in shorter acquisition and analysis times. Qualitative SPECT measures have been shown to correlate with measured hypoperfusion volumes, and both stroke severity and outcome.[60,61,62]

SPECT in stroke

With acute cerebral ischemia, up to 90% of SPECT scans will be abnormal within eight hours of symptom onset. SPECT may demonstrate the presence, location and degree of ischemia at a time when the changes on CT or MRI are subtle or inconclusive.[51,63] An exception to this is with lacunar infarction in which SPECT studies are often normal. The degree of hypoperfusion or volume of a hypoperfused region also correlate with clinical state, stroke outcome and final infarct size.[64–69] This prognostic information is over and above that provided by clinical scale scores alone.[60,70–72]

SPECT studies may facilitate patient targeted acute stroke therapy. Ueda et al.[73] found that ischemic tissue with CBF less than 35% of cerebellar flow may be salvaged if intra-arterial thrombolysis is initiated up to 5 hours after stroke onset, but is at risk of hemorrhagic transformation after this time. SPECT may help exclude patients from particular acute stroke therapies. For example, patients with increased isolated radioisotope uptake have a favourable outcome. These patients are likely to have reperfused at the time of imaging and should avoid thrombolytic therapy. Patients with a focal absence of perfusion are likely to have vessel occlusion without collateral flow and may be at risk of hemorrhagic transformation or death following thrombolytic therapy.[74–77] The feasibility of using SPECT to help decide acute stroke therapy has been demonstrated by a number of groups. Serial SPECT may also be used to monitor spontaneous changes or therapy-induced changes in perfusion over time (Fig. 2.5, see colour plate section).[62,75,78–81]

SPECT limitations

Perfusion SPECT is a generally safe and well-tolerated procedure. One of the major concerns is exposure to ionizing radiation. The International Commission on Radiological Protection has developed a measure, the effective dose equivalent (EDE), which takes into account the relative radio-sensitivity of each organ and tissue.[82] The EDE for ^{99}Tc-HMPAO of an injected dose of 500 MBq, with bladder voiding every 3.5 hours, is 6.9 mSv. This is similar to that received from a radionuclide bone scan and is 43% of the average annual background radiation in the United States.[51] SPECT is contraindicated in pregnancy.

A further major limitation of perfusion SPECT is poor image quality compared to CT or MR imaging. This is the result of the effects of photon attenuation and scatter, inadequate spatial resolution and partial volume effects. Structural imaging with CT or MRI must also be performed to exclude intracranial hemorrhage and other non-stroke pathologies. Thus two separate imaging sessions, usually in different hospital departments, are required. This adds to the time needed for acute investigation and delays the institution of any therapy.

SPECT is more operator dependent than CT or MRI. Thus, the interpretation of results often requires a close collaboration between nuclear medicine physicians and clinicians.[51] There is also no widespread and standardized SPECT image acquisition or analysis protocol. This has made it difficult to compare results obtained by different centres. As a consequence, the use of SPECT in large multicentre acute stroke therapy trials has been limited.[80]

SPECT is unable to assess cerebral metabolism. It is therefore unable to determine the presence of hypoperfused yet still potentially viable penumbral tissue (Fig. 2.6, see colour plate section). This information can only be inferred in retrospect by determining whether any reperfusion was maintained at outcome (nutritional reperfusion). Thus, SPECT cannot be used to limit therapy to only those with potentially salvageable ischemic tissue.

Positron emission tomography

Positron emission tomography (PET) has provided major insights into the response of cerebral tissues to reduced cerebral perfusion. In stroke, PET enables the simultaneous measurement of regional CBF, the consumption of oxygen with the cerebral metabolic rate of oxygen ($CMRO_2$), the consumption of glucose with the cerebral metabolic rate of glucose (CMR_{glc}), and the oxygen extraction fraction (OEF). These measures permit the delineation of CBF thresholds for electrical and structural failure and as such PET has enabled the characterization of the ischemic penumbra. The role of PET in imaging the ischemic penumbra will be discussed in more detail in Chapter 15. However, while it has been a useful research tool, PET is not well suited to the acute investigation of stroke patients (Table 2.4).

Acquisition of PET images

With PET imaging, patients are given radionuclide tracers that are radioisotope *labelled* biological molecules, e.g. ^{11}C-CO_2, ^{15}O-O_2, ^{15}O-H_2O, ^{18}F-fluorodeoxyglucose (^{18}F-FDG), or drugs, e.g. ^{18}F-fluoromisonidazole (^{18}F-FMISO). As these tracer isotopes decay, a positron is emitted. A positron is a subatomic particle with the same mass as an electron but with a positive, rather than negative,

Table 2.4. Advantages and limitations of positron emission tomography (PET) in stroke

Advantages of PET in stroke	Limitations of PET in stroke
Quantification of cerebral blood flow	Expensive
Demonstration of cerebral metabolism	Exposure to ionizing radiation
Enables mapping of neuroreceptors	Technically and logistically complex
Demonstration of the ischemic penumbra	Limited to research or large tertiary institutions
	Still require CT or MRI imaging
	No standardized image acquisition or analysis protocols
	PET has no established clinical role in stroke

charge. The positron then interacts with an electron in a matter–antimatter reaction, resulting in the annihilation of both particles and the release of two gamma rays (photons). The gamma rays diverge from the site in opposite directions and are detected by one of a large number of external detector pairs configured in one or more rings.

By configuring the system so that only the near simultaneous arrival of these photons is detected (coincidence detection), only those photons arising from between the detectors will be recorded. Not all photon pairs will reach the detectors because of a change in direction (Compton scatter), or absorption by intervening tissues. Accurate quantification of images requires correction for this absorption and scatter of photons. Two- or three-dimensional images can then be generated according to the distribution of regional radioactivity. Mathematical models that relate radionuclide tissue concentration to the physiological variable under study are then used. These models attempt to account for tracer delivery to tissues, tracer distribution and metabolism within the tissues, the effects of recirculation of both metabolized and non-metabolized tracer, and the amount of tracer remaining within the bloodstream.

Cerebral blood flow

Cerebral blood flow (CBF) is the most useful physiological parameter to be measured by PET in stroke (Fig. 2.7, see colour plate section). The measurement of CBF is based on the principles of inert, freely diffusible tracers.[83] Most PET CBF studies are performed using either intravenously injected $^{15}O-H_2O$ or inhaled $^{15}O-CO_2$; where $^{15}O-CO_2$ is rapidly converted to $^{15}O-H_2O$ by red blood cell carbonic anhydrase. However, $^{15}O-H_2O$ based techniques may underestimate CBF as a result of the incomplete permeability of the blood–brain barrier to H_2O and incomplete tissue extraction of H_2O at high flow rates.[84]

The two main techniques for measuring CBF are the steady state and autoradiographic methods. In the steady state method, tracer is administered until an equilibrium is reached. At this point, the amount of $^{15}O-H_2O$ entering the brain in arterial blood is equal to the amount lost to radioactive decay and venous outflow. Simultaneous measurement of arterial blood radioactivity enables quantification of regional CBF from PET imaging. The autoradiographic method of CBF measurement utilizes a single bolus of tracer ($^{15}O-H_2O$ or $^{15}O-CO_2$) followed by PET scanning.[85–87] Tracer activity in the arterial blood is also measured, with CBF values determined assuming a constant blood:brain partition coefficient for the tracer. Each of these techniques have advantages and disadvantages which are beyond the scope of this chapter and will not be discussed further.

Cerebral blood volume

Cerebral blood volume (CBV) can be measured using ^{11}C or ^{15}O labelled CO. The CO binds irreversibly to hemoglobin forming labelled carboxyhemoglobin. Once equilibrium is reached, the measured peripheral blood radioactivity will be proportional to the regional carboxyhemoglobin concentration, red cell mass and CBV. This enables quantification of CBV after adjustments are made for the hematocrit in peripheral blood and cerebral microvessels. CBV can then be used to correct other PET measurements such as the $CMRO_2$ and OEF, for radiotracer not extracted by the tissues.

Cerebral metabolic rate of oxygen and oxygen extraction fraction

Measures of cerebral oxygen metabolism are usually measured using a steady-state method after the inhalation of ^{15}O–O_2.[88] Tissue radioactivity is proportional to the amount of oxygen extracted from the blood (OEF). The $CMRO_2$ can then be calculated from the relationship between OEF and CBF, described by the equation:

$$CRMO_2 = CBF \times OEF \times \text{arterial } O_2 \text{ content}$$

Tracer that remains bound to hemoglobin can result in an overestimation of OEF and $CMRO_2$. This error is greatest at where CBF is low, such as ischemic or infarcted regions but can be corrected by the independent measurement of CBV. Cerebral oxygen metabolism can also be measured using a single breath inhalation method,[89] and a dynamic method in which dynamic PET scans are obtained after single breath, multiple breath, or continuous inhalation of labelled oxygen.[90]

Other PET techniques used to study cerebral ischemia

Additional PET techniques used to study cerebral ischemia have included the measurement of glucose metabolism (CMR_{glc}) using a modification of the autoradiographic method described by Sokoloff and colleagues.[91] Benzodiazepine receptors can be mapped using ^{11}C-flumazenil.[92] Studies using the hypoxia marker ^{18}F-fluoromisonidazole have been reported as a potential method for directly identifying the ischemic penumbra.[93]

Limitations of PET

PET is a generally safe procedure. The radiation exposure in a typical study is similar to that received in many other routine imaging studies.[94] A moderate degree of patient cooperation is required, which can be a problem in unwell, aphasic or unconscious patients. Protocols typically require the placement of an arterial catheter to monitor plasma concentrations of radiolabelled tracers. Difficulties related to the use of inhalational tracers (e.g. ^{15}O-labelled O_2 or CO_2) are common and may result from inability to comprehend the required task. Other problems arise from comorbidities affecting respiratory function and unstable blood pressure.

PET is expensive and requires specialized equipment and staff. The short half-life of the commonly used PET radioisotopes ($t_{1/2}$ for ^{15}O 2 min, ^{11}C 20 min, ^{18}F 110 min) mean that they must be generated by a cyclotron that is either at or near the PET scanner. This contributes to the significant technical and logistical complexities associated with scanning patients at the acute stage. As a result, PET scanners are limited to a small number of large tertiary hospitals and research centres. The acquisition and analysis of PET images is also time consuming. Additional time is needed with techniques such as ^{18}F-FMISO PET, which requires a delay between tracer injection and imaging.

As a result of these difficulties, it is unlikely that PET will have a place in the routine investigation of acute stroke patients in the foreseeable future. To date, there have been few studies investigating the potential role of PET in acute therapeutic intervention. Most of these have examined small numbers of patients with considerable variations in the time interval between symptom onset and PET studies.[95–97] The only data on the effect of thrombolysis in humans studied with PET comes from Heiss et al.,[98] who reported on 12 stroke patients studied with PET either before or during the administration of alteplase. None the less, PET has provided an invaluable contribution to our knowledge of stroke pathophysiology, particularly the characterization of the ischemic penumbra.

Conclusions

Of the imaging modalities described above, only CT and MRI have established roles in the clinical setting. However, both CT and MRI have low sensitivities for acute ischemia in the hyperacute phase and neither imaging modality is able to identify hypoperfused but potentially salvageable ischemic tissue. SPECT and PET have added significantly to our knowledge of the pathophysiology of stroke. However for logistic reasons, neither is particularly suited to the acute evaluation of stroke patients. PET is the only established method of identifying the penumbra but its cost, technical complexity and limited availability mean it is far from suitable for routine clinical use. While SPECT is certainly less expensive and more widely available than PET, there is no accepted standardized image acquisition and analysis protocol.

ACKNOWLEDGEMENTS

We thank Dr Stephen Read PhD, FRACP for his advice on the preparation of this chapter.

REFERENCES

1 Madden KP, Karanjia PN, Adams HP, Jr., Clarke WR. Accuracy of initial stroke subtype diagnosis in the TOAST study. Trial of ORG 10172 in acute stroke treatment. *Neurology* 1995; 45: 1975–1979.

2 Toni D, Fiorelli M, De Michele M et al. Clinical and prognostic correlates of stroke subtype misdiagnosis within 12 hours from onset. *Stroke* 1995; 26: 1837–1840.

3 Kidwell CS, Alger JR, Di Salle F et al. Diffusion MRI in patients with transient ischemic attacks. *Stroke* 1999; 30: 1174–1180.

4 Warlow CP, Dennis MS, van Gijn J et al. *Stroke: A Practical Guide to Management.* 2nd edn. Oxford: Blackwell Science Ltd; 2001.

5 Gilman S. Imaging of the brain. First of two parts. *N Engl J Med* 1998; 338: 812–820.

6 Royal College of Radiologists. *Making the Best Use of a Department of Clinical Radiology.* 3rd edn. London: Royal College of Radiologists; 1995.

7 Garcia JH. Experimental ischemic stroke: a review. *Stroke* 1984; 15: 5–14.

8 Unger E, Littlefield J, Gado M. Water content and water structure in CT and MR signal changes: possible influence in detection of early stroke. *Am J Neuroradiol* 1988; 9: 687–691.

9 Tomura N, Uemura K, Inugami A, Fujita H, Higano S, Shishido F. Early CT finding in cerebral infarction: obscuration of the lentiform nucleus. *Radiology* 1988; 168: 463–467.

10 von Kummer R, Nolte PN, Schnittger H, Thron A, Ringelstein EB. Detectability of cerebral hemisphere ischaemic infarcts by CT within 6 h of stroke. *Neuroradiology* 1994; 38: 31–33.

11 von Kummer R, Allen KL, Holle R. Acute stroke: usefulness of early CT findings before thrombolytic therapy. *Radiology* 1997; 205: 327–333.

12 Donnan GD, Tress B, Bladin P. A prospective study of lacunar infarction using computerised tomography. *Neurology* 1982; 32: 49–56.

13 Bamford J, Sandercock P, Jones L, Warlow C. The natural history of lacunar infarction: the Oxfordshire Community Stroke Project. *Stroke* 1987; 18: 545–551.

14 Lindgren A, Norrving B, Rudling O, Johansson BB. Comparison of clinical and neuroradiological findings in first-ever stroke. A population-based study. *Stroke* 1994; 25: 1371–1377.

15 Hakim AM, Ryder-Cooke A, Melanson D. Sequential computerized tomographic appearance of strokes. *Stroke* 1983; 14: 893–897.

16 Becker H, Desch H, Hacker H, Pencz A. CT fogging effect with ischemic cerebral infarcts. *Neuroradiology* 1979; 18: 185–192.

17 Skriver EB, Olsen TS. Transient disappearance of cerebral infarcts on CT scan, the so-called fogging effect. *Neuroradiology* 1981; 22: 61–65.

18 Horowitz SH, Zito JL, Dinnarumma R, Patel M, Alvir J. Computed tomographic-angiographic findings within the first five hours of cerebral infarction. *Stroke* 1991; 22: 1245–1253.

19 von Kummer R, Holle R, Gizyska U et al. Interobserver agreement in assessing early CT signs of middle cerebral artery infarction. *Am J Neuroradiol* 1996; 17: 1743–1748.

20 Schriger DL, Kalafut M, Starkman S, Krueger M, Saver JL. Cranial computed tomography interpretation in acute stroke: physician accuracy in determining eligibility for thrombolytic therapy. *J Am Med Assoc* 1998; 279: 1293–1297.

21 Marks MP, Holmgren EB, Fox A, Patel S, von Kummer R, Froehlich J. Evaluation of early computed tomographic findings in acute ischemic stroke. *Stroke* 1999; 30: 389–392.

22 Adams HP, Brott TG, Furlan AJ et al. Guidelines for thrombolytic therapy for acute stroke: A supplement to the guidelines for the management of patients with acute ischemic stroke. A statement for healthcare pro-

fessionals from a special writing group of the stroke council, American Heart Association. *Stroke* 1996; 27: 1711–1718.

23 Neurology Report of the Quality Standards Committee of the American Academy of Neurology. Practice advisory: Thrombolytic therapy for acute ischemic stroke – summary statement. *Neurology* 1996; 47: 835–839.

24 Mies G, Auer L, Ebhardt G, Traupe H, Heiss W. Flow and neuronal density in tissue surrounding chronic infarction. *Stroke* 1983; 14: 22–27.

25 Barber PA, Darby DG, Desmond PM et al. Identification of major ischemic change: diffusion-weighted imaging versus computed tomography. *Stroke* 1999; 30: 2059–2065.

26 Knauth M, von Kummer R, Jansen O, Hahnel S, Dorfler A, Sartor K. Potential of CT angiography in acute ischemic stroke. *Am J Neuroradiol.* 1997; 18: 1001–1010.

27 Shrier DA, Tanaka H, Numaguchi Y, Konno S, Patel U, Shibata D. CT angiography in the evaluation of acute stroke. *Am J Neuroradiol* 1997; 18: 1011–1020.

28 Na DG, Byun HS, Lee KH et al. Acute occlusion of the middle cerebral artery: early evaluation with triphasic helical CT–preliminary results. *Radiology* 1998; 207: 113–122.

29 Wildermuth S, Knauth M, Brandt T, Winter R, Sartor K, Hacke W. Role of CT angiography in patient selection for thrombolytic therapy in acute hemispheric stroke. *Stroke* 1998; 29: 935–938.

30 Muzelaar JP, Fatouros PP, Schroder ML. A new method for quantitative regional cerebral blood volume measurements using computed tomography. *Stroke* 1997; 28: 1998–2005.

31 Hunter GJ, Hamberg LM, Ponzo JA et al. Assessment of cerebral perfusion and arterial anatomy in hyperacute stroke with three-dimensional functional CT: early clinical results. *Am J Neuroradiol* 1998; 19: 29–37.

32 Gur D, Good WF, Wolfson SK, Jr., Yonas H, Shabason L. In vivo mapping of local cerebral blood flow by xenon-enhanced computed tomography. *Science* 1982; 215: 1267–1268.

33 Yonas H, Darby JM, Marks EC, Durham SR, Maxwell C. CBF measured by Xe-CT: approach to analysis and normal values. *J Cereb Blood Flow Metab* 1991; 11: 716–725.

34 Firlik AD, Kaufmann AM, Weschler LR, Firlik KS, Furkui MB, Yonas H. Quantitative cerebral blood flow determinations in acute ischemic stroke. Relationship to computed tomography and angiography. *Stroke* 1997; 28: 2208–2213.

35 Biller J, Yuh WTC, Mitchell GW, Bruno A, Adams HP, Jr. Early diagnosis of basilar artery occlusion using magnetic resonance imaging. *Stroke* 1988; 19: 297–306.

36 Yuh WTC, Crain MR, Loes DJ, Greene GM, Ryals TJ, Sato Y. MR imaging of cerebral ischemia: findings in the first 24 hours. *Am J Neuroradiol* 1991; 12: 621–629.

37 Schuier FJ, Hossmann K-A. Experimental brain infarcts in cats II: ischemic brain edema. *Stroke* 1980; 11: 593–601.

38 Spetzler RF, Zabramksi JM, Kaufman B, Yeung HN. Acute NMR changes during MCA occlusion: a preliminary study in primates. *Stroke* 1983; 14: 185–191.

39 Brant-Zawadzki M, Pereira B, Weinstein P et al. MR imaging of acute experimental ischemia in cats. *Am J Neuroradiol* 1986; 158: 701–705.

40 Patel R, Edelman R, Warach S. Detection of hyperacute primary intraparenchymal hemorrhage by magnetic resonance imaging. *Stroke* 1996; 27: 2321–2324.

41 Atlas SW, Thulborn KR. MR detection of hyperacute parenchymal hemorrhage of the brain. *Am J Neuroradiol* 1998; 19: 1471–1507.

42 Schellinger PD, Jansen O, Fiebach JB, Hacke W, Sartor K. A standardized MRI stroke protocol: comparison with CT in hyperacute intracerebral hemorrhage. *Stroke* 1999; 30: 765–768.

43 Linfante I, Llinas RH, Caplan L, Warach S. MRI features of intracerebral hemorrhage within 2 hours from symptom onset. *Stroke* 1999; 30: 2263–2267.

44 Ebisu T, Tanaka C, Umeda M et al. Hemorrhagic and nonhemorrhagic stroke: diagnosis with diffusion-weighted and T2-weighted echoplanar MR imaging. *Radiology* 1997; 203: 823–828.

45 Singer MB, Atlas SW, Drayer BP. Subarachnoid space disease: a diagnosis with fluid-attenuated inversion recovery MR imaging and comparison with gadolinium-enhanced spin-echo MR imaging – blinded reader study. *Radiology* 1998; 208: 417–422.

46 Mansfield P. Multi-planar image formation using NMR spin echoes. *J Phys C* 1977; 10: 349–352.

47 Turner R, Le Bihan D, Chesnick AS. Echo-planar imaging of diffusion and perfusion. *MRM* 1991; 19: 247–253.

48 Edelman R, Wielopolski P, Schmitt F. Echoplanar MR imaging. *Radiology* 1994; 192: 600–612.

49 Kanal E. An overview of electromagnetic safety considerations associated with magnetic resonance imaging. *Ann NY Acad Sci* 1992; 649: 202–224.

50 Athey T. Current FDA guidance for MR patient exposure and considerations for the future. *Ann NY Acad Sci* 1992; 649: 242–257.

51 Report of the Therapeutics and Technology Assessment Subcommittee of the American Academy of Neurology. Assessment of brain SPECT. *Neurology.* 1996; 46: 278–285.

52 Eberl S, Zimmerman RD. The computer and its application in nuclear medicine. In: Murray I, Ell P, eds. *Nuclear Medicine in Clinical Diagnosis and Treatment.* Edinburgh: Churchill Livingstone; 1994: 1299–1314.

53 Costa DC, Ell PJ, Cullum ID, Jarritt PH. The in vivo distribution of ^{99}Tc-HM-PAO in normal man. *Nucl Med Commun* 1986; 7: 647–658.

54 Lassen NA, Andersen AR, Friberg L, Paulson OB. The retention of [^{99}m-Tc]-D,L-HM-PAO in the human brain after intracarotid bolus injection: a kinetic analysis. *J Cereb Blood Flow Metab* 1988; 8: S13–S22.

55 Neirinck RD, Burke JF, Harrison RC, Forster AM, Andersen AR, Lassen NA. The retention mechanism of technetium-^{99}m-HMPAO: intracellular reaction with glutathione. *J Cereb Blood Flow Metab* 1988; 8: S4–S12.

56 Holman BL, Devous MD. Functional Brain SPECT: the emergence of a powerful clinical method. *J Nucl Med* 1992; 33: 1888–1904.

57 Masdeu JC, Brass LM, Holman BL, Kushner MJ. Brain single-photon emission computed tomography. *Neurology* 1994; 44: 278–285.

58 Fayad PB, Brass LM. Single photon emission computed tomography in cerebrovascular disease. *Stroke* 1991; 22: 950–954.

59 Infeld B, Binns D, Lichtenstein M, Hopper JL, Davis SM. Volumetric analysis of cerebral hypoperfusion on SPECT: validation and reliability. *J Nucl Med* 1997; 38: 1447–1453.

60 Alexandrov AV, Black SE, Ehrlich LE et al. Simple visual analysis of brain perfusion on HMPAO SPECT predicts early outcome in acute stroke. *Stroke* 1996; 27: 1537–1542.

61 Alexandrov AV, Bladin CF, Ehrlich LE, Norris JW. Noninvasive assessment of intracranial perfusion in acute cerebral ischemia. *J Neuroimaging* 1995; 5: 76–82.

62 Alexandrov AV, Grotta JC, Davis SM, Lassen NA. Brain SPECT and thrombolysis in acute ischemic stroke: time for a clinical trial. *J Nucl Med* 1996; 37: 1259–1262.

63 Baird AE, Austin MC, McKay WJ, Donnan GA. Sensitivity and specificity of ^{99}Tc-HMPAO SPECT cerebral perfusion measurements during the first 48 hours for the localization of cerebral infarction. *Stroke* 1997; 28: 976–980.

64 Rango M, Candelise L, Perani D et al. Cortical pathophysiology and clinical neurologic abnormalities in acute cerebral ischemia. A serial study with single photon emission computed tomography. *Arch Neurol* 1989; 46: 1318–1322.

65 Raynaud C, Rancurel G, Samson Y et al. Pathophysiologic study of chronic infarcts with I-123 isopropyl iodo-amphetamine (IMP): the importance of periinfact area. *Stroke* 1987; 18: 21–29.

66 Bushnell DL, Gupta S, Micoch AG, Barnes WE. Prediction of language and neurologic recovery after cerebral infarction with SPECT imaging using *N*-isopropyl-*p*-(I-123) iodoamphetamine. *Arch Neurol* 1989; 46: 665–669.

67 Launes J, Nikkinen P, Lindroth L, Brownell AL, Liewendahl K, Ivanainen M. Brain perfusion defect size in SPECT predicts outcome in cerebral infarction. *Nucl Med Commun* 1989; 10: 891–900.

68 Giubilei F, Lenzi GL, Di Piero V et al. Predictive value of brain perfusion single-photon emission computed tomography in acute ischemic stroke. *Stroke* 1990; 21: 895–900.

69 Davis SM, Chua M, Lichtenstein M, Rossiter SC, Tress BM, Hopper JL. Perfusion changes with recovery after stroke. *Aust NZ J Med* 1993; 23: 68.

70 Laloux P, Richelle F, Jamart J, De Coster P, Laterre C. Comparative correlations of HMPAO SPECT indices, neurological score, and stroke subtypes with clinical outcome in acute carotid infarcts. *Stroke* 1997; 26: 816–821.

71 Bowler JV, Wade DT, Jones BE, Nijran K, Steiner TJ. Single-photon emission computed tomography using hexamethylpropyleneamine oxime in the prognosis of acute cerebral infarction. *Stroke* 1996; 27: 82–86.

72 Lövblad K-O, Jakob PM, Chen Q et al. Turbo spin-echo diffusion-weighted MR of ischemic stroke. *Am J Neuroradiol* 1998; 19: 201–208.

73 Ueda S, Sakaki S, Yuh WTC, Nochide I, Ohta S. Outcome in acute stroke with successful intra-arterial thrombolysis and predictive value on initial single-photon emission-computed tomography. *J Cereb Blood Flow Metab* 1999; 19: 99–108.

74 Alexandrov AV, Black SE, Ehrlich LE, Caldwell CB, Norris JW. Predictors of hemorrhagic transformation occurring spontaneously and on anticoagulants in patients with acute ischemic stroke. *Stroke* 1997; 28: 1198–1202.

75 Ueda T, Hatakeyama T, Kumon Y, Sakaki S, Uraoka T. Evaluation of risk of hemorrhagic transformation in local intra-arterial thrombolysis in acute ischemic stroke by initial SPECT. *Stroke* 1994; 25: 298–303.

76 Davis SM, Chua M, Lichtenstein M, Rossiter SC, Hopper JL, Tress BM. Cerebral hypoperfusion in stroke prognosis and brain recovery. *Stroke* 1993; 24: 1691–1696.

77 Limburg M, van Royen EA, Hijdra A, de Bruine JF, Verbeeten B, Jr. Single-photon emission computed tomography and early death in acute ischemic stroke. *Stroke* 1991; 21: 1150–1155.

78 Hanson SK, Grotta JC, Rhoades H et al. Value of single-photon emission-computed tomography in acute stroke therapeutic trials. *Stroke* 1993; 24: 1322–1329.

79 Overgaard K, Sperling B, Boysen G et al. Thrombolytic therapy in acute ischemic stroke. A Danish pilot study. *Stroke* 1993; 24: 1439–1446.

80 Alexandrov AV, Masdeu JC, Devous MD, Black SE, Grotta JC. Brain single-photon emission CT with HMPAO and safety of thrombolytic therapy in acute ischemic stroke. Proceedings of the meeting of the SPECT safe thrombolysis study collaborators and the members of the brain imaging council of nuclear medicine. *Stroke* 1997; 28: 1830–1834.

81 Grotta JC, Alexandrov AV. tPA-associated reperfusion after acute stroke demonstrated by SPECT. *Stroke* 1998; 29: 429–432.

82 Eberl S, Zimmerman RD. Radiation protection and dosimetry in clinical practice. In: Murray I, Ell P, eds. *Nuclear Medicine in Clinical Diagnosis and Treatment*. Edinburgh: Churchill Livingstone; 1994: 1367–1388.

83 Kety SS, Schmidt CF. The nitrous oxide method for the quantitative determination of cerebral blood flow in man: theory, procedure and normal values. *J Clin Invest* 1946; 25: 476–482.

84 Eichling JO, Raichle ME, Grubb RL, Jr., Ter-Pogossian MM. Evidence of the limitations of water as a freely diffusible tracer in brain of the rhesus monkey. *Circ Res* 1974; 35: 358–364.

85 Kety SS. Measurement of local blood flow by the exchange of an inert, diffusible substance. *Med Res* 1960; 8: 228–236.

86 Herscovitch P, Markham J, Raichle ME. Brain blood flow measured with intravenous H2(15)O. I. Theory and error analysis. *J Nucl Med* 1983; 24: 782–789.

87 Raichle ME, Martin WR, Herscovitch P, Mintun MA, Markham J. Brain blood flow measured with intravenous H2(15)O. II. Implementation and validation. *J Nucl Med* 1983; 24: 790–798.

88 Frackowiak RS, Lenzi GL, Jones T, Heather JD. Quantitative measurement of regional cerebral blood flow and oxygen metabolism in man using ^{15}O and positron emission tomography: theory, procedure, and normal values. *J Comput Assist Tomogr* 1980; 4: 727–736.

89 Mintun MA, Raichle ME, Martin WR, Herscovitch P. Brain oxygen utilization measured with O-15 radiotracers and positron emission tomography. *J Nucl Med* 1984; 25: 177–187.

90 Ohta S, Meyer E, Thompson CJ, Gjedde A. Oxygen consumption of the living human brain measured after a single inhalation of positron emitting oxygen. *J Cereb Blood Flow Metab* 1992; 12: 179–192.

91 Sokoloff L, Reivich M, Kennedy C et al. The [14C]deoxyglucose method for the measurement of local cerebral glucose utilization: theory, procedure, and normal values in the conscious and anesthetized albino rat. *J Neurochem* 1977; 28: 897–916.

92 Heiss WD, Graf R, Fujita T et al. Early detection of irreversibly damaged ischemic tissue by flumazenil positron emission tomography in cats. *Stroke* 1997; 28: 2045–2051; discussion 2051–2052.

93 Read SJ, Hirano T, Abbott DF et al. The fate of hypoxic tissue on 18F-fluoromisonidazole positron emission tomography after ischemic stroke. *Ann Neurol* 2000; 48: 228–235.

94 Assessment: positron emission tomography. Report of the Therapeutics and Technology Assessment Subcommittee of the American Academy of Neurology. *Neurology* 1991; 41: 163–167.

95 Hakim AM, Evans AC, Berger L et al. The effect of nimodipine on the evolution of human cerebral infarction studied by PET. *J Cereb Blood Flow Metab* 1989; 9: 523–534.

96 Yamauchi H, Fukuyama H, Ogawa M, Ouchi Y, Kimura J. Hemodilution improves cerebral hemodynamics in internal carotid artery occlusion. *Stroke* 1993; 24: 1885–1890.

97 Heiss W-D, Holthoff V, Pawlik G, Neveling M. Effect of nimodipine on regional cerebral glucose metabolism in patients with acute ischemic stroke as measured by positron emission tomography. *J Cereb Blood Flow Metab* 1990; 10: 127–132.

98 Heiss WD, Grond M, Thiel A, von Stockhausen HM, Rudolf J. Ischaemic brain tissue salvaged from infarction with alteplase. *Lancet* 1997; 349: 1599–1600.

Clinical efficacy of CT in acute cerebral ischemia

Rüdiger von Kummer

Department of Neuroradiology, University of Technology, Dresden, Saxonia, Germany

Patients with acute cerebral ischemia represent with hemiparesis, hemianopia, speech disturbance, or impairment of consciousness. The differential diagnosis is intracranial hemorrhage, cerebral venous thrombosis, focal encephalitis, demyelination disorder or tumour. Brain imaging is necessary to assess the exact diagnosis and the acute pathophysiological state of the brain. Both pieces of information will guide treatment and will finally determine the clinical outcome of the patient.

Kent and Larson proposed five levels of clinical efficacy for assessing diagnostic technology: (i) technical capacity; (ii) diagnostic accuracy; (iii) diagnostic impact; (iv) therapeutic impact; and (v) patient outcome.[1] In this chapter, I will study the question what unenhanced CT is able to assess in patients with acute stroke; how accurate this information is; and whether imaging with CT has any impact on stroke diagnosis, stroke treatment and, finally, on the clinical outcome of patients.

Level 1 of clinical efficacy: technical capacity of CT in acute cerebral ischemia

Technical capacity is the capability of CT to reproducibly display recognizable images that demonstrate pathology with good intra- and interobserver reliability.[2] Based on changes in X-ray attenuation, CT is capable of detecting intracranial hemorrhage, thrombo-embolic occlusion of major brain arteries, brain tissue swelling without edema, and ischemic brain edema. Intra- and interobserver reliability was not studied for all of these findings. Generally, it seems as if hyperattenuating lesions are easier to detect than hypoattenuating lesions.

CT detection of intracranial blood

In patients with acute stroke, blood may be present in one or more cranial compartments: brain parenchyma, ventricles, subarachnoid space, and subdural or epidural space. Clinically, an acute parenchymal hemorrhage cannot reliably be distinguished from ischemic stroke. After acute hemorrhage, blood appears as a hyperattenuated, often space-occupying mass. The degree of hyperattenuation depends on the amount of blood, whether it is clotted or not, and whether the blood is intermixed with cerebrospinal fluid (CSF) or brain tissue. Hemorrhages related to coagulopathies or treatment with anticoagulants or thrombolytics are often inhomogeneous with fluid levels (Fig. 3.1). The sensitivity of CT for detection of parenchymal hemorrhage is considered to be almost 100%, but small hemorrhages into the brain parenchyma or subarachnoid space can be missed. The investigators of the European Cooperative Acute Stroke Studies (ECASS I and II) rarely missed a small parenchymal hemorrhage and a subarachnoid hemorrhage (SAH) in 1420 patients (0.1%) that was later detected by neuroradiologists. Emergency physicians in another study had an error rate in stroke detection by CT twice that of neurologists and radiologists, and only 17% of emergency physicians, 40% of neurologists and 52% of radiologists achieved a 100% sensitivity for the identification of intracranial hemorrhage.[3] This observation underlines that some hemorrhages

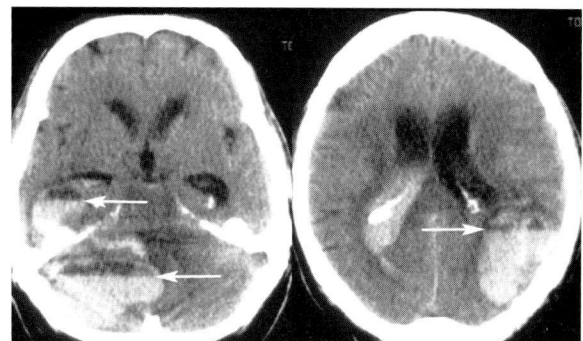

Fig. 3.1. CT of a 79-year-old man with a stroke after myocardial infarction and thrombolytic therapy shows multiple hematomas with fluid levels (arrows).

are subtle, interobserver reliability does not only depend on the technical capacity of CT, and that CT reading requires special training and experience.

Acute hemorrhages usually show hyperattenuation without surrounding edema. If marked edema is present under those circumstances, underlying neoplasm or venous obstruction should be suspected. The location of the hematoma often provides clues about its underlying etiology. Multiple hemorrhagic lesions should make one think about metastatic disease, coagulopathy or cerebral amyloid angiopathy.

CT is 90% sensitive for the detection of SAH within the first 24 hours of bleeding. When blood later intermixes with cerebrospinal fluid, the density will be similar to the adjacent brain and difficult to visualize. If the hemorrhage is small, it may be missed entirely by the scan, necessitating lumbar puncture for definitive diagnosis in patients with a history and a syndrome highly suspicious for SAH. The sensitivity of CT in detecting subarachnoid blood declines to approximately 50% at 1 week after SAH.[4]

Calcification of the basal ganglia can occasionally be mistaken for a deep intraparenchymal hemorrhage. It has a similar degree of attenuation to acute blood, but may be distinguished by its characteristic location and tendency to be bilateral.

CT detection of arterial obstruction

Thrombo-embolic occlusion of major brain arteries may be represented as a hyperattenuating arterial segment in comparison to other arterial segments

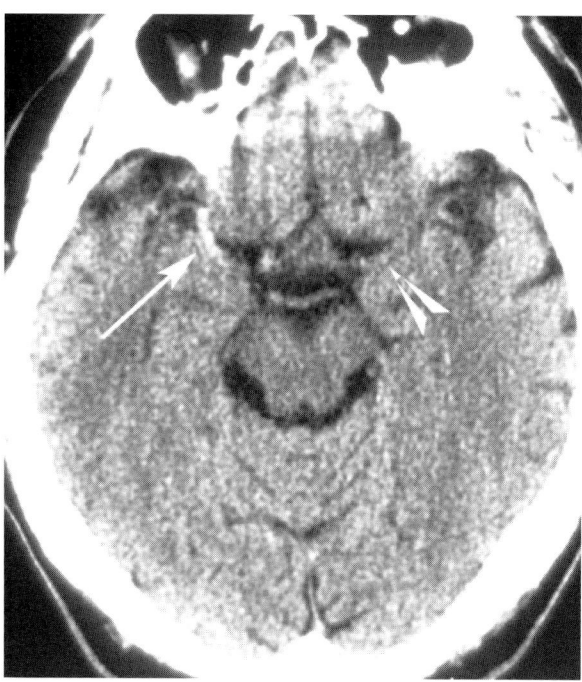

Fig. 3.2. Patient with left-sided hemiparesis since less than 5 hours. CT depicts hyperattenuating right middle cerebral artery (MCA) trunk (arrow). The left MCA trunk (arrowhead) is not hyperattenuating.

on unenhanced CT (Fig. 3.2). The interobserver agreement on such 'hyperdense artery signs' varied between poor and moderate ($\kappa = 0.20$ and 0.63).[5-7]

CT detection of brain tissue swelling

The enlargement of anatomical structures like the cerebral cortex and the effacement of cerebral spinal fluid spaces suggest brain tissue swelling. CT may detect brain tissue swelling without hypoattenuation for a short period early after arterial or venous obstruction (Fig. 3.3). Compensatory arterial dilatation due to low perfusion pressure[8] or passive arterial dilatation due to high venous pressure[9] cause this type of swelling. Six neuroradiologists agreed on tissue swelling in 45 CT of acute stroke patients with a $\kappa = 0.56 - 0.59$.[6]

CT detection of ischemic brain edema

Brain tissue swelling with hypoattenuation is best explained by ischemic edema (Fig. 3.4). Cerebral

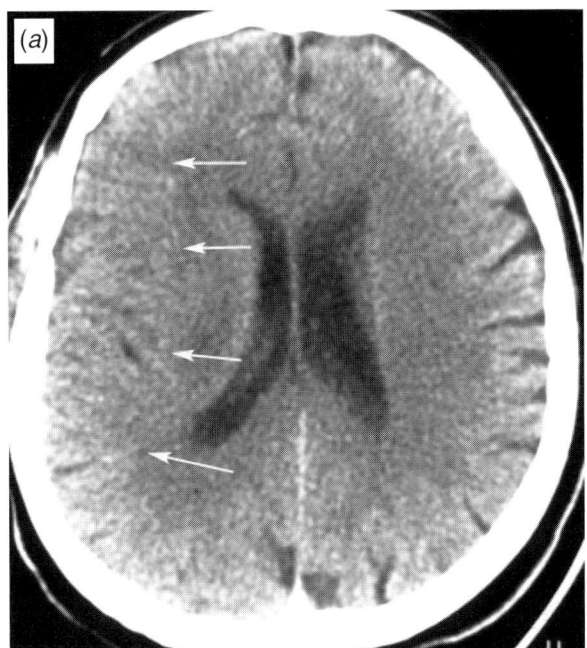 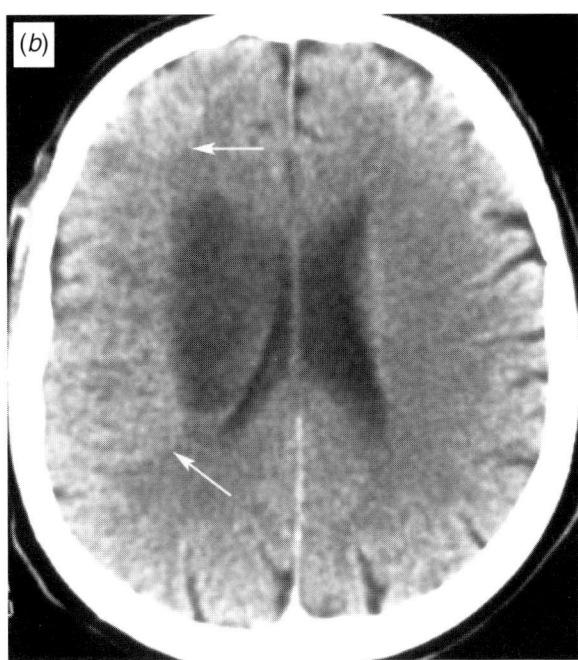

Fig. 3.3. (*a*) CT obtained 2 hours after symptom onset in a 58-year-old man with hyperattenuating right MCA trunk (not shown) shows swelling of the cortical layer within the right MCA territory (arrows). (*b*) 6 days later the swelling is still present in addition to a subcortical ischemic infarct. The patient was treated with IV rt-PA. His NIH stroke Score improved from 17 at baseline to 11 at day 90 after stroke. (Courtesy of Professor Otto Busse, Minden, Germany).

blood flow (CBF) of 8–12 ml /100 g per min is accepted as the flow threshold for structural integrity.[10] A sudden decrease in cerebral perfusion below 8–12 ml/100 g per min causes the grey matter to immediately take up water.[11–14] (The CBF threshold that triggers a decrease in the ADC is considerably higher: 30–40 ml/100 g per min.[15]) The amount of water accumulating during ischemia is significantly correlated to the duration of ischemia. The mean ischemic blood flow was 5.8 ± 0.4 ml per 100 g and min.[16] Significant resolution of brain edema occurred only if ischemia lasted less than 15 minutes.[13] This early type of ischemic edema thus indicates the tissue with flow values below the threshold of structural integrity and may herald ischemic necrosis. Imaging of ischemic edema could then identify the proportion of ischemic brain tissue that is irreversibly damaged.[17]

CT attenuation is linearly proportional to specific gravity and thus allows monitoring of tissue water content.[18,19] An increase by 1% of tissue water content causes a decrease of X-ray attenuation by 2.6 HU in gels[20] and by 2.1 HU in experimental cryogenically induced brain edema.[19] Co-registration of CT attenuation and CBF revealed that hypoattenuation develops only in areas of critically hypoperfused brain tissue.[21] The mean CBF in the affected MCA territory of patients with hypoattenuation of the basal ganglia (7 ml per 100 g and min) was significantly lower than that of patients who did not have these findings (17 ml per 100 g and min).[22] A decline in cerebral blood volume (CBV) may add to the decrease in X-ray attenuation.

Using a CT window width of 80 HU, the minimal visible contrast is at about 4 HU, which corresponds with an increase in brain tissue water content of about 1.5%. This suggests that the very first and potentially reversible stage of the developing ischemic edema cannot be seen on CT because the decline of attenuation has not reached the contrast resolution of 4 HU. In other words: a normal CT in a patient with stroke excludes hemorrhage and other disease, but cannot exclude ischemic edema at a very early stage. This insensitivity of CT for the very first

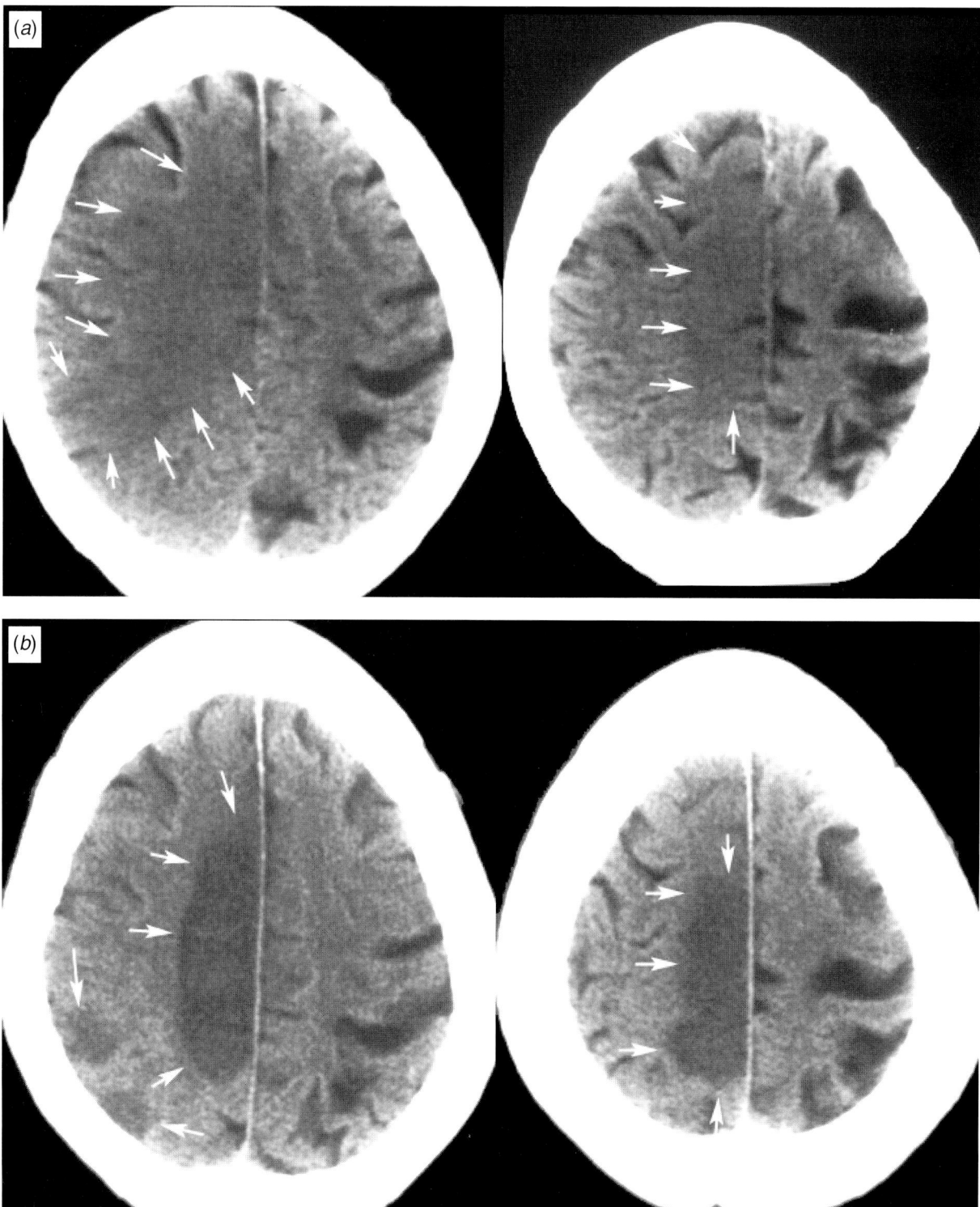

Fig. 3.4. CT within 6 hours of the sudden onset of left-sided hemiparesis. (*a*) The two sections show hypoattenuating tissue (arrows) within the territory of the pericallosal artery and of an MCA branch and in addition marked effacement of sulci due to ischemic brain tissue swelling. (*b*) Three days later the follow-up CT shows a well-marked cerebral infarct in the same territory. Tissue swelling is still present.

stage of ischemic edema may have an advantage: edema at that stage may be potentially reversible, so that CT depicts ischemic edema only at its irreversible stage. Hypoattenuation of brain parenchyma on CT after arterial occlusion indicates severe ischemia under the critical level of structural integrity for 1 to 3 hours. Under clinical conditions, hypoattenuation may appear by 22 minutes after the onset of symptoms.[17] It has not yet been studied, however, whether hypoattenuation of ischemic brain tissue can disappear if the tissue is reperfused less than 30–60 minutes after stroke onset and to what extent changes in CBV contribute to changes in CT attenuation.

Because of its subtlety, early ischemic edema is recognized with only moderate interobserver reliability.[6,7,23] The National Institute of Neurological Disorders and Stroke rt-PA stroke trialists and others demonstrated that training in CT reading considerably affects the sensitivity to detect ischemic edema.[23,24] Attempts were made to improve the capability of CT in detecting ischemic edema by performing a density-difference analysis between both cerebral hemispheres, by varying window width and centre level, and by using a quantitative score.[25–27]

The frequency of positive CT findings in acute stroke may also be diminished by the prejudice that CT is negative within the first 24 to 48 hours after stroke that is still discussed in review articles[28] and books.[29] In contrast, many studies have described positive findings within the first 3–6 hours of stroke onset: Tomura et al. studied 25 patients with embolic cerebral infarction between 40 and 340 minutes after the onset of symptoms.[30] Twenty-three CT scans (92%) were positive with 'obscuration of the lentiform nucleus' caused by hypodensity.[30] Bozzao et al. observed parenchymal hypodensity in 25 of 36 patients (69%).[31] A 'loss of the insular ribbon' was reported in 23 of 27 (85%) patients.[32] Horowitz et al. reported on hypodensity and mass effect in 56% of 50 scans.[33] When comparing MR vs. CT imaging in identical patients within 3 hours of symptom onset, CT was positive in 19 patients (53%) and MRI in 18 (50%) patients with hemispheric stroke.[34] We reported 17 positive CT scans (68%) performed in a series of 25 patients with MCA trunk occlusion during the first 2 hours. The incidence of positive CT findings increased to 89% in the third hour after symptom onset and to 100% thereafter.[35] In another series of patients with hemispheric stroke, the incidence of early CT signs of infarction was 82%.[36] In patients selected for thrombolytic therapy, 12 of 23 patients (52%) had a parenchymal hypodensity on the CT performed within 3 hours of stroke onset.[21] In a series of 100 consecutive patients with MCA infarction, CT detected hypodensity of the lentiform nucleus in 48% and of the insular cortex in 59% of the patients within 14 hours of stroke onset.[37] In a recent randomized trial on pro-urokinase in patients with MCA occlusions, the investigators detected infarct signs in 125 of 171 patients (73%) on CT within the first 6 hours.[38]

In summary, CT has the capacity to identify different pathophysiological states that all results in the same clinical picture of an acute stroke syndrome: intracranial hemorrhage, ischemic edema and ischemia without ischemic edema. In addition, arterial occlusion is detected in some patients. Because these CT findings represent different pathophysiological states, it is incorrect to address them all as 'early infarct signs'. Moreover, it makes no sense, to study and count certain 'CT signs', like 'obscuration of the lentiform nucleus', 'loss of the insular ribbon', 'loss of grey–white matter distinction', 'hypodensity', because all these phenomena are caused by hypoattenuating grey matter due to ischemic edema.

Level 2 of clinical efficacy: diagnostic accuracy of CT in acute cerebral ischemia

Diagnostic accuracy is the accuracy in detecting and classifying pathology, measured in true and false positive ratios.[2] The optimal design for assessing the diagnostic accuracy of CT is a prospective, blinded comparison to a reference standard in a consecutive series of patients from a relevant clinical population.[39] Because CT was the first modality that could image the brain in vivo, a reference standard for CT findings in acute cerebral ischemia has seldom been available.

Table 3.1. Cerebral hemorrhagic events in the placebo groups of randomized trials on thrombolysis

Trial	n	Cerebral hemorrhagic events		
		All (%)	'Symptomatic' (%)	fatal (%)
ECASS I	307	37	3	2
NINDS I and II	312	4	1	0.3
MAST E	154	40	3	n.a.
MAST I	156	10	1	n.a.
ASK	166	17	3	2
ECASS II	391	40	6	1
PROACT II	59	57	4	n.a.

Notes: ECASS, European Cooperative Acute Stroke Study; NINDS, National Institute of Neurological Disorder and Stroke rt-PA Study; MAST-E, Multicentre Acute Stroke Trial–Europe; MAST-I, Multicentre Acute Stroke Trial – Italy; ASK, Australian Streptokinase Trial; PROACT, Prolyse in Acute Cerebral Thromboembolism Trial.

Diagnostic accuracy of CT in detecting intracranial hemorrhage

Surgery or autopsy regularly confirms the CT finding of intracranial hemorrhage. To my knowledge, the rate of false negative CT in brain hemorrhage has not been extensively studied. Presumably, CT does not detect subtle and small hemorrhages into the brain parenchyma or CSF space. The frequency of post-ischemic hemorrhagic transformations is higher in pathological series than with serial CT[40] and varies among the placebo groups of major stroke trials (Table 3.1). The latter observations support the impression that the frequency of post-ischemic transformation is affected by the CT technique, the time and frequency of CT studies, the definition of a hemorrhage on CT, the experience in CT assessment and the patient population under study.

Diagnostic accuracy of CT in detecting arterial obstruction

The determination of the specificity of a hyperattenuating arterial segment requires the comparison with digital subtraction angiography (DSA) as a gold-standard for the assessment of arterial occlusion. We studied the 'hyperdense middle cerebral artery sign' (HMCAS) in 53 patients with DSA proven unilateral MCA trunk occlusions.[35] The HMCAS was positive in 25 patients (sensitivity: 47%) and 100% specific (no false-positive findings). Tomsick et al.[47] described a sensitivity of 79% and a specificity of 93% in 25 patients. The HMCAS may be false-positive in patients with calcification of the arterial wall or high hematocrit (Fig. 3.5).

Diagnostic accuracy of CT in detecting ischemic brain tissue swelling

For the discussion of 'false-negative' CT in acute stroke, it is important to recognize that no reference standard exists to determine the accuracy of CT in assessing brain tissue swelling with and without edema. A normal CT without any hypoattenuation of the brain parenchyma in a patient with acute stroke may be true negative and represent a disturbance of brain perfusion above the level that induces edema. Such a CT could be false negative if the hypoattenuation is too subtle or too small to be detected by CT. Another issue is whether hypoattenuation of tissue on early CT in stroke patients is specific for irreversible damage. This was recently prospectively studied in 786 patients.[17] In this study, CT predicted ischemic necrosis in 449 patients that was confirmed by follow-up CT in 433 patients (positive predictive value = 96%, specificity = 85%). The false-positive findings in 16 patients were explained in retrospect by image artefacts due to poor technique. A true normalization of prior hypoattenuating tissue was not observed.

Level 3 of clinical efficacy: diagnostic impact of CT in acute cerebral ischemia

It seems as if advances in imaging are being made faster than the ability to fully evaluate their diagnostic and therapeutic impact. Diagnostic impact is the accuracy and clinical value compared with existing alternatives.[2] MRI was introduced into clinical practice as the second modality that can image brain parenchyma, and is now considered as an evolving standard of care in acute stroke.[41] It is an unresolved

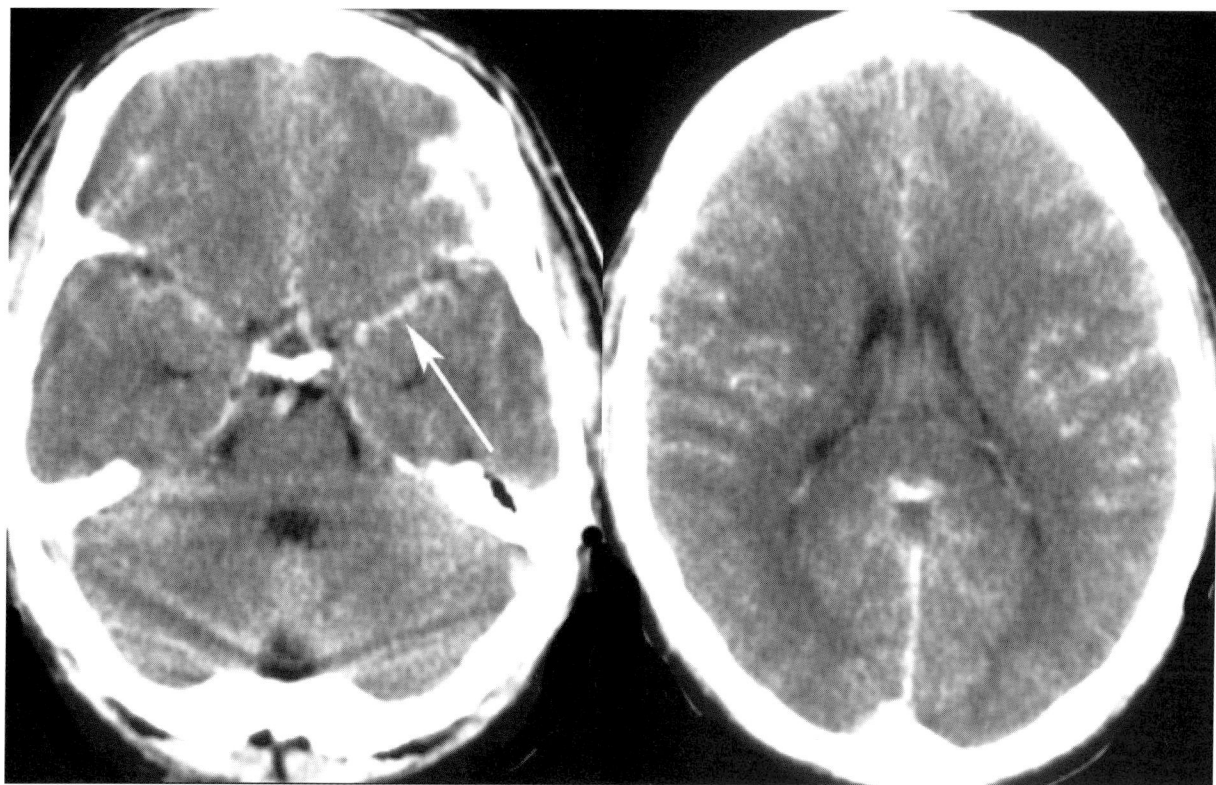

Fig. 3.5. CT of a 19-year-old man with Down syndrome, heart failure, and a hematocrit of 71% shows a hyperattenuating left MCA (arrow) and hyperattenuating other vessels, although contrast was not given.

issue, however, whether CT or MRI has a higher clinical efficacy in patients with acute stroke.

Diagnostic impact on intracranial hemorrhage

CT was the first imaging modality that could reliably differentiate between hemorrhagic and ischemic stroke. It seems as if susceptibility weighted MR sequences have the same sensitivity to detect brain hemorrhage in acute stroke.[42] Again, no randomized comparison has been done so far, to my knowledge, to decide whether CT can be completely replaced by MRI in acute stroke. It is another controversy, whether special MR sequences like FLAIR, have the same accuracy as CT in detecting SAH.[43–45]

Diagnostic impact on ischemic edema

The diagnostic accuracy and clinical value of both techniques have rarely been properly compared. In a gelatin model, there was a linear relationship between water content, CT attenuation, T_1–, and T_2 relaxation time. An increase in water content of 6%, however, resulted in only a 19% increase in signal intensity of gel on the T_2-weighted image, but in a 25% change in CT attenuation in the same specimens.[20] In an experiment with boiled eggs, Unger et al. demonstrated that T2 relaxation is not only affected by water content. Egg hardening caused dramatic T_2 shortening and modest T_1 shortening, but had no effect on CT attenuation,[20] suggesting that the proportion of bound or structured water affects T_2 relaxation. It is still unclear, however, whether the effects of water structure play a role in the acute ischemic brain. Typical flaws of studies comparing CT with MRI were no reference standard, or a poorly defined one,[46–49] and MRI performed considerably later than CT.[47,49] To our knowledge, no study compared CT and MRI in a randomized manner. Not surprisingly, some studies

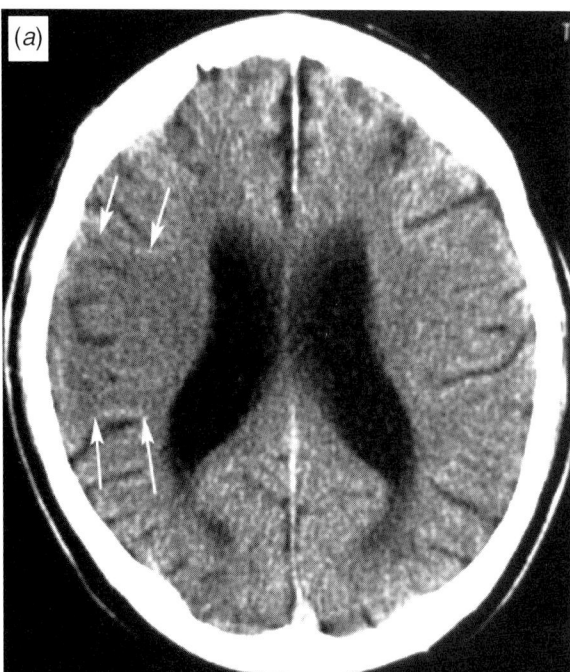

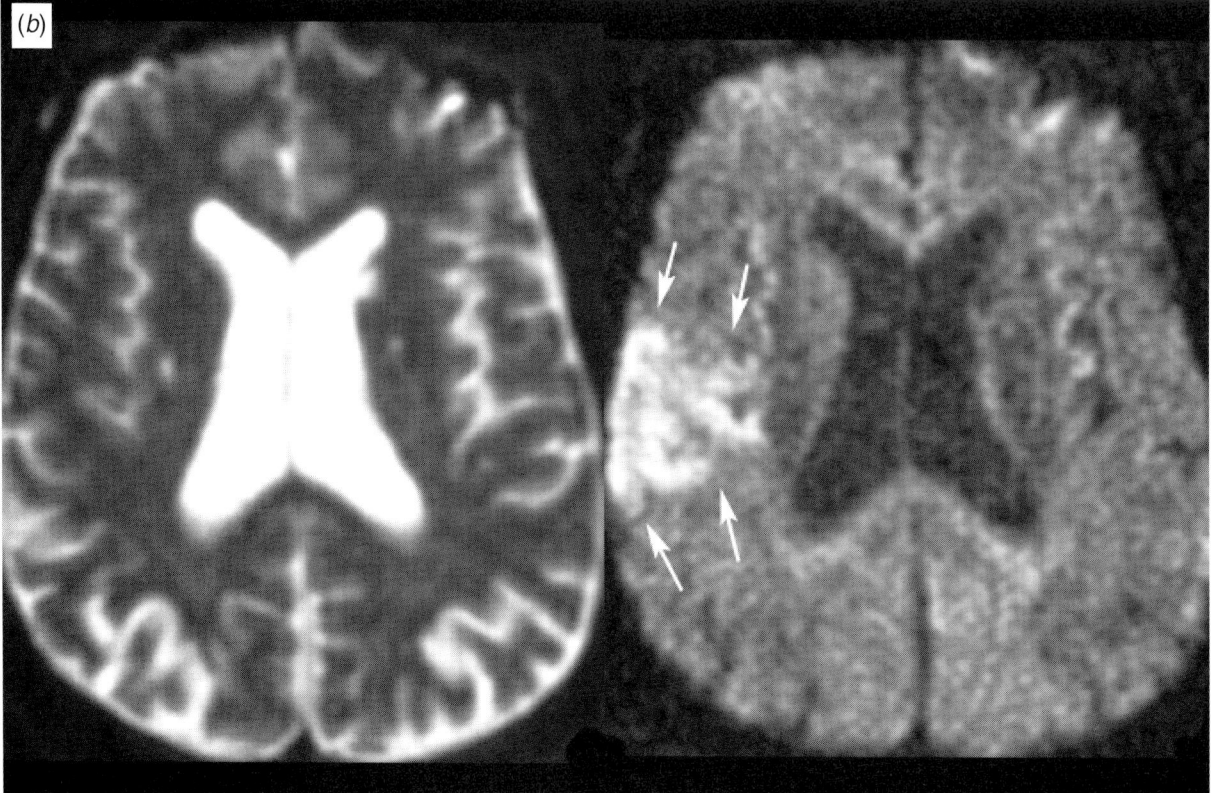

Fig. 3.6. (*a*) CT performed 90 minutes after onset of left-sided hemiparesis shows a wedge shaped area of hypoattenuating brain tissue (arrows). (*b*) The MRI was performed 2 hours after symptom onset. The T_2W image does not show any pathology in this area. The DWI shows disturbed diffusion within the area depicted by CT 30 minutes earlier.

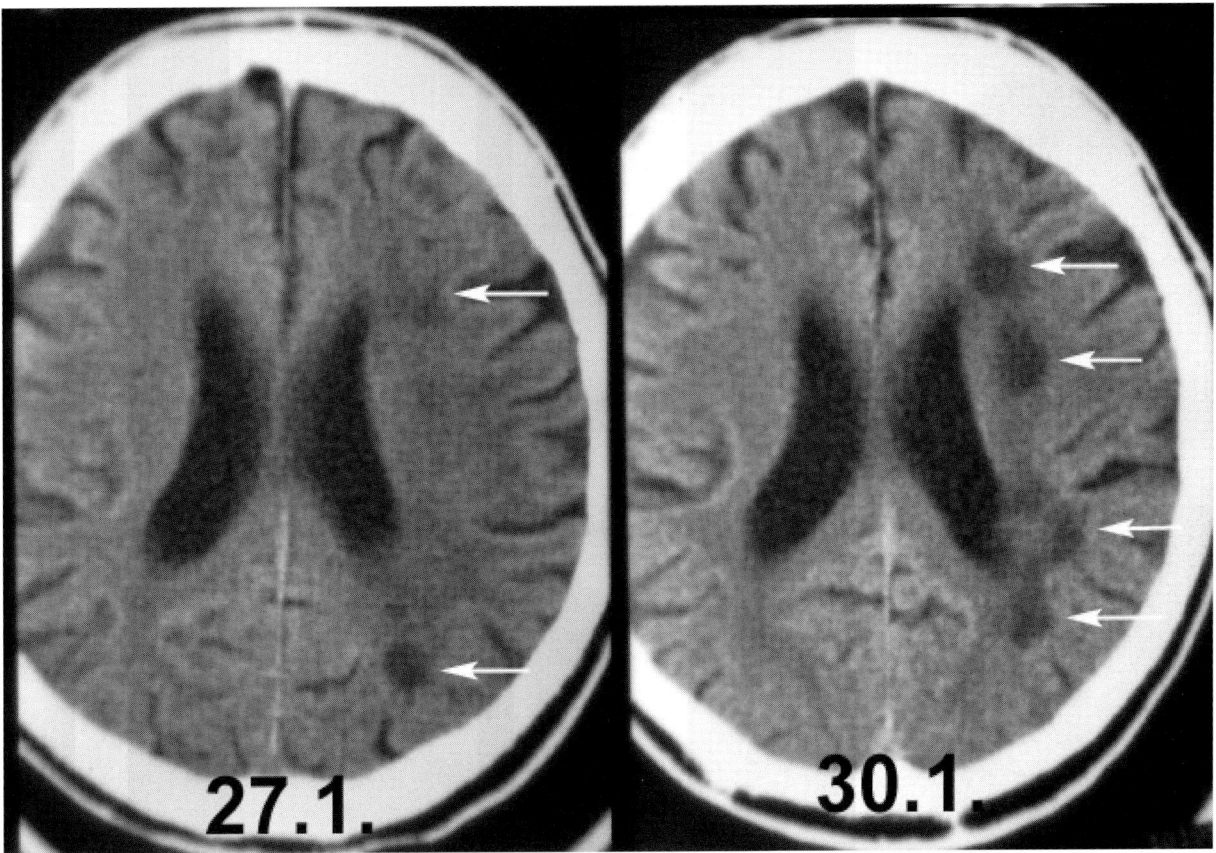

Fig. 3.7. Two CT scans within 4 days of a 73-year-old man with occlusion of the left internal carotid artery and progressive right-sided hemiparesis and aphasia. The ischemic lesions are mainly located in the end-supply area of the left MCA (arrows).

found that MRI including diffusion-weighted imaging (DWI) is more sensitive than CT[46–49], whereas other studies did not show that MRI is superior to CT in detecting ischemic changes of cerebral parenchyma.[34,50]

CT was used to differentiate among types of cerebral ischemia like territorial infarcts (Fig. 3.6) caused by emboli, infarcts in end-supply areas or 'watershed areas' (Fig. 3.7) often associated with major artery occlusion or stenosis, and disseminated small infarcts (Fig. 3.8) caused by small vessel disease.[51] Others have challenged the concept that stroke mechanisms can be inferred from interpretation of lesion patterns on brain scans.[52,53]

Another approach to the diagnostic impact of CT is the interpretation of the extent of ischemic edema detected by CT. We showed that the extent of hypoattenuating brain tissue due to ischemic edema is associated with the neurological score and with clinical outcome.[17,35,54–56] Fiorelli et al. concluded from their experience with emergency CT in acute ischemic stroke that it adds significantly to the prediction of clinical outcome made on clinical grounds.[57]

Level 4 of clinical efficacy: therapeutic impact of CT in acute cerebral ischemia

Therapeutic impact is the effect of the diagnostic test on patient care, on prognostic information, on treatment selection, and on the costs and risks of the diagnostic process.[2]

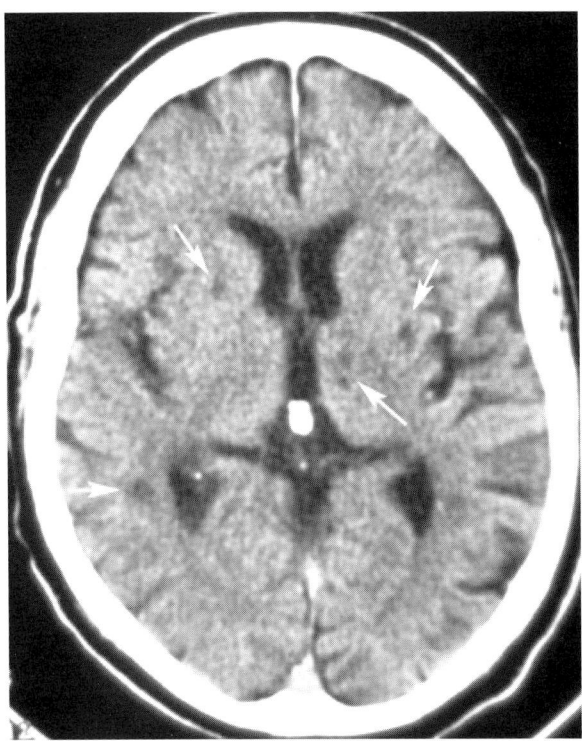

Fig. 3.8. 59-year-old man with acute mild stroke since 3 hours. CT shows multiple small subcortical ischemic lesions (arrows) typical for dissiminated small vessel disease.

For the first time in history, CT enabled the identification of patients suffering from cerebral ischemia. As a consequence, specific treatment like thrombolysis could be tested. CT has thus an enormous therapeutic impact just by differentiating between ischemic and hemorrhagic stroke.

In acute cerebral ischemia, the only treatment that is proved to improve clinical outcome is intravenous thrombolysis with rt-PA applied within 3 hours of symptom onset or intra-arterial infusion of pro-urokinase in patients with MCA occlusion if applied within 6 hours of symptom onset.[38,58] Whereas the NINDS rt-PA Study Group used CT to exclude patients with intracranial hemorrhage, the PROACT investigators excluded patients from the study who had a hypoattenuated area on CT exceeding one third of the MCA territory. The first ECASS study supported the hypothesis that patients with such a region of extensive ischemic edema did not benefit from rt-PA treatment and

has an increased risk for brain hemorrhage.[55,59] This hypothesis was confirmed by ECASS II.[60,61] Moreover, the ECASS II data showed, that acute stroke patients with a normal CT have a less severe neurological deficit and a better clinical course compared to patients with hypoattenuated brain tissue. This is illustrated in Fig. 3.9 showing the NIHSS over time in the ECASS I and II populations in relationship with the findings on their baseline CT.

Level 5 of clinical efficacy: impact on patient outcome of CT in acute cerebral ischemia

Impact on patient outcome is the most important criterion for the usefulness of a diagnostic test showing that it leads to a change in patient management that improves patient outcome.[2] ECASS I and II are the only studies with prospectively defined categories for the extent of ischemic edema on baseline CT. We will use here the combined dataset of both trials to study whether the response to rt-PA treatment was different in patients with a normal CT compared to patients with a small region of edema (≤ 33% of MCA territory) (Fig. 3.10) and compared to patients with more extensive edema (> 33% of MCA territory) (Fig. 3.11). This dataset includes 1350 patients. According to the common assessment of 3 neuroradiologists, 688 patients had a normal CT at baseline, 618 patients had a small ischemic edema, and only 89 patients had extensive ischemic edema. (Such large edema was an exclusion criterion in ECASS I and II.) Figure 3.9 shows that only patients with small ischemic edema had benefit from rt-PA treatment. The odds ratio for a beneficial outcome without a functional deficit (Rankin 0 and 1) at 3 months was 1.20 (95% CI, 0.89 – 1.63) for patients with normal CT, 1.47 (95% CI, 1.03 – 2.09) for patients with small ischemic edema, and 0.71 (95% CI, 0.21 – 2.41) for patients with large edema. This suggests that rt-PA treatment may enhance the chance for stroke patients by almost 50% to not be disabled after 3 months. In contrast, rt-PA treatment did not demonstrate a beneficial effect in patients with

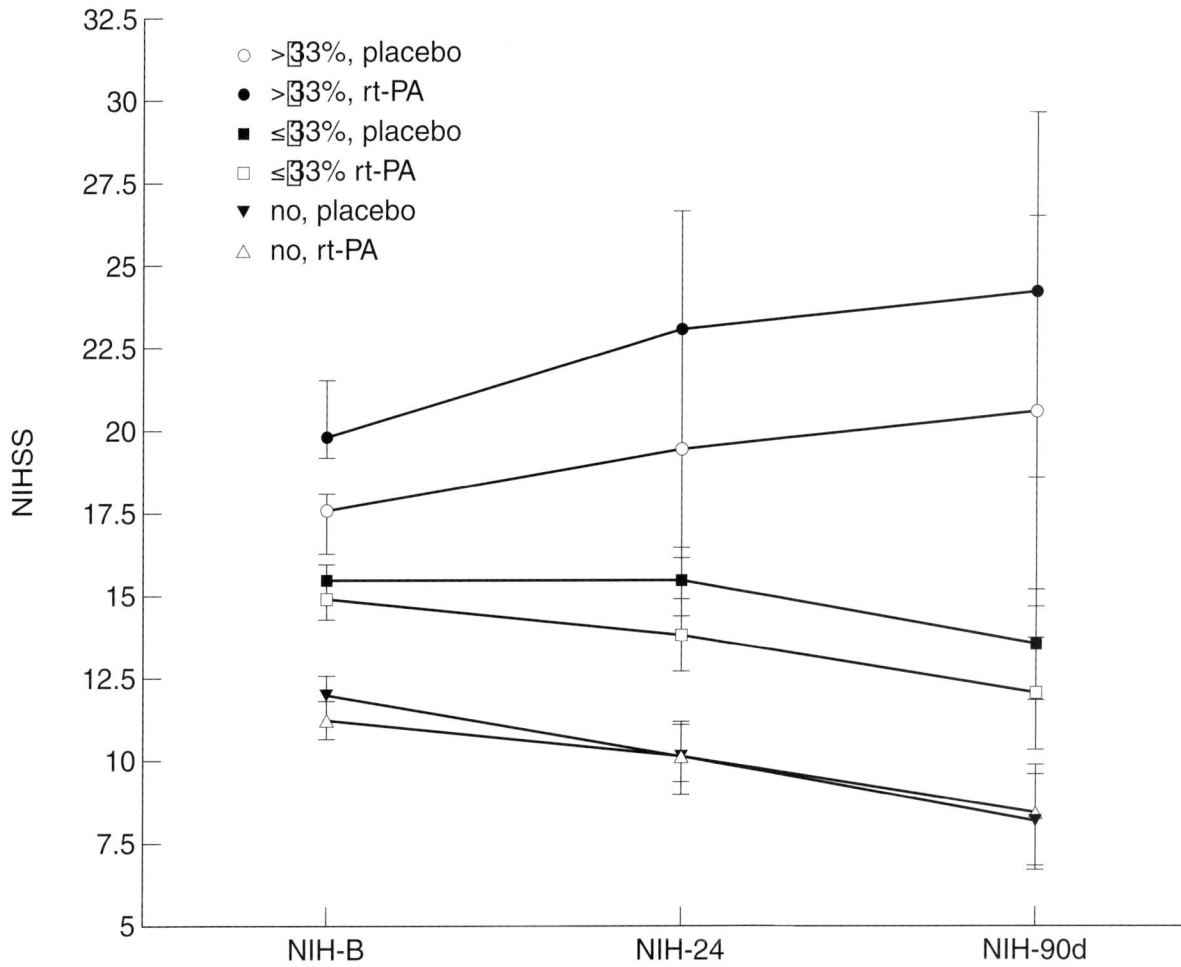

Fig. 3.9. Baseline CT findings in ECASS I and II and the response to rt-PA. NIHSS, National Institute of Health Stroke Scale; NIH-B, NIHSS at baseline; NIH-24, NIHSS at 24 hours after stroke onset; NIH-90d, NIHSS at 3 months after stroke onset.

normal CT, and may be deleterious in patients with a large region of ischemic edema. The last group was, however, too small to really prove the impact of this CT finding on patient outcome.

Kent and Larson proposed four grades of methodologic quality for studies of diagnostic tests:[1] (a) studies with broad generalizability to a variety of patients and no significant flaws in research methods; (b) studies with a narrower spectrum of generalizability and with only a few flaws that are well described so that their impact on conclusions can be assessed; (c) studies with several flaws in research methods, small sample sizes, or incomplete reporting; (d) studies with multiple flaws in research methods or reports of opinion unsubstantiated by data.

ECASS II was a double-blinded randomized multicentre-controlled trial with a prospective protocol of CT assessment. This trial provides high-quality evidence (grade B evidence) that the CT finding of hypoattenuating brain tissue in less than one-third of the MCA territory is associated with a beneficial effect of rt-PA treatment in ischemic stroke.

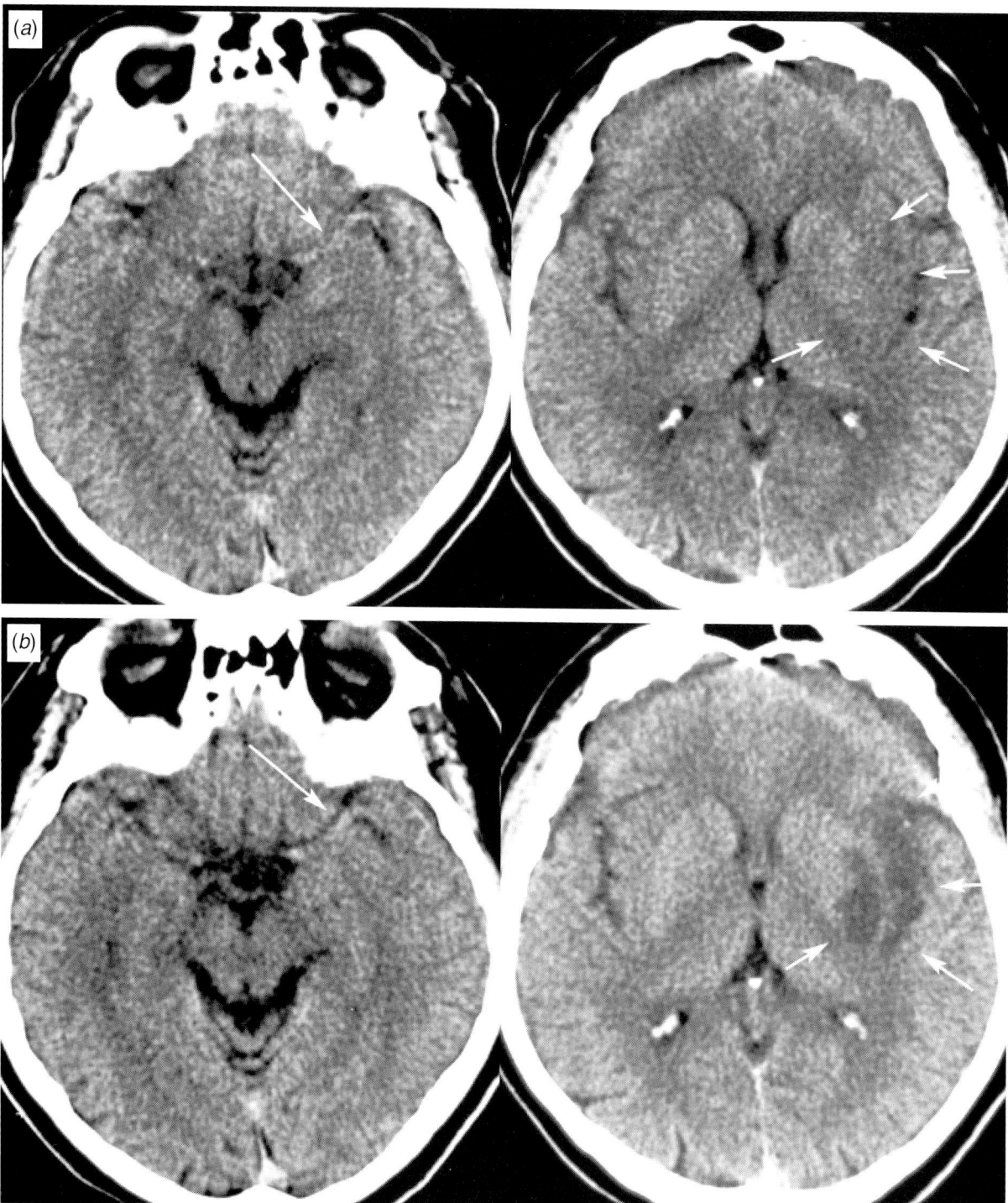

Fig. 3.10. Two CT scans in a 42-year-old man. (*a*) The first scan was obtained 2 hours after stroke onset and shows a hyperattenuated left MCA trunk (long arrow) and branches and a hypoattenuating left insular cortex and putamen (short arrows). (*b*) The second scan was obtained 24 hours later. The hypoattenuating brain tissue is still restricted to the left insular cortex and putamen (short arrows) despite a hyperattenuated left MCA (long arrow).

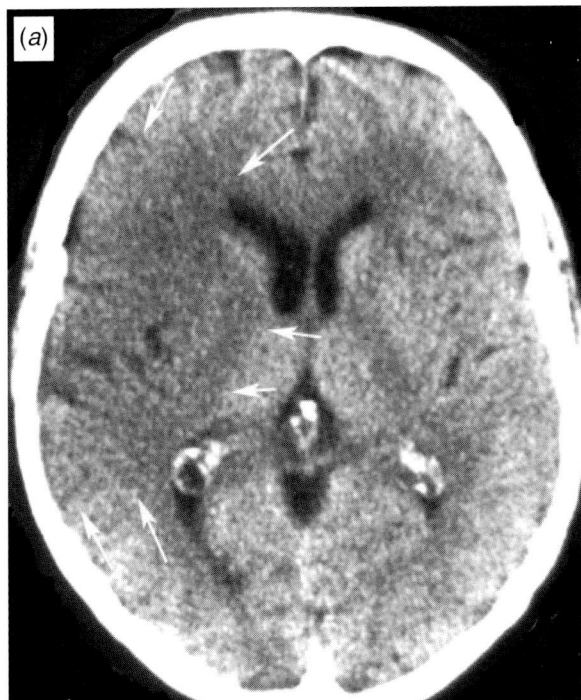 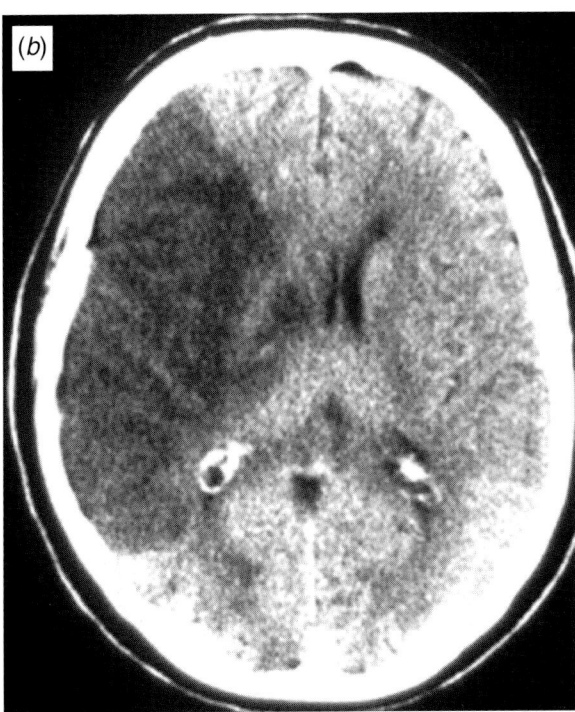

Fig. 3.11. Two CT scans in a 68-year-old man. (*a*) The first scan obtained 140 minutes after stroke onset shows an extended area of hypoattenuated brain tissue (arrows) covering the entire right MCA territory in this section. (*b*) Seven days later and after placebo treatment, the follow-up scan shows a complete right MCA infarction with slight hemorrhagic transformation.

REFERENCES

1. Kent D, Larson E. Disease, level of impact, and quality of research methods; three dimensions of clinical efficacy assessment applied to magnetic resonance imaging. *Invest Radiol* 1992; 27: 245–254.
2. Powers W. Testing a test. A report card for DWI in acute stroke. *Neurology* 2000; 54: 1549–1551.
3. Schriger D, Kalafut M, Starkman S, Krueger M, Daver J. Cranial computed tomography interpretation in acute stroke. Physician accuracy in determining eligibility for thrombolytic therapy. *J Am Med Assoc* 1998; 279: 1293–1297.
4. Schievink W. Intracranial aneurysms. *N Engl J Med* 1997; 336: 28–40.
5. Tomsick T, Brott T, Chambers A, et al. Hyperdense middle artery sign on CT: efficacy in detecting middle cerebral artery thrombosis. *Am J Neuroradiol* 1990; 11: 473–477.
6. von Kummer R, Holle R, Grzyska U et al. Interobserver agreement in assessing early CT signs of middle cerebral artery infarction. *Am J Neuroradiol* 1996; 17: 1743–1748.
7. Marks M, Holmgren E, Fox A, Patel S, von Kummer R, Froehlich J. Evaluation of early computed tomographic findings in acute ischemic stroke. *Stroke* 1999; 30: 389–392.
8. Gibbs J, Wise R, Leenders K, Jones T. Evaluation of cerebral perfusion reserve in patients with carotid-artery occlusion. *Lancet* 1984; 8372: 310–314.
9. Yuh W, Simonson T, Wang A et al. Venous sinus occlusive disease: MR findings. *Am J Neuroradiol* 1994; 15: 309–316.
10. Hossmann KA. Viability thresholds and the penumbra of focal ischemia. *Ann Neurol* 1994; 36: 557–565.
11. Watanabe O, West C, Bremer A. Experimental regional cerebral ischemia in the middle cerebral artery territory in primates. Part 2: Effects on brain water and electrolytes in the early phase of MCA stroke. *Stroke* 1977; 8: 71–76.
12. Schuier FJ, Hossmann KA. Experimental brain infarcts in cats. II. Ischemic brain edema. *Stroke* 1980; 11: 593–601.
13. Todd N, Picozzi P, Crockard A, Ross Russel R. Duration of ischemia influences the development and resolution of ischemic brain edema. *Stroke* 1986; 17: 466–471.

14 Gotoh O, Asano T, Koide T, Takakura K. Ischemic brain edema following occlusion of the middle cerebral artery in the rat. I: The time courses of the brain water, sodium, and potassium contents and blood–brain-barrier permeability to ^{125}I-Albumin. *Stroke* 1985; 16: 101–109.

15 Wang Y, Hu W, Perez-Trepichio A et al. Brain tissue sodium is a ticking clock telling time after arterial occlusion in rat focal cerebral ischemia. *Stroke* 2000; 31: 1386–1392.

16 Todd N, Picozzi P, Crockard A, Ross Russel R. Reperfusion after cerebral ischemia: Influence of duration of ischemia. *Stroke* 1986; 17: 460–465.

17 von Kummer R, Bourquain H, Bastianello S et al. Early prediction of irreversible brain damage after ischemic stroke by computed tomography. *Radiology* 2001; 219: 95–100.

18 Phelps M, Gado M, Hoffman E. Correlation of effective anatomic number and electron density with attenuation coefficients measured with polychromatic X-rays. *Radiology* 1975; 117: 585–588.

19 Rieth KG, Fujiwara K, Di Chiro G et al. Serial measurements of CT attenuation and specific gravity in experimental cerebral edema. *Radiology* 1980; 135: 343–348.

20 Unger E, Littlefield J, Gado M. Water content and water structure in CT and MR signal changes: Possible influence in detection of early stroke. *Am J Neuroradiol* 1988; 9: 687–691.

21 Grond M, von Kummer R, Sobesky J, Schmülling S, Heiss W-D. Early computed-tomography abnormalities in acute stroke. *Lancet* 1997; 350: 1595–1596.

22 Firlik A, Kaufmann A, Wechsler L, Firlik K, Fukui M, Yonas H. Quantitative cerebral blood flow determinations in acute ischemic stroke. Relationship to computed tomography and angiography. *Stroke* 1997; 28: 2208–2213.

23. Grotta J, Chiu D, Lu M et al. Agreement and variability in the interpretation of early CT changes in stroke patients qualifying for intravenous rtPA therapy. *Stroke* 1999; 30: 1528–1533.

24 von Kummer R. Effect of training in reading CT scans on patient selection for ECASS II. *Neurology* 1998; 51 (Suppl 3): S50–S52.

25 Bendszus M, Urbach H, Meyer B, Schultheiss R, Solymosi L. Improved CT diagnosis of acute middle cerebral artery territory infarcts with density-difference analysis. *Neuroradiology* 1997; 39: 127–131.

26 Lev M, Farkas J, Gemmete J et al. Acute stroke: improved nonenhanced CT detection–benefits of soft-copy interpretation by using variable window width and center level settings. *Radiology* 1999; 213: 150–155.

27 Barber P, Demchuk A, Zhang J, Buchan A. Validity and reliability of a quantitative computed tomography score in predicting outcome of hyperacute stroke before thrombolytic therapy. *Lancet* 2000; 355: 1670–1674.

28. Gilman S. Imaging of the brain. *N Engl J Med* 1998; 338: 812–820.

29 Sorensen A, Reimer P. *Cerebral MR Perfusion Imaging.* Stuttgart, New York: Thieme; 2000.

30 Tomura N, Uemura K, Inugami A, Fujita H, Higano S, Shishido F. Early CT finding in cerebral infarction. *Radiology* 1988; 168: 463–467.

31 Bozzao L, Bastianello S, Fantozzi LM, Angeloni U, Argentino C, Fieschi C. Correlation of angiographic and sequential CT findings in patients with evolving cerebral infarction. *Am J Neuroradiol* 1989; 10: 1215–1222.

32 Truwit C, Barkovich A, Gean-Marton A, Hibri N, Norman D. Loss of the insular ribbon: Another early CT sign of acute middle cerebral artery infarction. *Radiology* 1990; 176: 801–806.

33 Horowitz SH, Zito JL, Donnarumma R, Patel M, Alvir J. Computed tomographic – angiographic findings within the first five hours of cerebral infarction. *Stroke* 1991; 22: 1245–1253.

34 Mohr J, Biller J, Hilal S et al. Magnetic resonance versus computed tomographic imaging in acute stroke. *Stroke* 1995; 26: 807–812.

35 von Kummer R, Meyding-Lamadé U, Forsting M et al. Sensitivity and prognostic value of early computed tomography in middle cerebral artery trunk occlusion. *Am J Neuroradiol* 1994; 15: 9–15.

36 von Kummer R, Nolte PN, Schnittger H, Thron A, Ringelstein EB. Detectability of hemispheric ischemic infarction by computed tomography within 6 hours after stroke. *Neuroradiology* 1996; 38: 31–33.

37 Moulin T, Cattin F, Crépin-Leblond T et al. Early CT signs in acute middle cerebral artery infarction: Predictive value for subsequent infarct locations and outcome. *Neurology* 1996; 47: 355–375.

38 Furlan A, Higashida R, Wechsler L et al. Intra-arterial prourokinase for acute ischemic stroke. *J Am Med Assoc* 1999; 282: 2003–2011.

39 Lijmer J, Mol B, Heiserkamp S et al. Empirical evidence of design-related bias in studies of diagnostic tests. *J Am Med Assoc* 1999; 282: 1061–1066.

40 Hornig C, Dorndorf W, Agnoli A. Hemorrhagic cerebral infarction: a prospective study. *Stroke* 1986; 17: 179–185.

41 Hacke E, Warach S. Diffusion-weighted MRI as an evolving standard of care in acute stroke. *Neurology* 2000; 54: 1548–1549.
42 Schellinger P, Jansen O, Fiebach J, Hacke W, Sartor K. A standardized MRI stroke protocol: comparison with CT in hyperacute intracerebral hemorrhage. *Stroke* 1999; 30: 1974–1975.
43 Ogawa T, Inugami A, Shimosegawa E et al. Subarachnoid hemorrhage: Evaluation with MR imaging. *Radiology* 1993; 186: 345–351.
44 Atlas S. MR imaging is highly sensitive for acute subarachnoid hemorrhage ... Not! *Radiology* 1993; 186: 319–322.
45 Noguchi K, Ogawa T, Inugami A et al. Acute subarachnoid hemorrhage: MR Imaging with fluid-attenuated inversion recovery pulse sequences. *Radiology* 1995; 196: 773–777.
46 Kertesz A, Black S, Nicholson L, Carr T. The sensitivity and specificity of MRI in stroke. *Neurology* 1987; 37: 1580–1585.
47 Bryan N, Levy L, Whitlow W, Killian J, Preziosi T, Rosario J. Diagnosis of acute cerebral infarction: Comparison of CT and MR Imaging. *Am J Neuroradiol* 1991; 12: 611–620.
48 Barber P, Darby D, Desmond P et al. Identification of major ischemic change: diffusion-weighted imaging versus computed tomography. *Stroke* 1999; 30: 2059–2065.
49 Lansberg M, Albers G, Beaulieu C, Marks M. Comparison of diffusion-weighted MRI and CT in acute stroke. *Neurology* 2000; 54: 1557–1561.
50 Barber P, Demchuk A, Hill M et al. A comparison of CT versus MR imaging in acute stroke using ASPECTS: Will the 'new' replace the 'old' as the preferred imaging modality? *Stroke* 2001; 32: 325 (abstract).
51 Ringelstein E, Biniek R, Weiller C, Ammeling B, Nolte P, Thron A. Type and extent of hemispheric brain infarctions and clinical outcome in early and delayed middle cerebral artery recanalization. *Neurology* 1992; 42: 289–298.
52 Caplan L, Hennerici M. Impaired clearance of emboli (washout) is an important link between hypoperfusion, embolism, and ischemic stroke. *Arch Neurol* 1998; 55: 1475–1482.
53 Hennerici M, Daffertshofer M, Jakobs L. Failure to identify cerebral infarct mechanisms from topography of vascular territory lesions. *Am J Neuroradiol* 1998; 19: 1067–1074.
54 von Kummer R, Bastianello S, Bozzao L, Manelfe C, Hacke W. Early prediction of fatal ischemic brain edema. *Stroke* 1996; 27: 181.
55 von Kummer R, Allen K, Holle R et al. Acute stroke: usefulness of early CT findings before thrombolytic therapy. *Radiology* 1997; 205: 327–333.
56 von Kummer R, Bourquain H, Manelfe C, Bastianello S, Bozzao L, Meier D. Predictive value of early CT in acute ischemic stroke. *Stroke* 1999; 30: 250.
57 Fiorelli M, Toni D, Bastianello S et al. Computed tomography findings in the first few hours of ischemic stroke: implications for the clinician. *J Neurol Sci.* 2000; 173: 10–17.
58 NINDS Stroke Study Group. Tissue plasminogen activator for acute ischemic stroke. *N Engl J Med* 1995; 333: 1581–1587.
59 Larrue V, von Kummer R, del Zoppo G, Bluhmki E. Hemorrhagic transformation in acute ischemic stroke. Potential contributing factors in the European Cooperative Acute Stroke Study. *Stroke* 1997; 28: 957–960.
60 Hacke W, Kaste M, Fieschi C et al. Randomised double-blind placebo-controlled trial of thrombolytic therapy with intravenous alteplase in acute ischaemic stroke (ECASS II). *Lancet* 1998; 352: 1245–1251.
61 Larrue V, von Kummer R, Müller A, Bluhmki E. Risk factors for severe hemorrhagic transformation in ischemic stroke patients treated with rt-PA. *Stroke* 2001; 32: 438–441.

Computerized tomographic-based evaluation of cerebral blood flow

Lawrence R. Wechsler, Steven Goldstein and Howard Yonas

University of Pittsburgh Health System, Stroke Institute, Departments of Neurology and Neurosurgery, PA, USA

Introducton

Functional neuroimaging in the form of cerebral blood flow (CBF) measurement continues to be a rapidly expanding tool in the care of patients with cerebrovascular disease, head trauma, seizure disorders and many other disease states involving the central nervous system. Computerized tomographic (CT)-based assessment of cerebral blood flow (CBF) offers many advantages in the care of patients with disorders of the central nervous system. CT-based technology capable of evaluating CBF can be readily combined with routine CT scanning equipment thus increasing the availability and decreasing the costs of this technology. Monitoring of patients with respiratory and hemodynamic instability is also more easily done using CT based technology. In addition, patients with mechanical heart valves, permanent cardiac pacemakers and other ferromagnetic devices can be safely studied. Two primary CT-based imaging techniques are clinically available to evaluate CBF; stable xenon enhanced CT (XeCT) and dynamic CT perfusion imaging (CTP). These techniques are based upon two entirely different mathematical models. XeCT is based upon the well-established diffusable tracer model, while CTP is based upon a non-diffusable tracer kinetic model that can be applied to both CTP and magnetic resonance perfusion (MRP).

Xenon CT cerebral blood flow

Xenon (Xe) is a naturally occurring element that is an inert gas at room temperatures. Like iodine, Xe is effective in attenuating X-rays and can therefore be employed as a contrast agent. Unlike iodine, Xe is not reactive and is freely diffusible throughout most tissues in our body including the blood–brain barrier. These properties which are not dependent on radioactivity have led to a commercially available product that can interface with most modern CT scanners and is capable of measuring blood flow quantitatively.[1,2]

After inhalation, Xe diffuses into the circulation through the pulmonary capillary bed then rapidly crosses the blood–brain barrier into brain tissue. The CT scanner is able to detect small changes in attenuation due to the presence of Xe and the change in density is directly proportional to the concentration of Xe in the tissues. Since the Xe concentration in the blood can be measured indirectly by monitoring the end expiratory Xe concentration, and the change in density is measured directly by the sequential CT images, computation of cerebral blood flow on a pixel by pixel basis can be calculated.[3] The actual arterial concentration can be estimated based on the end expiratory concentration, and this allows the calculation of quantitative CBF values. CBF for all pixels is displayed in a colour-coded flow map and areas of interest can be drawn to outline vascular territories.

A series of images are obtained throughout the brain over a 6-minute interval. This includes two baseline images at each slice location followed by six additional images at each level during 4½ minutes of Xe inhalation. Only 28% Xe concentrations are required currently, which is well below the 80% dose usually associated with anesthesia.

This method has the advantage in stroke patients of allowing CBF measurements without moving from the CT table. Since most stroke patients undergo CT scanning to detect hemorrhage, CT based CBF measurements eliminate the need to move the patient and reduce overall time to acquire physiological data, a point that is particularly important in treatment of patients with acute stroke. Set-up time for XeCT CBF studies requires only a few minutes and the entire study is completed in 5–10 minutes. Processing data and construction of CBF maps adds another 5 minutes so that the time from completion of the standard head CT to obtaining clinically useful CBF information is only 15–20 minutes.

Some technical pitfalls exist. The major problem encountered is related to patient motion. Since the technique requires a series of sections to be obtained at precisely the same locations, any movement between slice acquisitions can be a source of error. That is, if a patient moves between images then the pixels are misaligned and the accuracy of the calculations is decreased. With attention to gaining the trust of the patient, careful positioning and securing the head, and occasional intravenous sedation, greater than 90% of awake studies yield useful information. If a patient is paralysed and intubated, the yield of excellent studies approaches 100%. Gas leaks in the administration set or in the mouth piece can also occur, though the monitoring systems usually detect these quickly. Finally, in theory, pulmonary disease sufficient to cause poor diffusion of the Xe gas across the capillary membranes from the alveoli to the bloodstream could impair the uptake and alter the apparent equilibrium, although in over 9000 studies at our institution, this has rarely been a problem. The one issue related to pulmonary disease that occasionally has been problematic occurs in patients who require high percentages of oxygen in a ventilator in order to maintain oxygenation. Then, the addition of Xe gas may require decreasing the percentage of oxygen during the blood flow examination and, in some clinical situations, this may be intolerable to the patient. Agitation or vomiting occurs rarely, particularly with the use of lower Xe concentrations associated with current CT scanning technology. In the vast majority of patients, the technical limitations are easily overcome and cerebral blood flow data can be obtained expeditiously.

Clinical applications of XeCT

The primary goal of thrombolytic therapy in acute stroke is to re-establish tissue perfusion before the onset of irreversible ischemia. Two major determinants of irreversible cerebral ischemia leading to tissue infarction include the duration and severity of reduced CBF.[4] In a review of thresholds of ischemia in different animal models, Hossmann demonstrated a distinct rank order of susceptibilities to eventual infarction.[5] The sodium–potassium ratio of brain tissue, an important marker of anoxic depolarization, increases at CBF values below 10–15 ml/100 g per min[6] and extracellular ion changes occur at CBF values between 6 and 15 ml/100 g per min.[7–9] In the baboon, Yonas et al. demonstrated that selective occlusion of the lenticulostriate arteries caused reduction of CBF to < 8 ml/100 g/min. At this level of CBF tissue infarction was consistently produced after 60 minutes.[10,11] This suggests that the early extent of severe ischemia defines the final extent of infarction.

Acute stroke

In patients with acute stroke, direct measurement of CBF is potentially helpful to maximize the benefit of acute stroke therapy and reduce the complications. To accomplish these goals, an imaging method must distinguish brain already infarcted or destined to infarct from reversibly ischemic brain capable of returning to normal functioning with reperfusion. In addition, some patients recanalize in the first few hours after stroke despite persistent neurological deficits. In such cases, normal CBF values suggest that reperfusion therapy is not necessary, possibly avoiding angiography or thrombolytic therapy.

Xenon CT provides quantitative CBF values that can potentially be used to triage acute stroke patients. CBF values below 6 cm^3/100 g per min measured in the setting of acute stroke correlated with subsequent infarction on follow-up CT whether or not reperfusion had occurred following thrombolytic therapy.[12] Patients with occlusion of the M1 segment of the middle cerebral artery (MCA) had significantly lower mean CBF values in the MCA territory than those without MCA occlusion.[13] All patients with M1 occlusions had mean MCA CBF values less than 20 cm^3/100 g per min. Thus Xe CT may identify within the first few hours after stroke areas of brain already infarcted as well as predict the presence of proximal arterial occlusion.

Reperfusion of infracted brain does little to improve neurological function but may cause neurological worsening due to hemorrhage or cerebral edema with herniation. Mean CBF values in the MCA territory less than 15 ml^3/100 g per min were associated with a greater risk of hemorrhage or herniation in patients treated with thrombolytic therapy after acute stroke.[14] CBF values were also shown to more accurately predict complications of symptomatic hemorrhagic conversion or herniation due to edema than initial NIHSS (Figs. 4.1, 4.2, see colour plate section).[15]

Initial CBF values may also predict long-term outcome in patients with acute stroke. Mean CBF measured within 6 hours of stroke onset was significantly lower in patients with severe deficits or death 1 year or more after stroke compared to those with mild deficits.[16] CBF also predicted long-term outcome better than time to treatment which correlated poorly with long-term deficits. Similarly, CBF measured by XeCT in the first few hours after stroke was more predictive of subsequent infarction on CT than time from onset of symptoms to CBF measurement.[17]

In some patients, despite significant neurological deficits, CBF in the affected vascular territory is normal. This suggests reperfusion has already occurred and that there is little to gain by attempting thrombolysis. In many such patients, neurological deficits resolve over the ensuing 24 hours without acute stroke interventions.[18] The ability to avoid therapy with the potential to cause intracerebral hemorrhage in patients destined to improve may be a valuable contribution of quantitative CBF measurements in the setting of acute stroke.

Intermediate levels of CBF measured by XeCT may predict brain regions that can be salvaged with acute stroke therapy. Ultimately, the optimal CBF technique in acute stroke will be able to consistently identify areas of brain potentially recoverable by reperfusion or other acute stroke therapies. CBF values less than 20 ml/100 g per min indicating ischemia but greater than 6 ml/100 g per min, the level at which irreversible ischemia occurs even within the first few hours after stroke, hold the promise of identifying such reversibly ischemic areas. This must be confirmed by prospective studies showing that brain regions with this level of CBF go on to infarction if untreated, but recover after acute stroke intervention.

A possible problem with using CBF measurement in acute stroke is that measurements represent only one point in a time continuum from the moment of stroke onset. The CBF value obtained may vary with time and may not be representative of CBF values over the entire time since onset.[19] Studies performed in a primate model of middle cerebral artery stroke suggests, however, that without reperfusion there is little fluctuation in CBF within the first few hours. For each individual animal, the probability of an MCA qCBF value remaining within the 0–10 ml/100 g per min range at any point in time over 6 hours range was 95% (see Fig. 4.3). Clinically, this would suggest that qCBF determination in ischemic stroke, demonstrating the presence of an ischemic core measured within the first 6 hours after symptom onset, is unlikely to be significantly different if measured before, or after, the clinical study upon which treatment decisions may potentially be based.

Chronic cerebral ischemia

The role of hemodynamic factors in the risk of recurrent stroke in patients with extracranial carotid occlusive disease remains controversial. From 1977 to 1985, The International Cooperative Study of Extracranial–Intracranial Arterial Anastomosis compared the efficacy of the STA–MCA bypass procedure to medical management with aspirin therapy in a group of patients with minor strokes or TIAs within 3 months prior to surgery.[20] Despite its negative results some clinicians believe that patients with compromised hemodynamics may benefit from revascularization

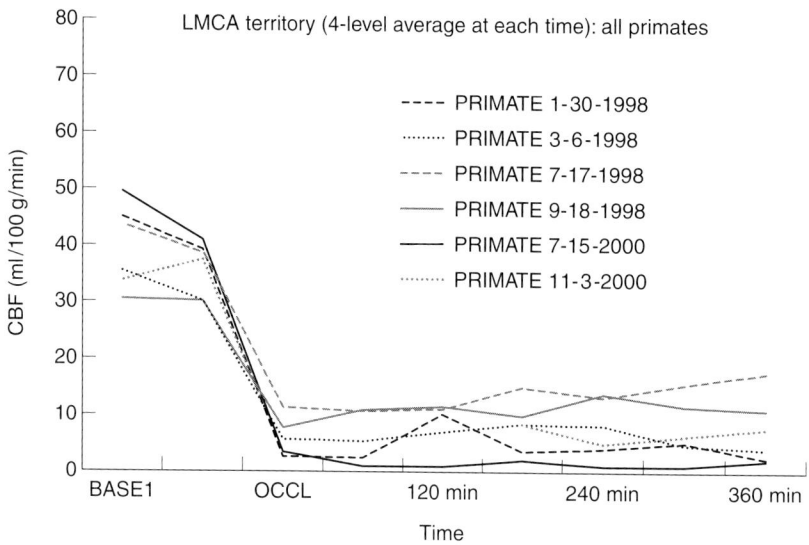

Fig. 4.3. Left MCA qCBF over time after MCA occlusion in a primate model of MCA infarction. Note that when qCBF approaches 10 cm³/100 g per min there is little variation of flow over time.

procedures. Recent data suggests that patients demonstrated to have compromised cerebrovascular reserve may define a subgroup at high risk for recurrent stroke. Increased oxygen extraction fraction (OEF) as measured by positron emission tomography (PET) has been reported to be associated with a statistically higher incidence of prior ischemic events (42%) than those patients with normal OEF (16%) in patients with carotid occlusive disease.[21,22] Using XeCT before and after an intravenous acetazolamide challenge both Yonas[23] and Webster[24] identified a group of patients with carotid occlusive disease and evidence of hemodynamic compromise or 'steal' defined as a 5% decrease in qCBF measured after acetazolamide challenge. These patients subsequently had a stroke rate of 36% within 6 months. This demonstrates that measurement of cerebrovascular reserve after vasodilatory challenge as well as increased OEF as measured by PET may identify patients at high risk of recurrent cerebral ischemic after symptomatic carotid occlusive disease. Planning of prospective trials are under way to reassess the utility of intracranial bypass in patients with carotid occlusion and compromised hemodynamic profile based on increased OEF and cerebrovascular reserve.

Intracerebral hemorrhage (ICH)

XeCT may provide valuable insights into the optimal blood pressure management of patients with ICH. Parenchymal ICH, commonly associated with hypertension, remains the most common form of hemorrhagic stroke and is an important cause of morbidity and mortality.[25] Substantial growth in the overall volume of ICH occurs in 26% of patients from baseline exam to a 1 hour CT and an additional 12% of all patients experience further growth in the volume of ICH between a 1 and 20 hour CT scan.[26] Volume expansion is a potentially important contributor to overall patient morbidity and mortality. Blood pressure reduction may reduce this rate of early volume expansion;[27] however, regional or global cerebral ischemia may be precipitated in brain areas surrounding the hemorrhage by decreasing CBF.[28] In an attempt to address these issues, investigators have begun to monitor global and regional CBF during attempts at aggressive blood pressure reduction in ICH. Powers and colleagues studied CBF changes after blood pressure reduction in nine patients with hypertensive ICH with PET. Intravenous labetolol or nicardipine were used to achieve a 15% reduction in mean arterial pressure (MAP). These nine patients did not demonstrate a significant change in mean hemispheric or regional CBF at the lower blood pressure.[29] Gebel et al. used XeCT to examine the effect of aggressive blood pressure reduction on CBF in a retrospective series of six hypertensive patients with ICH. Five of the six patients tolerated reduction to normotensive blood pressure levels without a significant decline in global or regional quantitative CBF.[30] In one patient, blood pressure reduction caused CBF values in the surround of the hemorrhage to fall into the ischemic range suggesting that aggressive blood pressure reduction may not be tolerated in all patients. Further efforts are under way, designed to demonstrate the utility of CBF monitoring during blood pressure reduction in ICH, and the efficacy of this strategy to improve outcome in these critically ill patients.

Subarachnoid hemorrhage (SAH) and vasospasm

Symptomatic vasospasm results in decreased cerebral perfusion at the parenchymal level leading to tissue ischemia and in some cases irreversible necrosis. Although transcranial Dopper (TCD) velocities measured in large conductance vessels correlate well with angiographic evidence of vasospasm, they may accurately reflect decreased CBF. Hyperemia also occurs in the setting of SAH and may also cause elevated TCD velocities.[31] TCD monitors blood flow velocity in the large arteries of the Circle of Willis. When leptomeningeal collateral is adequate, the brain may not be ischemic despite thre presence of vasospasm. The combination of TCD and a measure of tissue perfusion such as Xe CT may help avoid the pitfalls inherent in using TCD alone to monitor patients with SAH.[32] TCD is also insensitive to second- and third-order vessel spasm that can occur without significant involvement of the more proximal vessel examined by TCD. Although TCD generally correlates well with angiographic vasospasm it is likely that measurement of CBF yields the most important evidence of clinically significant vasospasm, that is, significant tissue hypoperfusion. XeCT provides a rapid and readily available technique for monitoring patients with SAH. When TCD velocities become elevated, CBF studies exclude hyperemia and identify regions of impending ischemia even before symptoms appear. In patients with neurological symptoms, measurement of CBF helps determine whether vasospasm is responsible for the symptoms.

CT perfusion

With the development of helical CT scanning technology it is now possible to track a bolus of intravenous contrast as it passes through the brain. Assuming there is a linear relationship between CT enhancement and the concentration of contrast material within the brain tissues and arteries, both a tissue enhancement curve and an arterial enhancement curve can be measured during the first pass of contrast following intravenous injection. From these curves, CBF, cerebral blood volume (CBV) and mean transit time (MTT) can be calculated. In addition, the ability to measure an arterial input function allows calculation of quantitative CBF.[33] However, current CT technology permits imaging of only a single slice compared with four slices imaged by XeCT. This is a considerable disadvantage in patients with stroke since the area of ischemia may extend across a much greater region of brain or a single slice may miss a small area of ischemia entirely. Quantitation of CBF using this method also has limitations. Values may change depending upon the artery chosen to be used as the arterial input function.[34] In one patient with recent stroke studied at our institution by CT perfusion and XeCT values correlated in areas of low flow, but in regions of normal CBF by XeCT there was poor correlation with CT perfusion values.

Clinical applications of CT perfusion

CT perfusion has only recently been introduced and only a few clinical studies assessing the utility of this technique have been published. Due to the problems with quantitation of CBF using this method, most studies used ratios comparing values in the affected regions with the contralateral hemisphere. Such comparisons also may introduce error since infarction in one hemisphere has been shown to be associated with decreased CBF values in the contralateral unaffected hemisphere.[35] Koenig et al.[36] found that CT perfusion studies in patients with stroke within 6 hours of onset predicted the development of infarction on follow-up CT scans. Since only a single slice was obtained, only infarction at this brain level was predicted. Other studies demonstrated a correlation between volume of hypoperfusion and angiographic data[37] as well as the clinical application of this technique in acute stroke patients.[38] Much more work is needed to establish the utility of CT perfusion in stroke patients. Quantitation also must be improved before it can rival XeCT for the measurement of ischemic levels of CBF. As CT technology improves, it is likely that multiple slice imaging will be possible, making this method more applicable to evaluation of stroke.

An alternative to bolus tracking CT perfusion is CT enhancement imaging of the brain parenchyma following a bolus of contrast for studies such as CT angiography.[39] In areas of ischemia there is less enhancement most likely reflecting reduced blood volume. This assessment can be easily accomplished in the acute stroke setting following CT angiography without the need for any additional contrast or injections. Although not quantitative it gives a rapid assessment of the localization and size of brain regions affected by ischemia and may predict areas of brain that are likely to go on to infarction.[40]

Conclusions

The need for quantitative physiologic information continues to expand as more emphasis is placed on acute therapeutic intervention in a host of disease states affecting the central nervous system. These techniques offer the possibility of improved patient selection and decreased complications from aggressive interventional techniques. However, in order to be of clinical usefulness these techniques must be capable of being rapidly performed with minimal delay in time to treatment. In addition, they must be widely available in order to have a true clinical impact. CT-based systems now offer the ability to provide exquisite tissue and vascular anatomy using conventional CT and CT angiography. In addition, CT-based perfusion techniques also provide physiologic information that is becoming increasingly important in clinical decision making. All this information (CT, CTA, XeCT and/or CTP) may be obtained in under 20–30 minutes using current technology.

REFERENCES

1 Good WF, Gur D. Xenon-enhanced CT of the brain: effect of flow activation on desired cerebral blood flow measurements. *Am J Neuroradiol* 1991; 12: 83–85.

2 Gur D, Yonas H, Wolfson SK Jr. et al. Xenon and iodine enhanced cerebral CT: a closer look. *Stroke* 1981; 12(5): 573–578.

3 Kety SS, Schmidt CF. The nitrous oxide method for the quantitative determination of cerebral blood flow in man: theory, procedure, and normal values. *J Clin Invest* 1948; 27: 476–483.

4 Jones TH, Morawetz RB, Crowell RM et al. Thresholds of focal cerebral ischemia in awake monkeys. *J Neurosurg* 1981; 54: 773–782.

5 Hossmann K-A. Viability thresholds and the penumbra of focal ischemia. *Ann Neurol* 1994; 36(4): 557–564.

6 Hossman K-A, Schuier FJ. Experimental brain infarcts in cats. Pathophysiological observations. *Stroke* 1980; 11: 583–592.

7 Astrup J, Symon L, Branston NM. Cortical evoked potential and extracellular K^+ and H^+ at critical levels of brain ischemia. *Stroke* 1977; 8: 51–57.

8 Branston NM, Strong AJ, Symon L. Extracellular potassium activity, evoked potential and tissue blood flow. Relationships during progressive ischaemia in baboon cerebral coretex. *J Neurol Sci* 1977; 32: 305–321.

9 Morawetz RB, Crowell RH, DeGirolami U. Regional cerebral blood flow thresholds during cerebral ischemia. *Fed Proc* 1979; 38: 2493–2494.

10 Yonas H, Gur D, Claassen D, Wolfson SKJ, Moosy J. Stable xenon enhanced computed tomography in the study of clinical and pathologic correlates of focal ischemia in baboons. *Stroke* 1988; 19: 228–238.

11 Yonas H, Gur D, Claassen D, Wolfson SKJ, Moosy J. Stable xenon-enhanced CT measurement of cerebral blood flow in reversible focal ischemia in baboons. *J Neurosurg* 1990; 73: 266–273.

12 Kaufaman AM, Firlik AD, Fukui MB, Wechsler LR, Jungreis CA, Yonas H. Ischemic core and penumbra in human stroke. *Stroke* 1999; 30(1): 93–99.

13 Firlik AD, Kaufmann AM, Wechsler LR, Firlik KS, Fukui MB, Yonas H. Quantitative cerebral blood flow determinations in acute ischemic stroke: relationship to computed tomography and angiography. *Stroke* 1997; 28: 2208–2213.

14 Firlik AD, Yonas H, Kaufmann AM et al. Relationship between cerebral blood flow and the development of swelling and life-threatening herniation in acute ischemic stroke. *J Neurosurg* 1998; 89: 67–73.

15 Goldstein S, Yonas H, Gebel JM et al. Acute cerebral blood flow as a predictive physiologic marker for symptomatic hemorrhagic conversion and clinical herniation after thrombolytic therapy. *Stroke* 2000; 31: 275. Accepted as oral presentation to the 25th AHA International Stroke Conference 2000.

16 Goldstein S, Jungreis CA, Wechsler LR et al. Time to treatment and cerebral blood flow as predictive measures of clinical outcome in patients treated with intra-arterial thrombolytic therapy. Accepted as an oral presentation at the American Society of Neuroradiology (ASNR) 39th Annual Meeting April 26, 2001.

17 Kilpatrick MM, Goldstein S, Yonas H et al. Sensitivity and specificity of quantitative cerebral blood flow vs. time from symptom onset as a predictor of cerebral infarction. Abstract accepted as a poster presentation to the 26th American Heart Association International Stroke Conference, February 14–16, 2001. *Stroke* 2001; 32 (1); 348.

18 Firlik AD, Rubin G, Yoans H, Wechsler LR. Relation between cerebral blood flow and neurologic deficit resolution in acute ischemic stroke. *Neurology* 1998; 51: 177–182.

19 Jovin TG, Goldstein S, Gebel J, Wechsler LR, Ott, M-B, Yonas H. Patterns of core and penumbra in acute M1 occlusion and their clinical correlates. Abstract accepted as a poster presentation to the 26th American Heart Association International Stroke Conference, February 14–16, 2001. *Stroke* 2001; 32 (1); 348.

20 The EC/IC Bypass Study Group. Failure of extracranial–intracranial arterial bypass to reduce the risk of ischemic stroke. Results of an international randomized trial. *N Engl J Med* 1985; 313: 1191–1200.

21 Derdeyn CP, Yundt KD, Videen TO, Carpenter DA, Grubb RL, Powers WL. Increased oxygen extraction fraction is associated with prior ischemic events in patients with carotid occlusion. *Stroke* 1998; 29: 754–758.

22 Grubb RL, Derdeyn CP, Fritsch SM et al. Importance of hemodynamic factors in the prognosis of symptomatic carotid occlusion. *JAMA* 1998; 280: 1055–1060.

23 Yonas H, Smith H, Durham S, Pentheny SL, Johnson DW. Increased stroke risk predicted by compromised cerebral blood flow reactivity. *J. Neurosurg* 1993; 79: 483–489.

24 Webster MW, Makaroun MS, Steed DL, Smith HA, Johnson DW, Yonas H. Compromised cerebral blood flow reactivity is a predictor of stroke in patients with symptomatic carotid artery occlusive disease. *J Vasc Surg* 1995; 21: 338–345.

25 Broderick JP, Brott T, Tomsick BT et al. Intracerebral hemorrhage is more than twice as common as subarachnoid hemorrhage. *J Neurosurg* 1993; 78: 188–191.

26 Brott T, Broderick J, Kothari R et al. Early hemorrhage growth in patients with intracerebral hemorrhage. *Stroke* 1997; 28: 1–5.

27 Dandapani BK, Suzuki S, Kelley RE, Reyes-Iglesias Y, Duncan RC. Relation between blood pressure and outcome in intracerebral hemorrhage. *Stroke* 1995; 26: 21–24.

28 Powers WJ. Acute hypertension after stroke: the scientific basis for treatment decisions. *Neurology* 1993; 43: 461–467.

29 Powers WJ, Adams RE, Yundt KD et al. Acute Pharmacological hypotension after intracerebral hemorrhage does not change cerebral blood flow. *Stroke* 1999; 30: 242; abstract.

30 Gebel JM, Kassam AB, Snyder JV et al. Effects of aggressive blood pressure reduction on cerebral blood flow in patients with acute intracerebral hemorrhage. *Stroke* 2000; 31: 283.

31 Iacopino DG, Todaro C, Alafaci C et al. Transorbital Doppler: an approach that increases transcranial Doppler sensitivity in the detection of SAH Vasospasm. *Stroke* 1993; 24: 519

32 Clyde BL, Resnick DK, Yonas H, Smith HA, Kaufmann AM. The relationship of blood velocity as measured by transcranial doppler ultrasonography to cerebral blood flow as determined by stable xenon computed tomographic studies after aneurismal subarachnoid hemorrhage. *Neurosurgery* 2001; 38: 896.

33 Cenic A, Nabavi DG, Craen RA, Gelb AW, Lee T-Y. Dynamic CT measurement of cerebral blood flow: A validation study. *Am J Neuroradiol* 1999; 20: 63–73

34 Wintermark M, Thiran J, Maeder P, Schnyder P, Meuli R. Simultaneous measurement of regional cerebral blood flow by perfusion CT and stable xenon CT: a validation study. *Am J Neuroradiol* 2001; 22: 905–914.

35 Firlik AD, Kaufmann AM, Wechsler LR et al. Quantitative cerebral blood flow determinations in acute ischemic stroke: relationship to computed tomography and angiography. *Stroke* 1997; 28: 2208–2213.

36 Koenig M, Kraus M, Theek C, Klotz E, Gehlen W, Heuser L. Quantitative assessment of the ischemic brain by means of perfusion-related parameters derived from perfusion CT. *Stroke* 2001; 32: 431–437.

37 Lee KH, Cho S, Byun HS et al. Triphasic perfusion computed tomography in acute middle cerebral artery stroke. *Arch Neurol* 2000; 57: 990–999.

38 Hunter GJ, Hamberg LM, Ponzo JA et al. Assessment of cerebral perfusion and arterial anatomy in hyperacute stroke with three-dimensional functional CT: early clinical results. *Am J Neuroradiol* 1998; 19: 29–37.

39 Hunter GJ, Hamberg LM, Ponzo JA et al. Assessment of cerebral perfusion and arterial anatomy in hyperacute stroke with three-dimensional functional CT: early clinical results. *Am J Neuroradiol* 1998; 19: 29–37.

40 Lev MH, Segal AZ, Farkas J et al. CT Blood volume imaging of hyperacute MCA stroke: prediction of final infarct volume and clinical outcome in response to intra-arterial thrombolysis. *Stroke* 2001; 32: 2021–2028.

Technical introduction to MRI

Rohit Sood and Michael Moseley

Department of Radiology, Stanford University, CA, USA

Introduction

Since the first image of the human wrist was obtained by Paul Lauterbur in 1972, magnetic resonance imaging (MRI) has developed significantly to a stage where it has found applications to most of the speciality branches in medicine. In the last decade there has been a rapid development in gradient and RF coil technology and this has resulted in the implementation of fast imaging techniques such as echo planar imaging (EPI), on clinical imaging systems. It is now possible to acquire a single image of the brain in less than 50 ms using EPI.[1] During this period, MR has been used for obtaining functional information about the different physiological processes in the brain, such as diffusion and perfusion. This has resulted in the development of newer techniques, with the MR systems being equipped with faster gradients. MRI has been used in the acute stroke setting over the past few years, due to the unique sensitivity of several new MRI techniques to rapidly detect cerebral ischemia. These new techniques include diffusion-weighted imaging (DWI), perfusion-weighted imaging (PWI), magnetic resonance spectroscopy (MRS) and high-speed MR-angiography (MRA). In this chapter, we will briefly outline the basic physical principles of MRI, which will lay a foundation for the following chapters. A brief overview of the MR techniques that have been developed for investigating stroke patients is provided. It is assumed, however, that the reader is familiar with the basic physics of MRI.

The integrated MR stroke 'protocol'

Because MRI can be made sensitive to many different tissue contrasts ranging from T_1 relaxation times to proton diffusion, and since many MRI sequences can be done in a few seconds to minutes scan time, stroke protocols using MRI have begun including many different sequences in order to maximize the amounts of information within a 20 to 30 minutes examination time. The following MRI methods that can be found in a typical MRI stroke protocol are described more fully below. The parameters that may be used in a typical stroke protocol are outlined in Table 5.1.

The T_1-weighted image

The time taken by the net nuclear magnetization vector to reach the thermal equilibrium with the surrounding environment (lattice) is called the spin-lattice relaxation time or T_1. The T_1 relaxation time depends on the environment of the relaxing spin nuclei. For example, proton spins in the cerebrospinal fluid (CSF) have a T_1 of 1900 ms (at 1.4 T static magnetic field) while the T_1 of protons in the thalamus is 700 ms.[2] Thus the thalamus has a shorter T_1 compared to the CSF due to the inherent property of the tissue. In general, proton spins that are not bound to molecules and exist in free form (as in the CSF, water) have longer T_1 relaxation times. The image generated from a signal with a greater T_1 dependence is called a T_1-weighted image (Figure 5.1 upper left). It is possible on the

Table 5.1. Typical stroke protocol[a]

1.	Sagittal scout	Scout
	Patient position:	Supine; Head First; Head Coil
	Imaging parameters:	Sagittal; 2D; GRE
	Scan timing:	1 echo; TE 20 ms; TR 500 ms
	Acquisition timing:	256 3 128; 1/2 NEX; Phase FOV 1; Autoshim; S/I
	Scanning range:	FOV 24; slice thickness 3 skip 1; 20 slices *Time: 0:36*
2.	FSE	FSE First and Second Echo
	Imaging parameters:	Oblique; 2D; Spin-echo (Fast)
	Scan timing:	1 echo; TE 17/100, TR 9000
	User CV:	Min Acquisitions 1
	Acquisition timing:	256 3 192; 1 NEX; A/P; Autoshim; Phase correct
	Scanning range:	FOV 24; 5 skip 2.5; 20 slices *Time: 3:00*
3.	Circle of Willis	MRA
	Imaging parameters:	Oblique; 3D; Vasc TOF SPGR; Flow Comp; MT; EDR
	Vascular options:	Collapse; 19 Projections; Ramp pulse I -> S
	Scan timing:	25°; MinTE; TR 5 44
	Scan setup:	Autoshim; Bandwidth ±15.63
	Scanning range:	FOV 20 cm; 2; 32 locations; overlap 4
	Saturation:	Explicit sat (S)
	Acquisition time:	256 3 128; A/P; Phase 0.75; 1 NEX; *Time: 2:17*
4.	Diffusion	DWI 1 DTI
	Imaging parameters:	Oblique; 2D; psd: DW-EPI
	User CV:	FLAIR 5 0, 1
	Diff options:	b-values 5 0–14,000 (2–8 NEX)
	Diff grad options:	0, x, y, z, then: xy, xz, yz, -xy, -xz, y-z
	Scan timing:	1 Shot; MinTE; TR 5 4000
	Acquisition timing:	128 3 128; Phase FOV 1; R/L;
	Scanning range:	FOV 24; 5 skip 2.5; 20 slices; GRx *Time 6:36*
5.	Bleed screen	GRE EPI
	Imaging parameters:	Oblique; 2D; GE-EPI; Multiphase
	Scan timing:	1 Shot; TE 5 60; TR 5 2000; Flip 60°
	Acquisition timing:	128x128; 1 NEX; Phase FOV 1; R/L; Autoshim; Phase correct
	Scanning range:	FOV 24; 5 skip 2.5; 20 slices *Time: 0:06*
6.	Perfusion	PWI
	Imaging parameters:	Oblique; 2D; GE-EPI; Multiphase
	Multiphase:	40 phases; Interleaved; Minimum delay
	Scan timing:	1 Shot; TE 5 60; TR 5 2000; Flip 60°
	Acquisition timing:	128x128; 1 NEX; Phase FOV 1; R/L; No Autoshim; Phase correct
	Scanning range:	FOV 24; 5 skip 2.5; 12 slices *Time: 1:21*

Note: [a] These parameters are listed for the GE Horizon Series and are meant for illustrative purposes only

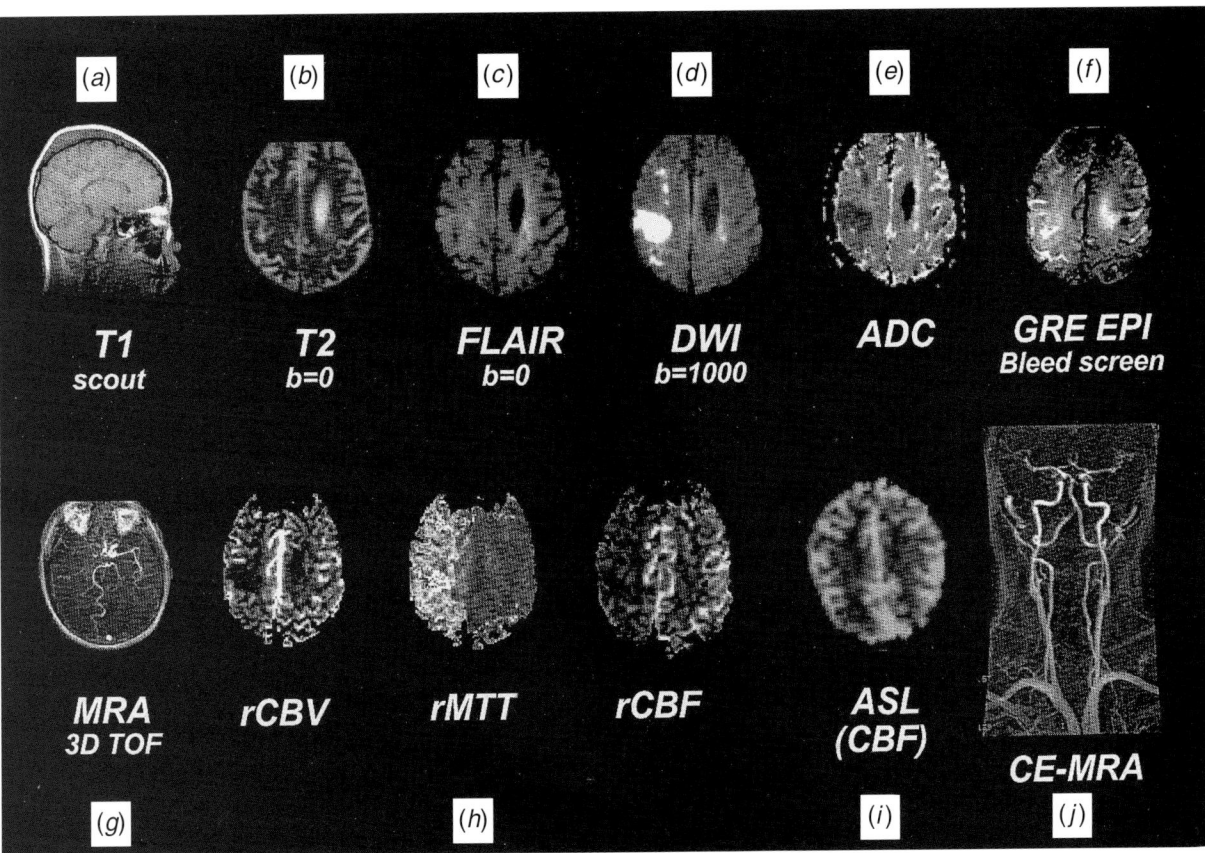

Fig. 5.1.
(a) T_1-weighted image of the brain (TR/TE 500/18.0 ms) used for scout.
(b) T_2-weighted axial image of the brain is commonly acquired using fast spin echo (FSE) sequence (TR/TE 4 s/100 ms). This can also be acquired as the b=0 image from the SE EPI series for DWI.
(c) Image acquired using FLAIR sequence from the FSE or SE EPI image.
(d) Diffusion-weighted image acquired at high b value. Note the right-sided lesion.
(e) ADC map obtained from the b=0 and the high b value images. Note the low ADC value in the lesion seen in the DW image.
(f) Upper right: A GRE EPI 'bleed screen' depicting possible bleed.
(g) Lower row – left: Time of Flight (3D TOF) MRA angiogram.
(h) Maps acquired from the PWI exam. rCBV, rMTT, and rCBF
(i) Arterial spin label (ASL) image (FAIR method) of normally perfused slice.
(j) CE-MRA image acquired during arterial phase of contrast bolus injection.

MR scanner to vary parameters such as TR (repetition time), TE (echo time) and T_1 (inversion time, if using an inversion recovery sequence) in order to obtain T_1 weighting. T_1-weighted images are typically obtained using spin echo sequences with short TR and short TE. On a T_1-weighted image of the brain, the CSF typically appears dark (no signal due to signal saturation because of the short TR and the long T_1 of CSF) while the white matter appears bright (high signal due to a relatively shorter T_1 than CSF). The T_1 property of tissue can also be modified due to the presence of a T_1 shortening agent (e.g. paramagnetic contrast agent such as gadolinium or the iron in methemoglobin).

MR sequences that generate a T_1-weighted image by virtue of adding an inversion recovery pulse to invert protons with a particular T_1 are STIR (short tau inversion recovery) and FLAIR (fLuid attenuated inversion recovery, Fig. 5.1(c)) FLAIR imaging has been particularly useful in imaging of patients with onset of cerebral ischemia[3] even though it is more properly an inversion recovery T_2-weighted spin echo sequence.

The T_1-weighted image is typically added to the stroke protocol usually as a pilot or scout image series for prescribing slices for subsequent image series, although T_1-weighted image series could also be acquired prior to and after gadolinium contrast injection to look for breakdowns in the blood–brain barrier or even as a quick depiction of evolving mass effects postischemia.

The T_2-weighted image

Due to mutual interaction between the spins, components of the magnetization vector get out of phase and result in decay of the net magnetization. The time for the components to decay is known as the T_2 or transverse relaxation time. Smaller molecules like water have longer T_2 relaxation times compared to large macromolecules and in general T_2 as well as T_1 are functions of water content, that is the higher the water content in the tissue, the longer the T_2 and T_1. CSF for example has a T_2 of 250 ms compared to thalamus whose T_2 is 75 ms (at 1.4T).[2] Hence on a T_2-weighted image of the brain (Fig. 5.1(b)) the CSF appears bright (due to longer T_2) as compared to cortical grey matter. Examples of MR sequences that are used for acquiring T_2-weighted images include conventional spin echo (CSE), rapid acquisition with relaxation enhancement (RARE) or fast spin echo/turbo spin echo and EPI-spin echo.

Paramagnetic contrast agents such as gadolinium (and its chelates) in high concentration have a T_2 (and T_2^*; discussed later under perfusion-weighted imaging) shortening effect (in addition to T_1 shortening).[4] On a T_2-weighted image this may result in loss of phase coherence and signal loss causing the tissue to appear dark. Compounds with paramagnetic properties found in the body also demonstrate T_2 shortening effects. For example, during the early subacute phase of a parenchymal hematoma the conversion of hemoglobin to methemoglobin has a T_2 shortening effect on the vascular lesion. This is due to the fact that methemoglobin, formed by the oxidative denaturation of hemoglobin, has five unpaired electrons on the heme iron making it paramagnetic and thus resulting in T_2 shortening (along with strong T_1 shortening).[5] As a result the lesion will appear dark on a T_2-weighted image due to spin related dephasing effects (or loss of phase coherence). However, T_2-weighted imaging techniques such as conventional and fast spin echo have not been very useful in the neurological assessment of acute ischemia due to subtle changes occurring in the parenchymal tissue on these images and the hyperintense signal from CSF masking the subtle pathological findings.

The T_2-weighted image is acquired, together with a proton density-weighted image in one integrated image series employing a long TR together with a short TE (the proton density weighted image) and long TE (the T_2-weighted image). The utility of the T_2-weighted image is to depict increases in water content due primarily to edema or inflammation. The use of the T_2 weighted image to detect hyperacute and acute ischemia, however, is hampered by the slow evolution of T_2 over the first 24 hours following an ischemic insult. The T_2 weighted image is largely considered to be the MRI gold standard for lesion volume at later time points beyond the first 24 hours.

Magnetic resonance angiography

Magnetic resonance angiography (MRA) is a major advance in application of MRI to imaging of patent blood flow in vessels. It is now used routinely with conventional MR studies of the brain for investigating ischemic lesions and arteriovenous malformations. The MRA techniques can be broadly classified as (i) the inflow of moving protons orthogonal to the slice that have not seen prior RF pulses producing a hyperintense 'time of flight' effect within the vascular walls and (ii) spins moving during the application of and in the direction of an imaging gradient that produce a signal phase shift (dependent on the type and direction of blood flow), so-called the 'phase contrast' technique.

Both two-dimensional[6] and three-dimensional[7] gradient echo TOF techniques have been popular for stroke-related MRA clinical utility. The two-dimensional TOF technique produces images with decreased spatial resolution in the slice select direction and has a longer TE compared to the three-dimensional technique. In the three-dimensional TOF MRA technique, a thick slab or volume of tissue is excited and extra phase encoding steps are applied along the slice select direction (in addition to those in the phase encoding direction) to divide the volume into multiple partitions or sections along the slice coverage. A three-dimensional Fourier transform is then performed to reconstruct the image. The three-dimensional data sets have voxel dimensions of less than $0.8 \times 0.8 \times 0.8$ mm, which is typically smaller than that can be achieved using two-dimensional techniques.[7] Other advantages of the three-dimensional over the two-dimensional technique are higher signal to noise ratio (SNR), improved slice profile and reduction in T_2^* effects[8] at the expense of the loss of inflow through deeper volumes.

A new MRA technique that acquires imaging data before, during and after administration of a single or double dose gadolinium contrast agent bolus injection is known as contrast-enhanced MRA (CE-MRA).[9] This technique has become very popular and is commonly used in stroke protocols today for investigating intracranial vascular diseases over large peripheral fields of view from typically the aortic arch to the circle of Willis. By injecting gadolinium, the blood T_1 can be shortened to a few tens of milliseconds and three-dimensional data sets can be longitudinally acquired with a very short examination time. This technique offers several advantages over non-contrast enhanced conventional MRA and offers useful information to the stroke protocol at the expense of a contrast bolus injection.

Diffusion-weighted imaging

The signal intensity in MRI depends on proton density, T_1, T_2 and T_2^* (explained later under perfusion-weighted imaging) relaxation process of any ensemble of the spins. Another important source of contrast in MRI is the signal loss caused by proton dephasing in the presence of coherent and incoherent flow. Random diffusion (Brownian motion of water molecules) of protons into areas of varying magnetic field strengths leads to random phase shifts (not seen in stationary tissue). There is a resultant loss of signal from these protons as a result of these phase shifts. In pure water, protons diffuse greater distances (20–25 microns) as compared to tissue water (7–15 microns) within an imaging time of 40 ms. Thus the process of diffusion, including rate and direction of diffusion reflect the hindered motion of water molecules in a given medium.[10] A parameter that quantitates the property of diffusion and proton displacement is called the apparent diffusion coefficient (ADC). A typical ADC value in human brain is 1×10^{-3} mm^2/s. The ADC value of water in tissue changes if the motion of protons is hindered along any one direction, resulting in the property of a non-random, anisotropic diffusion pathway, resulting in not a single average ADC, more appropriately in an ADC tensor. This property of anisotropic diffusion tensor imaging (DTI) is seen in myelin fibres in white matter, where the protons move faster along the direction of least resistance causing the ADC to be directionally dependent (anisotropic).[11] In such conditions the direction of the applied diffusion sensitizing gradient in the ST (Stejskal and Tanner) pulse sequence (see below) can be chosen by using one of the x, y or z axis field gradients or more. This allows assessment of the diffusion anisotropy tensor[12] and can be used to synthesize a diffusion tensor map (DTI map) the practice of which is becoming more popular in routine stroke MRI.

Building upon spin echo imaging techniques, it is possible to encode the ADC information by modifying pulse sequences to include extra 'diffusion sensitizing gradients' which are applied along typically six varying directions. This technique is known as the 'Stejskal–Tanner', ST technique or 'pulsed magnetic field gradient technique'.[13] The diffusion encoding gradients (noted in Fig. 5.2) are a set of matching gradient pulses played along the direction of diffusion of protons. The diffusion of

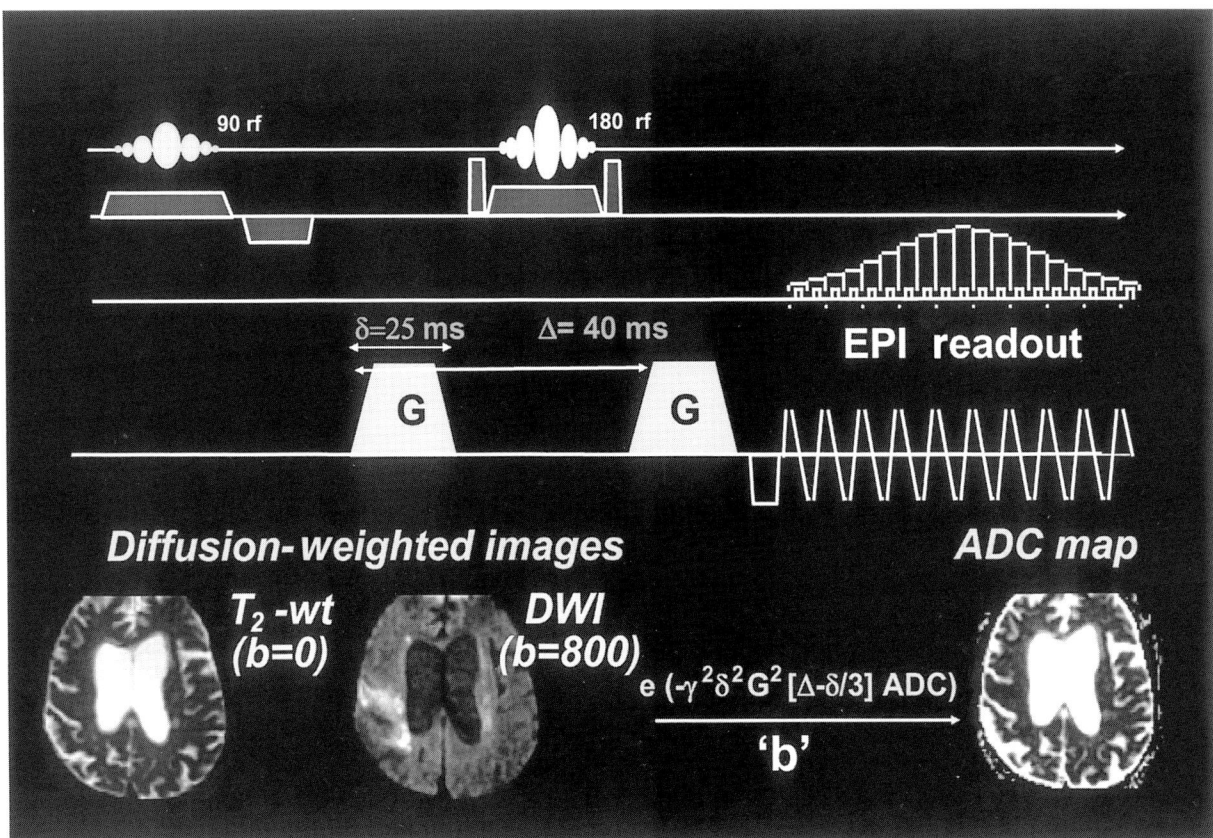

Fig. 5.2. Diffusion-weighted imaging using spin echo SE EPI sequence. The three main steps involved in obtaining a diffusion map of the brain are acquiring MR images with various b-values (typically $b=0$ and $b=800$–1000 s/mm^2), plot SI vs. b-values to obtain the ADC map.

protons during the application of pulsed gradients (Δ in Fig. 5.2) causes them to acquire a phase change (or dephase). As a result, the diffusion of protons causes incomplete spin rephasing and attenuation of spin echo signal during data acquisition. On the acquired DW (diffusion-weighted) images, relatively slow diffusion appears hyperintense while rapid diffusion appears hypointense. The signal intensity of the acquired signal (echo) depends on the following parameters which are known and can be varied:

(a) Δ: the time interval between the leading edges of the diffusion sensitizing gradients (DG),

(b) δ, G: the duration and amplitude of the diffusion sensitizing gradient pulses (DG)

(c) 'b' value is related to the above parameters and is given by $b = \exp[-\gamma^2 \delta^2 G^2 (\Delta - \delta/3)\, ADC]$.[13]

Given the typical parameters of Δ (53 ms), δ (45 ms), b values of up to 2500 s/mm^2 can be achieved depending upon the diffusion sensitizing gradient strength. The b value signifies the diffusion of protons under the influence of pulsed diffusion gradients. The differences between the slow and fast diffusion rates are best visualized at higher b values, however, at the cost of SNR. In order to maximize the b values, larger gradients than those commonly used are necessary, which has prompted improved design and commercial availability of stronger gradients.[14]

A typical diffusion examination consists of rapid acquisition (as shown in Fig. 5.2) of a DW image with $b=0$ (no diffusion weighting) followed by rapid acquisition of a DW image at a higher b value (typically 1000 s/mm^2). All the acquired images are then used to obtain the ADC value and to synthesize an ADC map (Fig. 5.1(e), 5.2) from the slope of the signal decrease with increasing the value. The calculation of b value is influenced somewhat by the interaction of diffusion encoding gradient with slice selective and frequency encoding gradients.[15] These gradients themselves act in a lesser way as dephase–rephase gradients and thus may contribute to the observed diffusion weighting.[16]

Patient motion and CSF pulsation during imaging using conventional spin echo imaging techniques results in motion degraded MR images. This is due to motion artefacts, also known as 'ghosting' artefacts, arising from motion during the long acquisition times seen with the conventional spin echo technique. With the development of fast imaging techniques such as single shot EPI and half Fourier RARE, it has been possible to suppress motion artefacts even with large diffusion gradients applied. Routine diffusion-weighted imaging is performed using DW–SE–EPI (diffusion weighted–spin echo–echo planar imaging) in regular clinical practice due to widespread availability of these techniques on commercial clinical MR systems (Fig. 5.2).

The role of diffusion-weighted imaging in clinical practice became clear when it was noted that the ADC of water was significantly slower in regions of ischemia compared with normally perfused regions of brain with ADC decreasing by 30% to 60% after the onset of stroke.[17] The ability of a non-invasive MR method such as DWI, to quickly and accurately detect and characterize cerebral ischemia occurred at a critical time in neuroimaging, when thrombolytic and neuroprotective agents were entering the clinical arena. The common use of DWI in stroke protocols is to provide the first look at the extent of the ischemic lesion, although more often than not, the DWI sequences used to rule out stroke in most CNS exams.

The concept of diffusion-weighted imaging was modified to account for these orientational variations in the ADC measurements and hence the concept of 'diffusion tensor'[18,19] involves the application of diffusion gradients in different directions and the data obtained is used to extract and characterize tissue microstructure such as the white matter tracts. The concept of DTI has been successfully applied to the study of white matter diseases such as multiple sclerosis,[20] which may provide better understanding about the underlying disease process. However, in routine stroke DWI, the trace ADC (the average of diagonal elements of the tensor matrix) images acquired from the DWI series is used. The trace averaging tends to remove the effects of anisotropic diffusion thus simplifying the detection of ischemic from normally perfused brain.

Perfusion-weighted imaging

Perfusion is the steady-state delivery of blood (nutrients and oxygen) to tissue parenchyma representing coherent motion of water and cellular material.[21] Since both perfusion-weighted imaging (PWI) and magnetic resonance angiography (MRA) map the flow of blood in vessels, there may be some confusion between the applications of these two techniques. MRA is useful in demonstrating the macroscopic vasculature (in both arteries and veins) and detecting morphological changes in blood vessels themselves such as stenosis, aneurysms, dissections and malformations. PWI detects microscopic flow at the capillary level and therefore is useful to investigate changes taking place at the cellular level.

Perfusion is typically measured in ml/100 g of tissue/min. The normal gray matter is perfused at the rate of 50–60 ml/100 g/min. There are three important parameters that are used to quantify and assess brain tissue perfusion: cerebral blood flow (CBF), cerebral blood volume (CBV) and mean transit time (MTT). CBV is defined simply as the amount of blood in a given amount of tissue at any time (ml/g) as compared to CBF, which represents the amount of blood moving through a certain amount of tissue per unit time (ml/g per min). The ratio of CBV and CBF is defined as the mean transit time (units minutes).

Perfusion imaging techniques can be divided into two broad groups, depending upon the type of contrast mechanism:
(i) signal monitoring using exogenous (injectable) contrast agents such as gadolinium DTPA (Gd-DTPA; T_1 shortening agent), oxygen 17 in H_2O[17]

(T_2 shortening agent) or superparamagnetic agents (T_2^* shortening). The technique that uses Gd-DTPA as the exogenous contrast agent will be discussed in greater detail, since it is the most commonly used technique in the clinical setup; and

(ii) Endogenous or inherent contrast agents such as arterial spin labelling technique (ASL).

The basic underlying concept of perfusion imaging involves visualizing (and quantifying) signal changes during the vascular transit of an injected contrast agent such as gadolinium (Gd), dysprosium (Dy) or iron (Fe) based compounds using rapid T_2^* sensitive imaging techniques such as EPI. These substances produce stronger magnetic field heterogeneity effects than other substances due to the inherent property of magnetic susceptibility (defined as the ratio of induced magnetic field in a substance to the applied static magnetic field). As a result, these substances cause perturbations in the local magnetic field, which influence water protons within a certain range. Water protons undergo dephasing as they diffuse through the sphere of influence of these contrast agent particles. The loss of phase coherence and signal loss occurs due to T_2^* relaxation and it follows an exponential decay similar to T_2. This effect can be reversed with spin echo based techniques and hence makes these techniques relatively insensitive to T_2^* effects. However, gradient echo based imaging techniques are very sensitive to small changes in magnetic susceptibilities, and as a result have proven to be useful in perfusion imaging.[22] The spheres of influence of these particles exists beyond immediate vicinity and have more significant long-range effects than do T_1 shortening effects (which exist around unpaired electron clouds only and hence are short-range effects). The long-range effects of these T_2^* sensitive agents are advantageous since a small concentration can greatly influence freely diffusing protons throughout the brain parenchyma.[23]

Regional blood flow in brain that is compromised due to a pathological process (such as stroke) can now be assessed by studying the dynamics of transit of T_2^* sensitive agents through the vasculature by synthesizing perfusion maps. PWI is performed by obtaining images at regular intervals before, during and after injection of a magnetic susceptibility contrast agent. For example, after injecting 0.1–2 mmol/kg of a gadolinium chelate at the rate of 5 ml/second, rapid imaging is performed using gradient echo EPI sequence and data sets (typically consisting of 12–15 slices) are acquired serially at 2-second (usually the TR) interval (Fig. 5.3 upper left). Once the data set is acquired, a plot of signal intensity change vs. time (Fig. 5.3 upper right) is obtained from each of these images using postprocessing techniques. Local change in relaxivity ($\Delta R_2^* = 1/T_2^*(t) - 1/T_2^*(0)$) is then obtained by creating a ΔR_2^* map using the signal intensity values from the images. The change in ΔR_2^* with time is fitted to a gamma variate curve[24] (so called because the curve resembles the plot of a mathematical function called gamma variate function). From this curve (Fig. 5.3 lower left) a number of parameters are then extracted such as relative CBF, relative CBV (Fig. 5.1(*h*)), relative MTT (Fig. 5.3, lower right), 'arrival time' (AT), peak height, 'time to peak' (TTP) and FWHM (full width at half maximum).[25] Thus it is the relation between the signal intensity vs. time plot and concentration of the tracer in the voxel over time that provides the necessary information about cerebral hemodynamics and perfusion.

A number of physiological factors influence the parameters that can be extracted from the signal vs. time or concentration vs. time plots. For example, hematocrit (Hct), which is defined as the ratio of cerebral red blood cell volume and cerebral blood volume and has units of percentage, which must be considered with MR techniques when using plasma markers.[26] Some other parameters that may indirectly influence perfusion imaging are heart rate and mean arterial blood pressure.

Perfusion imaging using endogenous contrast agents

Another popular technique used for perfusion MR imaging is the arterial spin labelling (ASL)

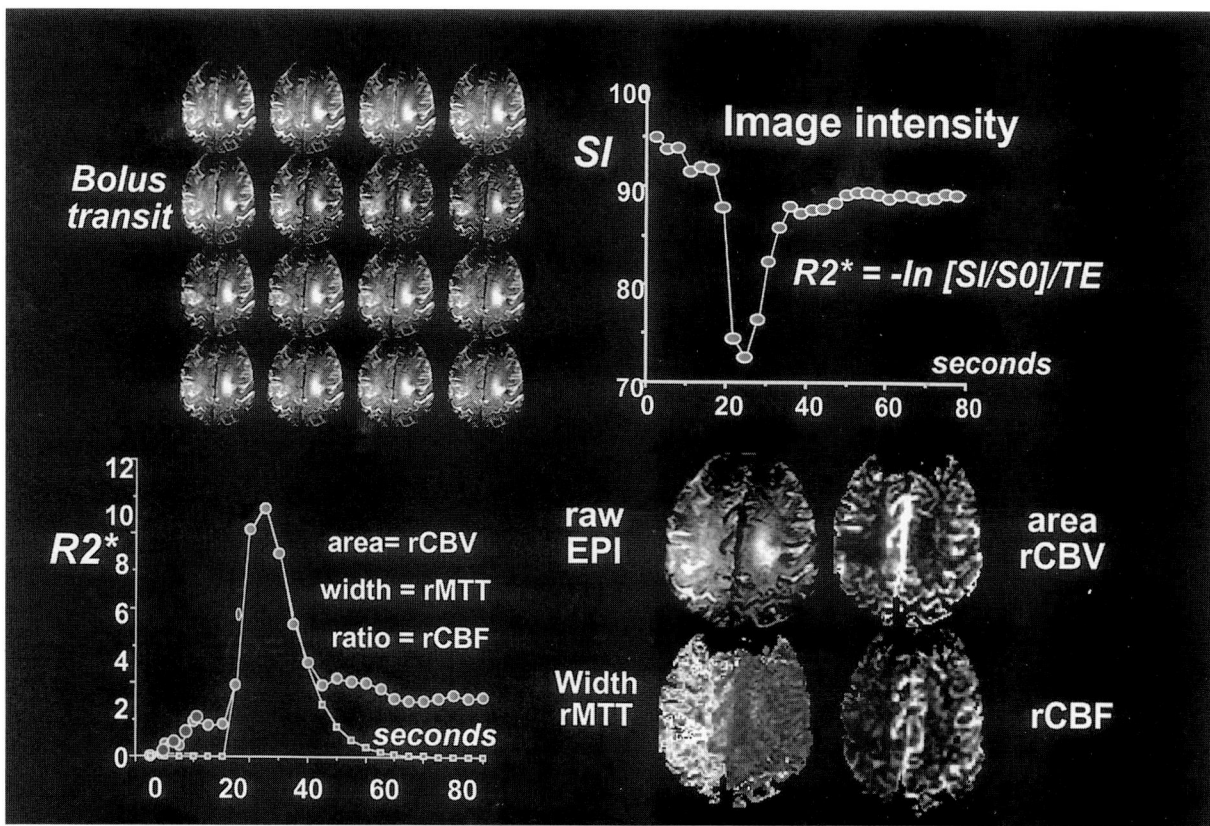

Fig. 5.3. Upper left: Series of GRE EPI images acquired from 12 slices every 2 seconds during a bolus injection of 0.1mmol/kg Gd. Upper right: Signal intensity vs. time curve for a given region of interest. (lower left) Relaxivity vs. time curve obtained from the perfusion-weighted images and the fit. Lower right: Synthesized maps of the hemodynamically weighted images from the R2 data fitting. Note the decrease in signal with time as the contrast agent reaches the region of interest.

technique. An advantage of this technique is that it is possible non-invasively, to obtain perfusion maps of the brain.

In this technique, protons in a slice proximal to the imaged slice are 'tagged' with an inversion 180° RF pulse. These saturated blood protons tagged in the proximal slice move in to the imaged slice due to arterial blood flow during the inversion time where the signal intensity is lowered relative to the control image acquired simultaneously. These images are then subtracted to obtain a perfusion map with hyperintense regions corresponding to the inflowing blood protons. This technique has been combined with EPI to enable fast imaging and is called EPISTAR.[27]

The ASL technique has found numerous applications to study and investigate various pathological conditions such as stroke,[28] traumatic brain injuries,[29] degenerative brain diseases[30] and brain tumours.[31]

Magnetic resonance spectroscopy

Magnetic resonance spectroscopy (MRS) of the brain also known as 'neurospectroscopy' is a non-invasive MR technique that gives the relative concentration of certain chemical compounds within 2 to 3 cm^3 of tissue.

MRS is based on principles similar to MRI. Each proton is shielded from the static magnetic field by electrons in the orbital (orbits around the proton in which the electrons are revolving) around it. This causes the precessional frequency of each proton to be different from its neighbours. The interaction of the static field and electrons causes the field at the nucleus to be slightly altered and is termed as chemical shift.[32] The chemical shift is measured as parts per million (ppm) and is proportional to the magnitude of the external static field. It is this property of chemical shift that allows the spectroscopist to detect a wide variety of individual protons linked to larger molecules such as proteins and carbohydrates. In a typical MRS spectrum obtained from brain tissue (Fig. 5.4), a number of peaks corresponding to frequencies of chemical nuclei will be seen, with the area under the peak representing the amount of chemical in the tissue.

^{1}H spectroscopy is the most commonly used technique in clinical practice. Localized proton spectroscopy has recently emerged as a useful tool for investigating brain diseases such as Alzheimer's disease,[33] stroke,[34] epilepsy,[35] multiple sclerosis,[36] and brain tumours[37] and is now available on commercial MR systems.

A typical MRS spectrum of adult brain (spectra vary for newborns, children under 8 years and elderly) is shown in figure (Fig. 5.4). The spectrum is read from right to left with the first and tallest peak assigned to neuronal marker NA (*N*-acetylaspartate) resonating at 2 ppm. The second tallest resonance is Cr (creatine including phosphocreatine) resonating at ~3 ppm. Adjacent to the Cr peak is the smaller but important Ch (choline) peak. The ratio Ch/Cr of about 0.5 is characteristic of brain gray matter. Peaks corresponding to glucose and myoinositol (ml) are also seen in the spectrum of the normal adult brain.

MRS has been suggested to be more sensitive than MRI in detecting hypoxic damage.[38] It has been proposed that MRS may be able to detect cerebral ischemia within seconds of its onset as compared to DWI that provides warning as early as 1 h after the onset. Research has shown that the metabolite profile obtained in patients with stroke is characteristic and correlates well with biochemical changes taking place during the disease process.[34]

Conclusion

Magnetic resonance imaging is now an established clinical imaging modality with applications extending from investigative radiology to functional imaging in neurosciences. The development of newer MR techniques such as diffusion- and perfusion-weighted imaging combined with fast imaging capabilities on commercial systems has revolutionized our understanding of the pathophysiological mechanisms involved in the many clinical conditions especially cerebral ischemia and stroke. Today, MRI is being increasingly used for investigating patients with stroke and in the evaluation of newer drugs, which may prove to be useful in the treatement and management of cerebral ischemic disorders.

REFERENCES

1 Edelman R, Wielopolski R, Schmitt F. Echo Planar Imaging. *Radiology* 1994; 192: 600.
2 Wehrli F, MacFall J, Prost J. Impact of the choice of the operating parameter on MR images. In: Partain C, Price R, Patton J, eds. *Magnetic Resonance Imaging*. Philadelphia: WB Saunders, 1988.
3 Rother J, De Crespigny A, D'Arceuil H et al. Recovery of apparent diffusion coefficient after ischemic induced spreading relates to cerebral perfusion gradient. *Stroke* 1996; 27: 980.
4 Gore J. Contrast agents and relaxation effects. In: Atlas S, ed. *Magnetic Resonance Imaging of the Brain and Spine*. New York: Raven Press, 1991.
5 Gomori J, Grossman R, Goldberg H. Intracranial hematomas: imaging by high field MR. *Radiology* 1985; 157: 87.
6 Gullberg G, Wehrli F, Shimakawa A et al. MR vascular imaging with fast gradient refocusing pulse sequence and reformatted images from transaxial sections. *Radiology* 1987; 165: 241.
7 Masaryk T, Modic M, Ross J et al. Three dimensional (volume) gradient echo imaging of the carotid bifurcation: preliminary clinical experience. *Radiology* 1989; 171: 801.
8 Haacke E, Tkach J, Parrish T. Reduction of T_2^* dephasing in gradient field echo imaging. *Radiology* 1989; 170: 457.

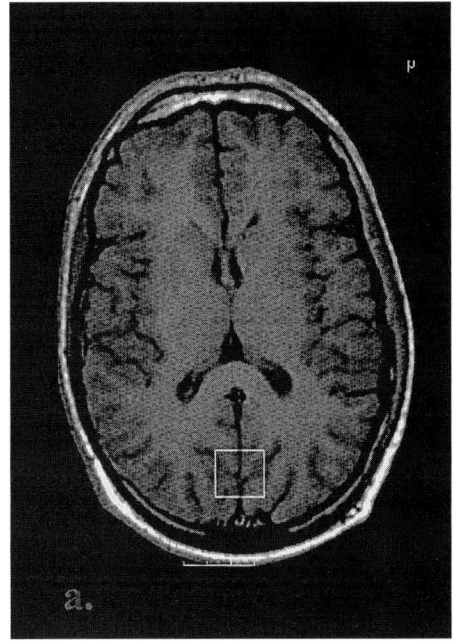
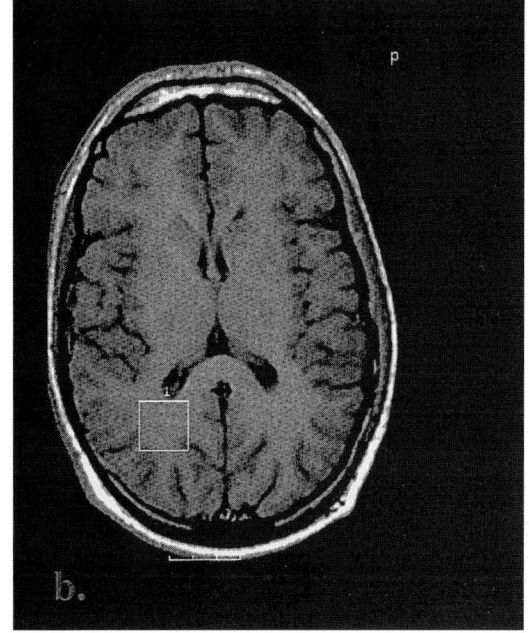

Fig. 5.4. Normal MR spectra of the adult male human brain. The magnetic resonance spectra of a 36-year-old normal male adult human brain have been produced by PROBE (GE's spectroscopy sequence) (TE 35 ms). The metabolite, NA is a neuronal marker, Creatine (Cr) is found in cell energy stores and Choline (Ch) is found in cell membranes. Normal variations in the spectral peaks are in the order of ±15 %. (Image courtesy: Daniel Spielman, Lucas MRIS, Stanford Radiology, Stanford University.)

9 Jung H, Chang K, Choi D et al. Contrast enhanced MR Angiography for the diagnosis of intracranial vascular disease. *Am J Roentgenol* 1995; 165: 1251.

10 Moseley M, Cohen Y, Kucharczyk J. Anisotropy in diffusion-weighted MRI. *Magn Reson Med* 1990; 14: 330.

11 Moseley M, Kucharczyk J, Mintorovitch J et al. Diffusion-weighted MRI of anisotropic water diffusion in cat CNS. *Radiology* 1990; 176: 439.

12 Basser P, Mattiello J, LeBihan D. MR imaging of fiber tract direction and diffusion in anisotropic tissues Twelfth annual meeting of the Society of Magnetic Resonance Imaging in Medicine. New York: Society of Magnetic Resonance in Medicine, 1993.

13 Stejskal E, Tanner J. Use of spin echo in pulsed magnetic field gradient to study anisotropic, restricted diffusion and flow. *J Chem Phys* 1965; 42: 288.

14 Benfield A, Prasad P, Edelman R et al. On the optimal b-value for measurement of lesion volumes in acute human stroke by diffusion-weighted imaging. Fourth annual scientific meeting of the International Society of Magnetic Resonance Imaging in Medicine. New York: International Society of Magnetic Resonance in Medicine, 1996.

15 Neeman M, Freyer J, Sillerud L. Pulsed-gradient SE studies in NMR imaging: effects of imaging gradients on the determination of diffusion gradients. *J Magn Reson* 1990; 90: 303.

16 LeBihan D, Breton E, Lallemand D. MR imaging of intravoxel incoherent motion: application to diffusion and perfusion in neurologic disorders. *Radiology* 1988; 161: 401.

17 Moseley M, Kucharczyk J, Mintorovitch J. Diffusion-weighted MR imaging of acute stroke: correlation with T_2 weighted and magnetic susceptibility-enhanced MR imaging in cats. *Am J Neuroradiol* 1990; 11: 423.

18 Basser P, Mattiello J, Le Bihan D. Estimation of the effective self-diffusion tensor from NMR spin echo. *J Magn Reson* 1994; 103: 247.

19 Le Bihan D, Mangin J, Poupon C et al. Diffusion tensor imaging: concepts and applications. *J Magn Reson Imaging* 2001; 13: 534.

20 Teivsky A, Ptak T, Farkas J. Investigation of apparent diffusion coefficient and diffusion tensor anisotropy in acute and chronic multiple sclerosis. *AJNR* 1999; 20: 1491.

21 Sorensen G, Reimer P. Cerebral hemodynamics-what are they. In: Sorensen G, ed. *Cerebral M_r Perfusion Imaging : Principles and Current Applications*. Theime Medical Publishers, 2001.

22 Villringer A, Rosen B, Believeau J. Dynamic imaging with lanthanide chelates on normal brain: contrast due to magnetic susceptibility effects. *Magn Reson Med* 1988; 6: 164.

23 Kucharczyk J, Roberts T, Moseley M et al. Applications of contrast enhanced perfusion sensitive MR imaging in the diagnosis of cerebrovascular disorders. *J Magn Reson Imaging* 1993; 3: 1.

24 Ostergaard L, Weisskoff R, Chesler D et al. High resolution measurement of cerebral blood flow using intra-vascular tracer bolus passages. Part I: Mathematical approach and statistical analysis. *Magn Reson Med* 1996; 36: 15.

25 Sorensen G, Reimer P. Perfusion MRI with dynamic susceptibility contrast imaging. In: Sorensen G, ed. *Cerebral MR Perfusion Imaging: Principles and Current Applications*. Theime Medical Publishers, 2001.

26 Barbier E, Lamalle L, Decorps M. Methodology of brain perfusion imaging. *J Magn Reson Imaging* 2001; 13: 496.

27 Edelman R, Siewert B, Darby D et al. Qualitative mapping of cerebral blood flow and functional localization with EPI and signal targeting with alternating radio frequency (EPISTAR). *Radiology* 1994; 192: 513.

28 Siewert B, Schlaug G, Edelman R, Warach S. Comparison of EPISTAR and T_2* weighted gadolinium enhanced perfusion imaging in patients with acute cerebral ischemia. *Neurology* 1997; 48: 673.

29 Forbes M, Hendrich K, Kochanek P et al. Assessment of cerebral blood flow and CO_2 reactivity after controlled cortical impact by perfusion magnetic resonance imaging using arterial spin labeling in rats. *J Cereb Blood Flow Metab* 1997; 17: 865.

30 Alsop D, Detre J, Grossman M. Assessment of cerebral blood flow in Alzheimer's disease by spin labeled magnetic resonance imaging. *Ann Neurol* 2000; 47: 93.

31 Gaa J, Warach S, Wen P, Thangaraj V, Weilopolski E. Noninvasive perfusion imaging of human brain tumors with EPISTAR. *Eur Radiol* 1996; 6: 518.

32 Brown T, Kincaid B, Ugurbil K. NMR chemical shift imaging in three dimensions. *Proc Natl Acad Sci USA* 1982; 79: 3523.

33 Meyerhoff D, MacKay S, Constans J et al. Axonal injury and membrane alternations in Alzheimer's disease suggested by in vivo proton magnetic resonance spectroscopy. *Ann Neurol* 1994; 36: 40.

34 Howe F, Maxwell R, Saunders D et al. Proton spectroscopy in vivo. *Magn Reson Q* 1993; 9: 31.

35 Cendes F, Andermann F, Dubeau F et al. Proton magnetic resonance spectroscopic images and MRI volumetric studies for lateralization of temporal lobe epilepsy. *Magn Reson Imaging* 1995; 13: 1187.

36 Arnold D, Mathews P, Franscis G et al. Proton magnetic resonance spectroscopy of human brain in vivo in the evaluation of multiple sclerosis: assessment of the load of disease. *Magn Reson Med* 1990; 14: 154.

37 Barker P, Glickson J, Bryan R. In vivo magnetic resonance spectroscopy of human brain tumors. *J Magn Reson Imaging* 1993; 5: 32.

38 Matson G, Weiner M. Spectroscopy. In: Stark D, Bradley W, eds. *Magnetic Resonance Imaging*. New York: Mosby, 1999: 182.

Clinical use of standard MRI

Brian M. Tress

The University of Melbourne Department of Radiology, and Department of Radiology The Royal Melbourne Hospital, Victoria, Australia

Introduction

MRI is supremely sensitive to the abnormal accumulation of water, much more so than is CT, so it might be expected that MRI is superior to CT in the detection of ischemic infarction. Although this principle is applicable to subacute infarction, it is not the case in the first 6 hours after the onset of the ischemic insult. A basic understanding of the pathological processes which precede infarction is necessary in order to understand their MRI manifestations.

Pathology of ischemic infarction

Deprivation of oxygen supply to neurones, whether as a result of embolus, thrombosis or prolonged hypotension, leads initially to malfunction in as little as a few seconds, e.g. a Stokes–Adams attack, in which brainstem ischemia induces unconsciousness within seconds of cardiac asystole. If the ischemic insult is prolonged the highly energy dependent sodium pump mechanism, which is responsible for maintaining a tenfold difference in extracellular to intracellular sodium concentration, begins to fail and sodium, water and calcium ions pass from the extracellular to the intracellular space. The cell swells, producing 'cytotoxic' edema and the extracellular space is simultaneously reduced. If the diminished oxygen supply is maintained, the less energy-dependent capillary endothelial cells start to lose their function and the normally tight junctions between them begin to lose their integrity. Intravascular fluid leaks into the extravascular space, producing 'vasogenic' edema.

Vasogenic edema spreads easily through the white matter due to its relatively less dense cellular density and more capacious extravascular space. The process of cytotoxic edema predominates in the first 6–8 hours. Subsequently, vasogenic edema becomes progressively more dominant and is largely responsible for the brain swelling in the first few days after the onset of infarction.

MRI technique

The basic standard MRI sequences which should be applied in screening for stroke are T_1 and T_2-weighted axial or sagittal scans through the whole brain. The type of T_2-weighted scans used is important. Conventional T_2-weighted spin echo sequences allow the acquisition of minimally T_2-weighted images or proton-weighted images as the first echo of a double echo sequence. Images acquired from the second echo of the spin echo sequence will be both heavily T_2-weighted and sensitive to the magnetic susceptibility effects of ferromagnetic blood products such as deoxyhemoglobin, intracellular methemoglobin and hemosiderin. The T_2-weighted multiple spin echo sequences used most commonly include 'fast spin echo', 'turbo spin echo' and 'rapid spin echo'. Although they provide exquisite T_2 weighting and spatial resolution, they suffer in that they are relatively insensitive to magnetic susceptibility effects and, hence, to hemorrhage. In the stroke context that is unacceptable. Therefore if one of these techniques is used, a further T_2-weighted magnetic susceptibility sensitive technique should be added. Appropriate sequences include echoplanar imaging

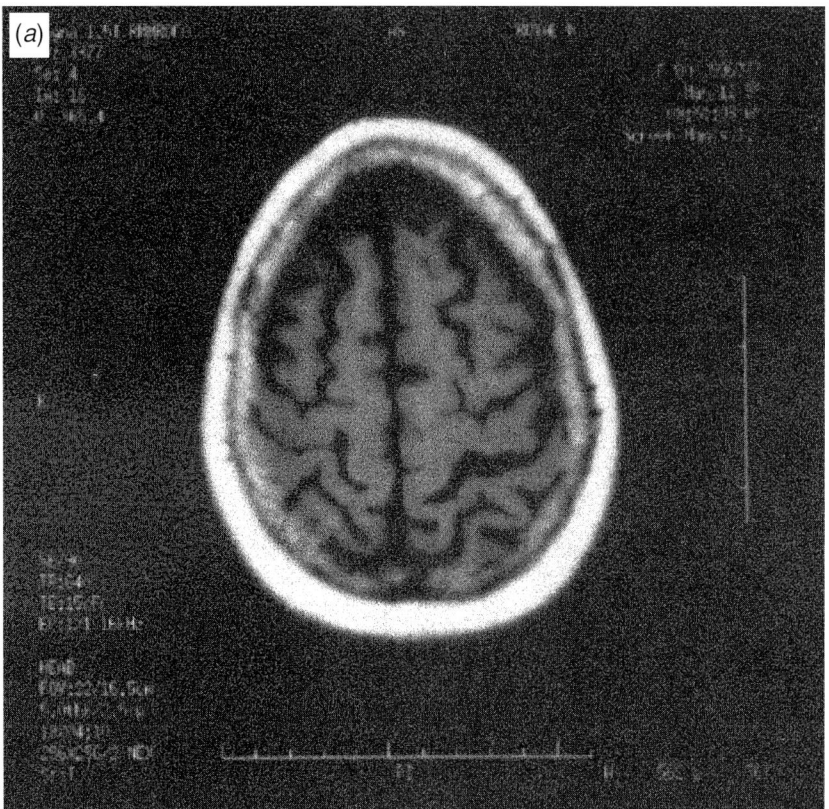

Fig. 6.1. Right middle cerebral artery territory infarct at 6 hours. T_1 and T_2-weighted scans through vertex (*a*), (*b*) show swollen right precentral and postcentral gyri, but no intrinsic signal abnormality. T_1-weighted post contrast scan (*c*) shows stasis in precentral and central arteries and pial enhancement from leptomeningeal collateral feeders.

spin echo (EPI SE) or T_2-weighted gradient echo (GE).

A very appropriate substitute for proton-weighted sequences is fluid attenuated inversion recovery (FLAIR). While retaining heavy T_2-weighting the cerebrospinal fluid is nulled, making any parenchymal abnormality more conspicuous. Furthermore, FLAIR sequences have been reported to be the only MRI sequence with high sensitivity and specificity in the detection of acute subarachnoid hemorrhage[1] and to be able to detect vessel occlusion and perfusion deficits more sensitively than conventional spin echo sequences[2,3]. FLAIR's drawback is its relative insensitivity to infratentorial intraaxial lesions.

In hyperacute stroke MRA sequences provide valuable and accurate information in respect to the patency of the major intracranial vessels. A rapid phase contrast MRA sequence can be obtained in restless patients in less than 2 minutes, while a more detailed time of flight (TOF) study of the intracranial circulation can be obtained in more cooperative patients.

Diffusion-weighted imaging (DWI), when available, should be a mandatory sequence in any protocol for stroke evaluation.

Plain MRI appearances of ischemic infarction

Conventional T_1- and T_2-weighted sequences

Appearances vary dramatically, according to the time at which imaging takes place after the ischemic insult. If imaging is initiated within the first 6 hours, during which time cytotoxic edema predominates, standard T_2- and T_1-weighted images are completely normal in the majority of cases. In a minority of cases careful scrutiny of the T_1-weighted images may show subtle evidence of mass effect (Fig. 6.1). This is in contrast to CT, the

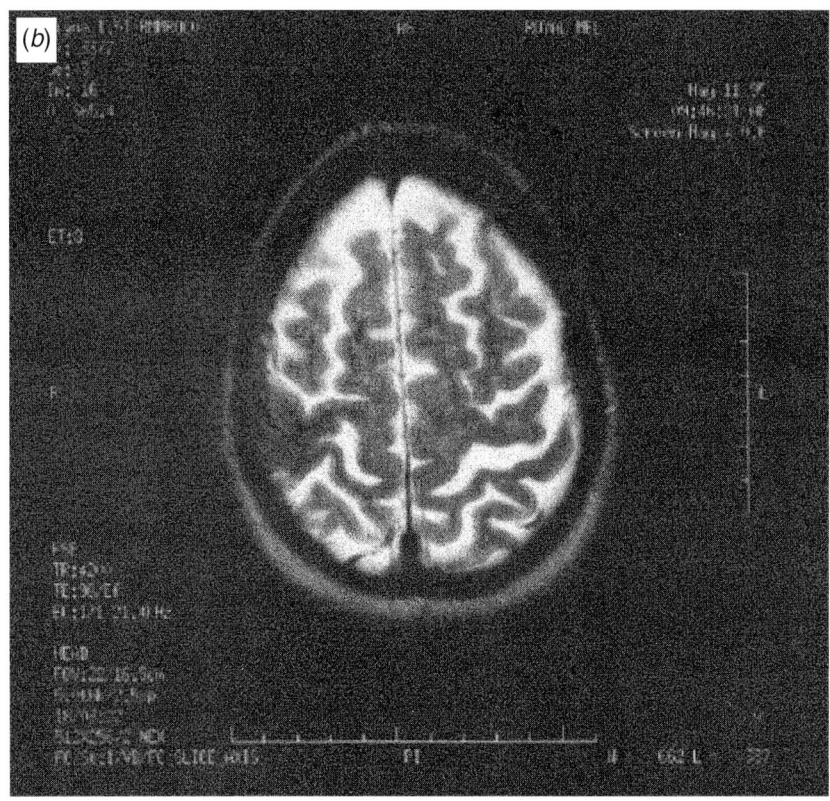

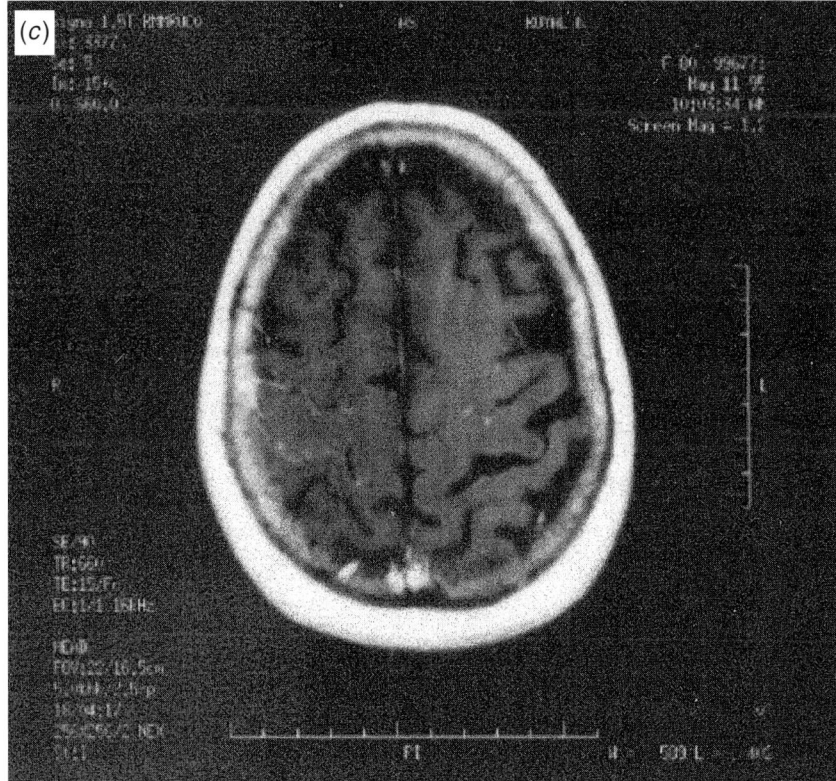

Fig. 6.1. *cont.*

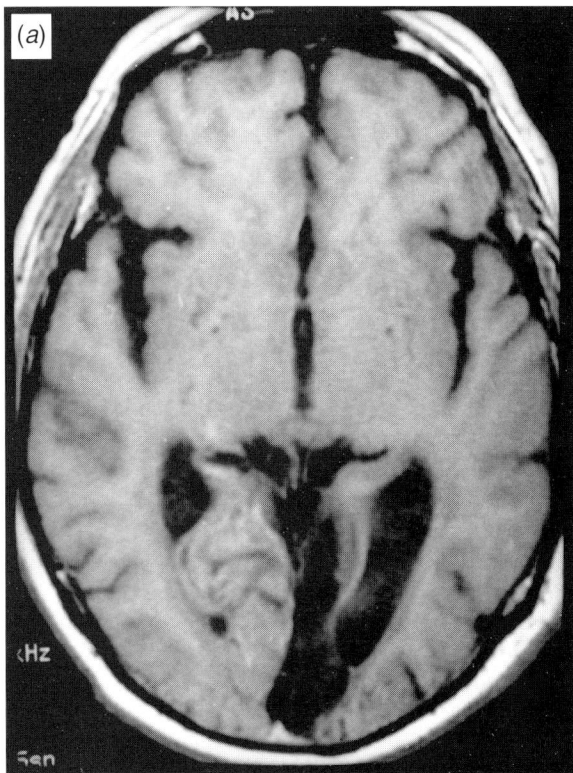 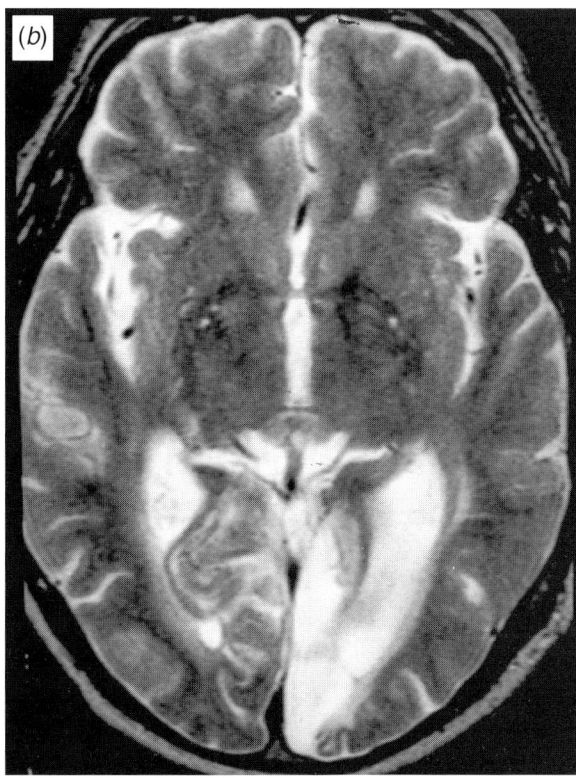

Fig. 6.2. Twelve-month-old infarct in left occipital lobe and 1-week-old infarct in right occipital lobe. (*a*) T_1-weighted and (*b*) T_2-weighted images show fluid filled gliotic area in left occipital lobe with compensatory dilatation of left occipital horn and slightly hemorrhagic and swollen right occipital lobe infarct.

sensitivity of which is variably reported from 30 to 80% within the first 12 hours.

By 12 hours, at which time a significant portion of the induced edema is of the vasogenic type, T_2-weighted scans show evidence of prolonged T_2 relaxation, manifested as increased signal in the affected area. In the case of classical peripheral embolic infarction the abnormal signal is characteristically within the cerebral cortex, as well as the underlying white matter, leading to a relative loss of grey/white differentiation. The peripheral portions of the abnormal signal are in some cases sharply defined, often clearly demarcating the border zones between classical vascular territories (Fig. 6.2). Occasionally peripheral vasogenic edema predominates. It is seen as finger like projections within white matter. Prolonged T_1 relaxation is often not as prominent in the first 24 hours, so that reduced signal intensity on T_1-weighted scans implies a less acute time frame. Sharply demarcated zones of hypointensity on T_1-weighted scans are particularly likely to represent older infarcts (Fig. 6.2).

Occasionally slowed flow within supplying arteries will be seen as hyperintensity within the vessels, particularly in T_1-weighted and FLAIR scans (Fig. 6.3). More commonly, absence of the normal flow void signal is seen in either or both T_1- and T_2-weighted scans. This sign is more easily identified in the larger vessels of the Circle of Willis and the M1 and M2 segments of the middle cerebral artery. When present in the middle cerebral artery, this sign can be regarded as the MRI equivalent of the dense middle cerebral artery sign, as seen with CT. Absence of flow void or even hyperintense signal is usually easily identified within the cavernous segment of the internal carotid artery, the internal carotid in the carotid canal and within the basilar artery. It is important to recognize that these

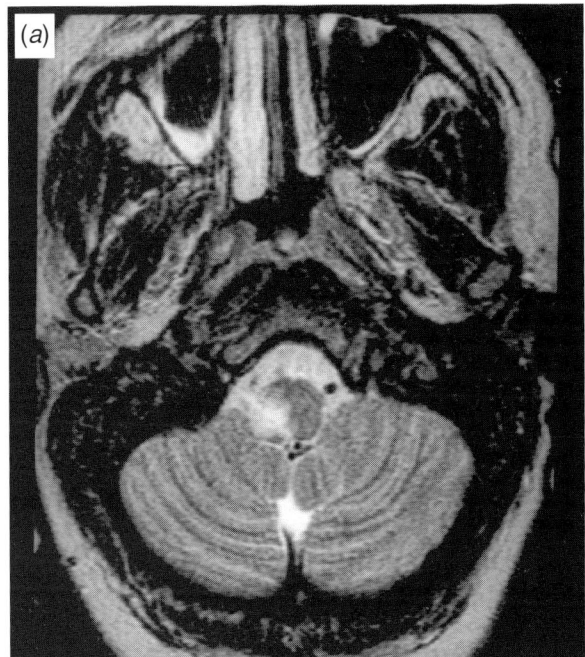 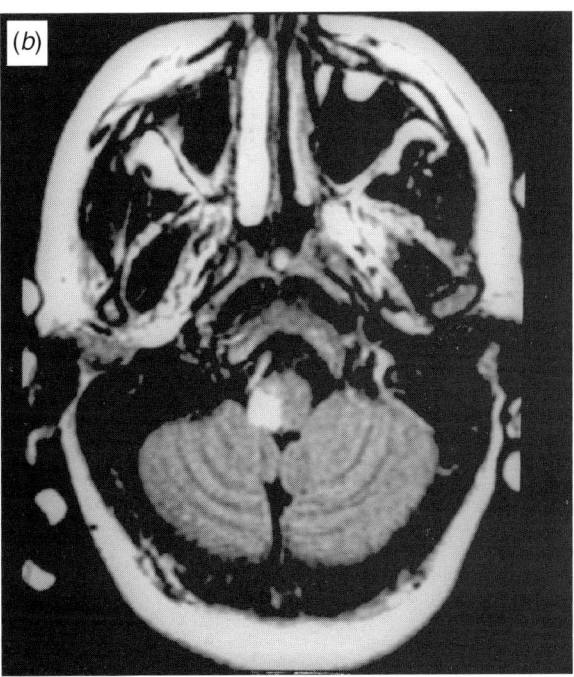

Fig. 6.3. Right-sided medullary infarct at 24 hours. (*a*) T_2-weighted scan shows hyperintense signal in right side of medulla, sharply delineated medially at the midline. Note markedly reduced signal void in right vertebral artery. FLAIR image (*b*) also shows right medullary infarct and right vertebral artery hyperintensity, indicating right vertebral occlusion or severe stenosis or markedly slowed flow.

signal changes can be the result of occlusion or severe stenosis and slow flow.

A second 'blind' period for conventional sequences has been described in the second week, when both T_1- and T_2-weighted sequences can revert almost to normality, even in the presence of a sizeable completed infarct (Fig. 6.4)[4]. This is attributed to revascularization and petechial hemorrhage effectively neutralizing the effect of vasogenic and any persistent cytotoxic edema. Even diffusion-weighted sequences may be negative if it happens that imaging is taking place at the point that diffusion is about to evolve from restriction to increase. At this stage contrast enhanced sequences are particularly valuable because the brain parenchyma will usually show vivid parenchymal contrast enhancement (Fig. 6.4). Sequences particularly sensitive to blood breakdown products, such as gradient echo T_2^* sequences, will usually detect even the small amount of blood associated with petechial hemorrhage (Fig. 6.5).

Contrast-enhanced T_1-weighted sequences

The injection of an intravenous contrast medium containing gadolinium significantly increases the ability of conventional sequences to diagnose infarction. Within the first 24 hours the signal intensity in arteries supplying the infarcted region is increased due to slow flow and T_1 shortening by the gadolinium in approximately 80% of cases (Fig. 6.1).[5] From day 2 to day 5 cortical surface contrast enhancement may result from leptomeningeal collaterals (Fig. 6.1).[5]

From approximately 4 days parenchymal enhancement commences as a result of revascularization by 'leaky' vessels. The phenomenon is seen in 100% of cases by day 7.[5,6] The contrast enhancement pattern is variable. A gyral pattern of enhancement is common (Fig. 6.4), but streaky, patchy and even ring patterns of enhancement may be seen. Some form of parenchymal enhancement is seen in almost 100% of infarcts during the second

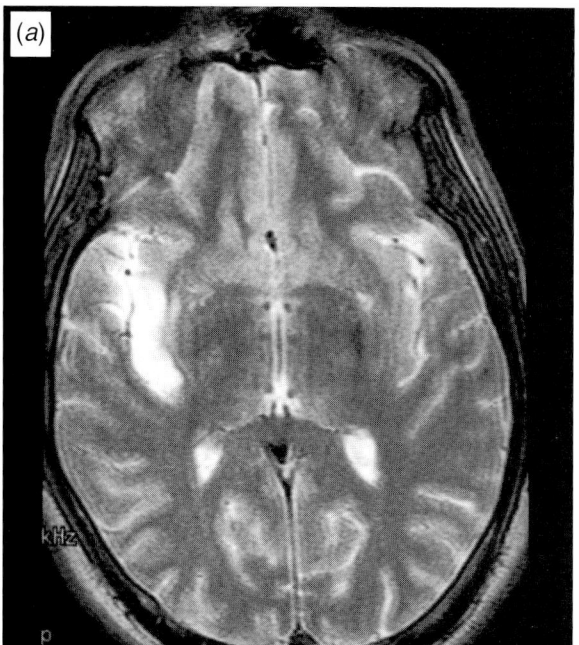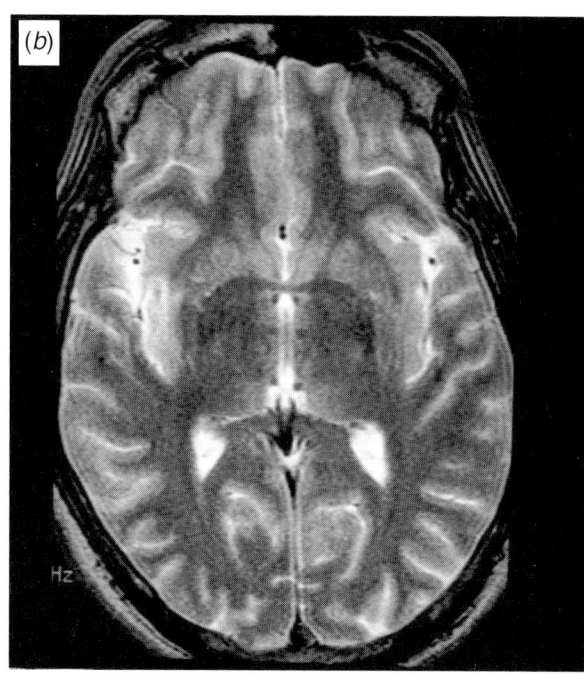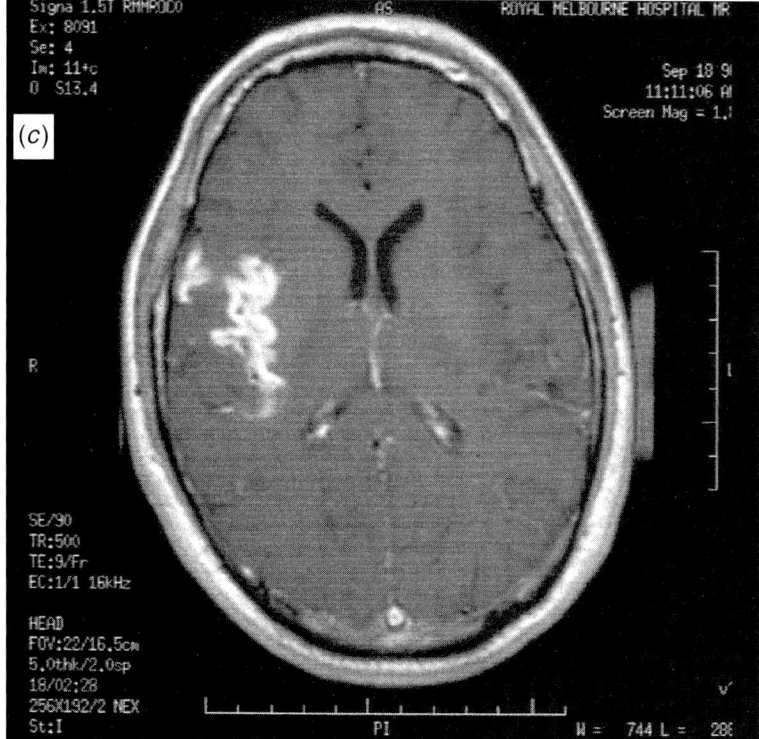

Fig. 6.4. Infarct involving right insular cortex.
(a) At 24 hours a T_2-weighted scan shows clearcut increased signal intensity within the right insular cortex.
(b) At 10 days the T_2-weighted scan shows only very subtle hyperintensity in the right insular cortex.
(c) Post-contrast T_1-weighted scan shows vivid parenchymal contrast enhancement in the insular cortex and adjacent right frontal cortex.

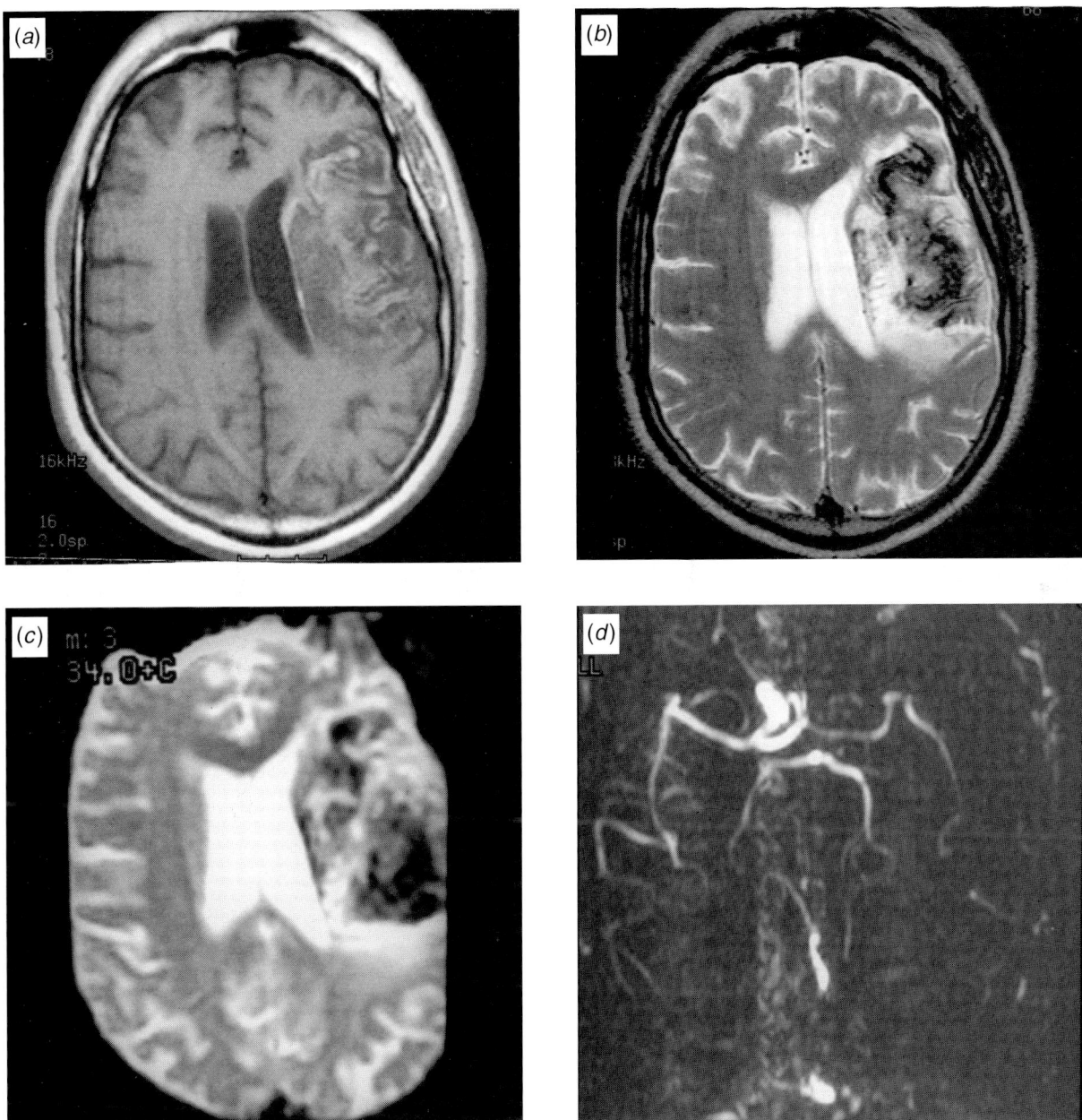

Fig. 6.5. Left frontal infarct at 12 days.
(a) T_1-weighted image shows serpentine hyperintense areas in infarct periphery.
(b) T_2-weighted fast spin echo image shows extensive areas of signal void within central portions of infarct.
(c) T_2-weighted EPI gradient echo image from diffusion weighted sequence without added gradients (Bo image), demonstrates far more extensive signal voids than T_2-weighted FSE image.
(d) Phase contrast MRA shows left internal carotid occlusion, with left middle cerebral artery patent via flow from the right internal carotid and anterior cerebral arteries.

and third weeks, but has largely disappeared by the second month.

All forms of contrast enhancement are seen in only a minority of small deep (lacunar) infarcts.

Fluid attenuated inversion recovery (FLAIR)

FLAIR is a routinely available technique which produces heavily T_2-weighted images, at the same time nulling or completely subtracting the normally bright cerebrospinal fluid signal. The technique is particularly suited to the identification of periventricular lesions such as demyelination plaques, and is often used as a substitute for minimally T_2-weighted ('proton weighted') sequences because of the relative conspicuity of any lesion with a prolonged T_2. Its sensitivity in the detection of supratentorial lesions is arguably greater than that of conventional T_2-weighted sequences. The major disadvantage of the sequence is its relative insensitivity to brainstem and cerebellar lesions.

Like conventional T_2-weighted sequences FLAIR shows no parenchymal signal abnormality in the first 6–8 hours after the ischemic insult. However, it has been observed that vessels in the ischemic region will show a hyperintense signal instead of the usual signal void in 10–96 % of cases (Figs. 6.3,6.6).[2,3] The hyperintense signal is associated particularly with large vessel occlusion or severe stenosis, slow flow and decreased perfusion. It corresponds to intravascular enhancement seen in contrast enhanced sequences.

Magnetic resonance angiography (MRA)

MRA is a very useful adjunct to conventional sequences. Middle cerebral or internal carotid occlusion can be confirmed in acute stroke patients, with appropriate impact on management. The various forms of MRA have been described in Chapter 7. Phase contrast MRA can be performed in less than 2 minutes to provide acceptable images of the terminal internal carotid arteries and the vertebrobasilar system and the Circle of Willis (Fig. 6.7). Time of Flight MRA provides more detailed anatomical images, often showing third order middle cerebral branches, but takes in excess of 4 minutes for data acquisition. This may result in degraded images due to movement induced artefact when scanning restless acute stroke patients.

MRA of the carotid arteries in the neck has been significantly improved by the development of contrast enhanced MRA[7] (see Chapter 7), which has increased the accuracy of the evaluation of the carotid bifurcation, particularly in regards to specificity. The addition of this technique to the standard evaluation means that information regarding the condition of brain parenchyma and the major arteries of supply from arch to circle of Willis can be evaluated in one examination, provided the patient is able to co-operate. Even non-contrast-enhanced MRA is at least equal to duplex Doppler ultrasound in the evaluation of the carotid bifurcation.[8] Its major advantage is in the demonstration of atherosclerotic disease in Asian and black ethnic groups, in whom the intracranial arteries are more frequently involved than in caucasian populations.

Magnetization Transfer Contrast (MTC)

This technique exploits the cross-relaxation between mobile water protons and the restricted proton pool, which includes protons in or around macromolecules such as myelin. The application of a broad frequency, off resonance pulse reduces the magnetization of the restricted proton pool to zero, while only partly reducing the free proton magnetization. Contrast enhancement after intravenous contrast medium injection can be maximized by this technique.[9] The ratio of signal intensity before and after application of the off resonance pulse (magnetization transfer ratio, or MTR) provides an indicator of demyelination, which has lead to its use in multiple sclerosis. In subacute and chronic stroke MTR has been found to be closely related to axonal damage and to correlate well with motor deficit.[10]

The principal use for MTC in the stroke context is in TOF MRA, where it suppresses background parenchymal signal, increasing the conspicuity of small vessels.

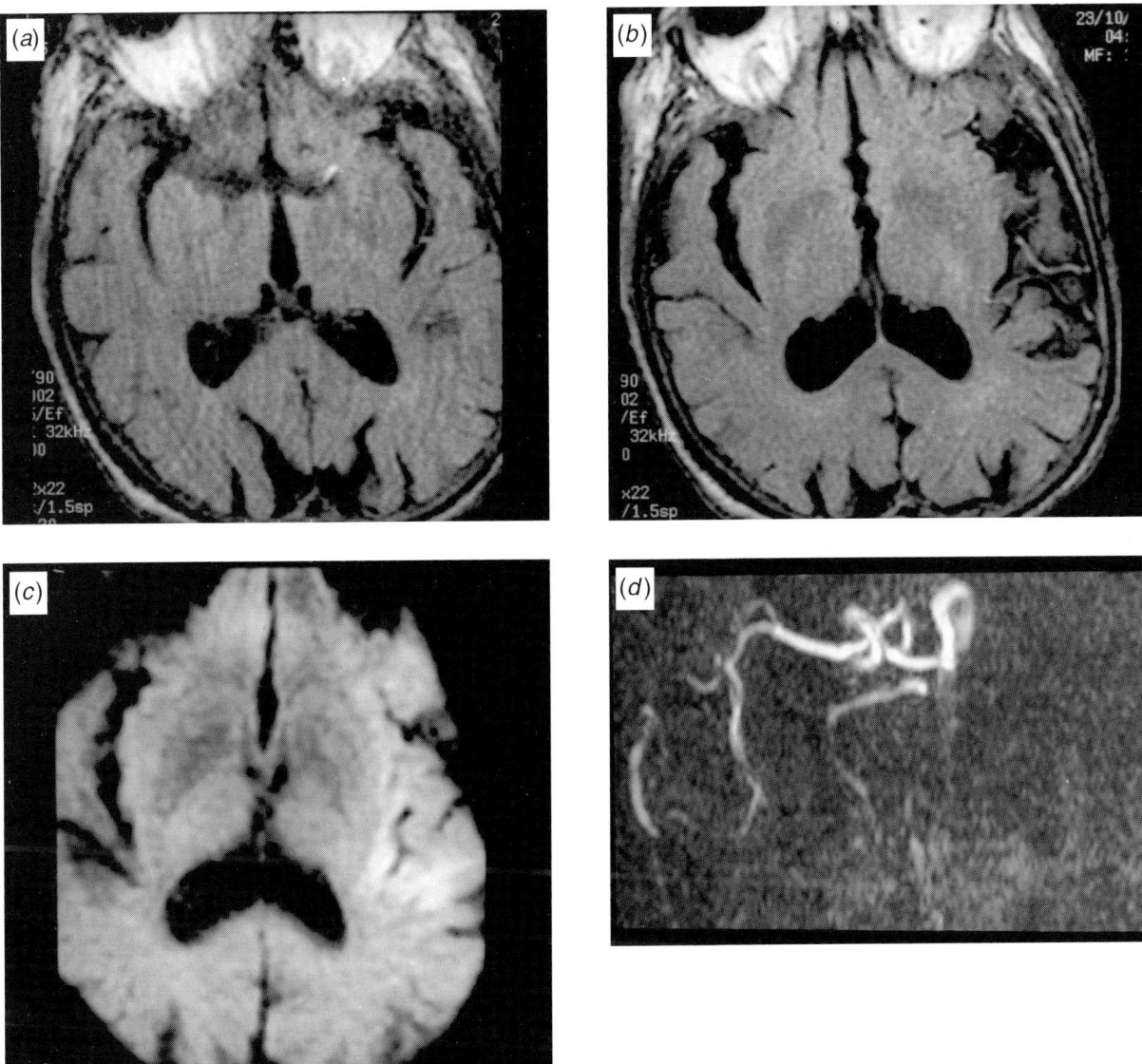

Fig. 6.6. FLAIR images of 4-hours-old infarct, showing high signal intensity within stem of left middle cerebral artery (a) and Sylvian branches (b) but no parenchymal signal change. Diffusion-weighted image (c) demonstrates restricted diffusion in left middle cerebral artery territory, indicating early infarct. Phase contrast MRA (d) shows left middle cerebral artery occlusion at its origin.

Hemorrhagic infarction

Approximately 60% of ischemic or bland infarcts develop evidence of petechial hemorrhage in the second and subsequent weeks. This is seen as patchy small, multifocal areas of signal loss within the infarcted cortex on T_2-weighted sequences (Fig. 6.5). These hemorrhages are not sufficiently large to be seen in most CT scans performed at the same time. They are normal sequelae of bland infarction and should not be considered part of the spectrum of true hemorrhagic infarction.

True hemorrhagic infarction is most often secondary to initially bland infarcts in which the feeding arteries have recanalized, either spontaneously, or as a result of therapeutic thrombolysis, allowing high pressure blood flow into irreversibly damaged capillaries. It is also a frequent sequel to venous

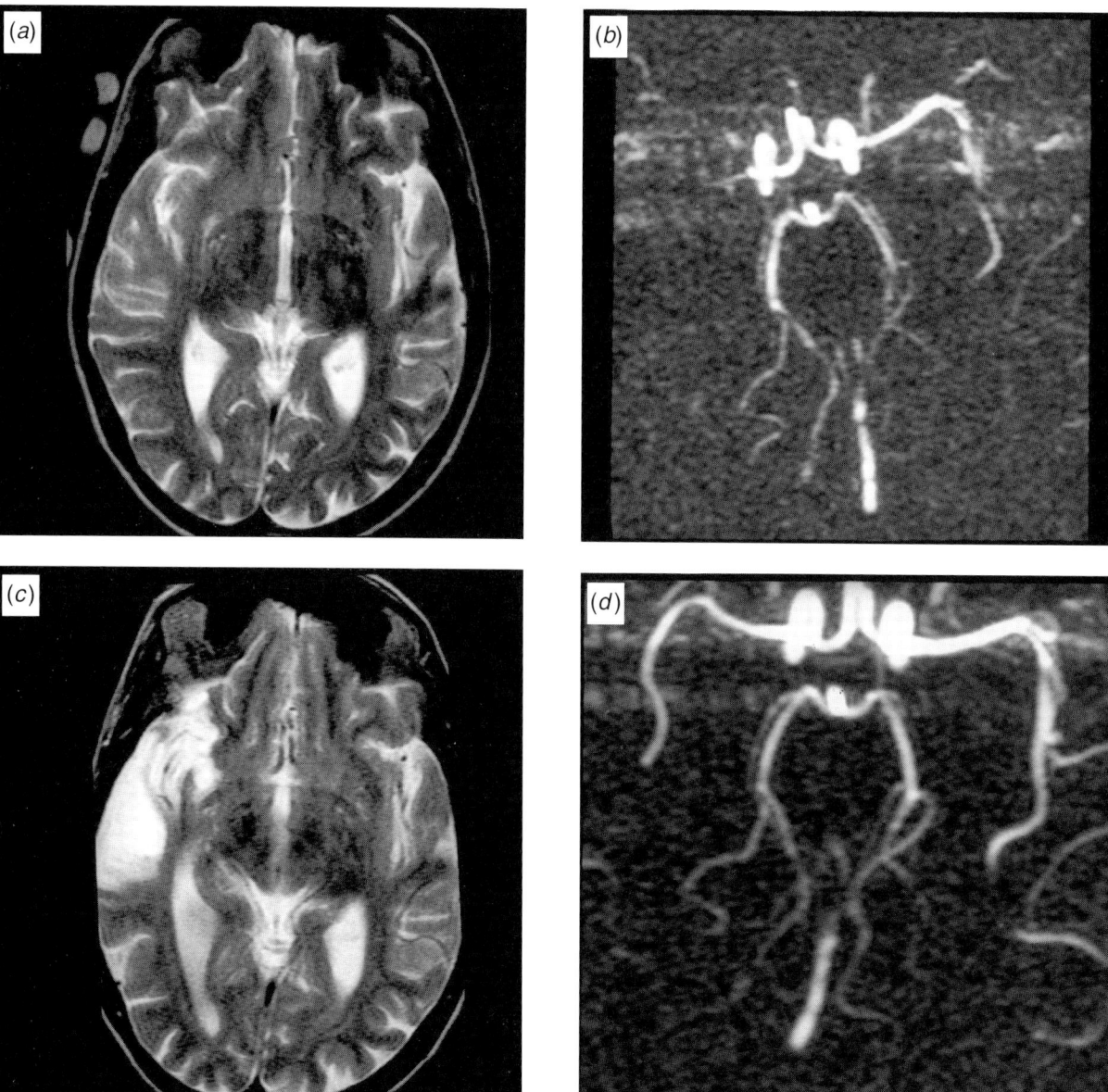

Fig. 6.7. Right middle cerebral artery territory infarct at 6 hours.
(a) T_2-weighted scan shows no abnormality
(b) Phase contrast MRA shows right middle cerebral artery occlusion.
(c) T_2-weighted scan shows clearcut infarct in right temporal lobe at 3 days.
(d) Phase contrast MRA demonstrates restoration of right middle cerebral artery patency.

thrombosis, usually after thrombus has retrogradely propagated into cortical veins from the venous sinuses. The MRI appearance varies accordingly.

Hyperacute parenchymal hemorrhage can be detected by MRI by utilizing one of the T_2-weighted magnetic susceptibility sensitive sequences such as T_2-weighted GE.[11] The first images of diffusion-weighted sequences before the application of the superimposed gradients are appropriately magnetic susceptibility sensitive, as the diffusion sequences are usually EPI T_2-weighed GE or SE (Fig. 6.5(c)).

Arterial origin hemorrhagic infarcts usually have a background of characteristic bland infarct appearances. They are largely confined to an arterial vascular territory and involve the cortex as well as the deeper structures. Superimposed on this background are heterogeneous zones of soft tissue with the typical appearance of hematoma. The signal characteristics of the hematoma component are dependent on its age.

Venous infarcts, on the other hand, transgress arterial territorial boundaries (Fig. 6.8). Those venous infarcts secondary to superior sagittal sinus thrombosis are often bilateral in the superior convexities of the hemispheres. The hemorrhagic element is heterogeneous and contrast enhancement is often minimal or absent. If the hemorrhage is more than 3 days old the affected venous sinuses may be hyperintense on T_1-weighted scans (Fig. 6.8). Occasionally the involved cortical veins may be similarly hyperintense. If the thrombotic process has propagated into the medullary veins, subependymal veins such as the internal cerebral veins and the great vein of Galen may also be hyperintense, or contain no flow void. Extension to the deep venous system produces an almost pathognomonic pattern of ischemic edema, involving both thalami and the upper brainstem.

Magnetic resonance venography (MRV), which is basically MRA with arterial flow suppressed, will often provide the definitive diagnosis of sinus thrombosis, but there are pitfalls. There may be gaps in up to 31% of non-dominant transverse sinuses in normal subjects.[12] Acute thrombus may produce signal voids on T_2-weighted sequences, due to the presence of deoxyhemoglobin or intracellular methemoglobin. The voids can simulate patency. This 'artefact' can be overcome by carefully perusing the sinuses in all sequences.[13] Subacute thrombus may appear hyperintense on T_1-weighted images. The maximal pixel intensity algorithm used to construct two and three dimensional images from time of flight MRA source images cannot distinguish between the hyperintensity of flowing blood and subacute thrombus. The MRV images may then appear normal. Phase contrast MRV is more reliable as only moving protons are included in the final image (Fig. 6.8).[13]

Differential diagnosis

Normal anatomical variants

Virchow–Robin spaces are perivascular spaces surrounding perforating arteries. They represent extensions of the subarachnoid space into the brain and are particularly prominent in the region of the anterior perforated substance, where the lenticulostriate arteries enter the base of the brain in the middle cranial fossae. The only consistent association is with increasing age.[14] They are virtually always visible in T_1- and T_2-weighted spin echo images of the lentiform nuclei and internal capsule, where they occasionally reach sizes of more than one centimetre (Fig. 6.9). They are characteristically sited in close relation to the anterior commissure. They can be differentiated from lacunar infarcts in that they are round or linear and follow the signal intensities of cerebrospinal fluid on all sequences.[15] It is important to perform proton-weighted sequences or FLAIR, as heavily T_1- and T_2-weighted sequences alone cannot distinguish between the two entities.

Brain tumours

In the vast majority of cases mass effect, enhancement pattern, surrounding vasogenic edema and transgression of more than one arterial territory easily differentiates tumour from infarct, even in the absence of a characteristic history. Occasionally, an infarct can be truly simulated by tumour in an isolated examination. Gliomas of low or intermediate grade are most often responsible. Protoplasmic, non-enhancing astrocytomas can be confined to the cortex and underlying medulla in an apparent single vascular territory and have sharp margins. Alternatively, an infarct can sometimes induce abundant vasogenic edema and vivid contrast enhancement, occasionally with a 'ring' pattern to simulate a malignant tumour. If MRS and diffusion-weighted imaging are not immediately available the simplest method of differentiating between tumour and infarct is simply to rescan in 1 to 2 weeks' time. An infarct will have significantly changed in

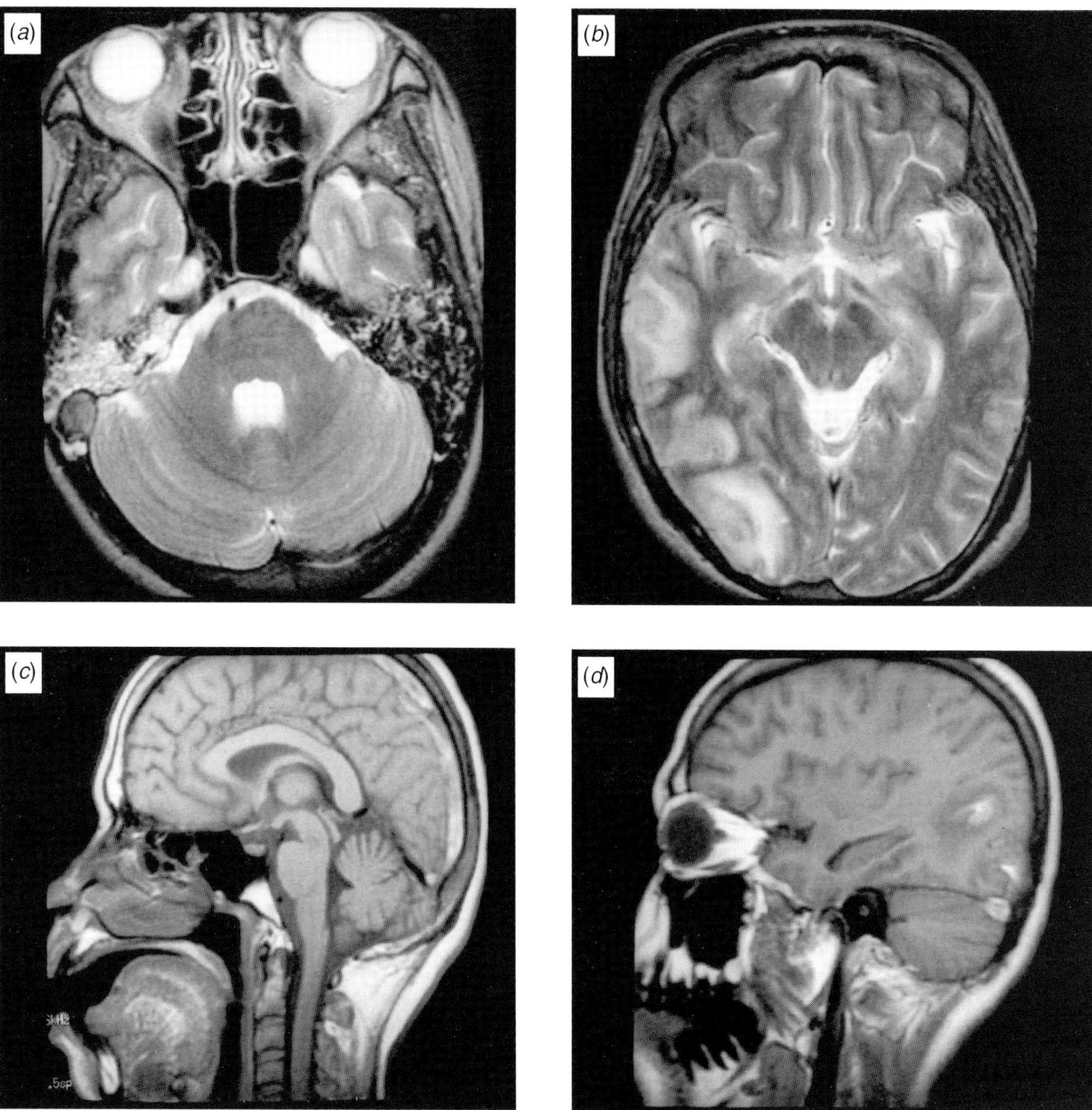

Fig. 6.8. Axial T$_2$-weighted image (*a*) through posterior fossa structures shows mottled signal within the right sigmoid sinus. Note inflammatory changes in the adjacent mastoid air cells. Axial T$_2$-weighted image through occipital lobes (*b*) shows irregular lobulated zones of abnormal signal in lateral temporal and occipital lobes.

Sagittal and lateral sinus thrombosis. Sagittal T$_1$-weighted images show hyperintensity in superior saggittal sinus (*c*) and lateral sinus (*d*). Note hemorrhagic infact in adjacent occipital lobe. MRV studies confirm lack of flow in superior sagittal sinus (*e*) and right lateral sinus (*f*).

Clinical use of standard MRI

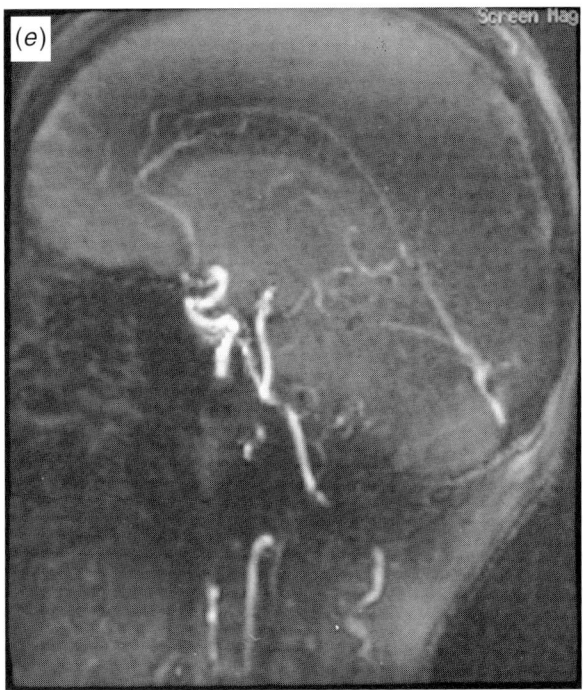

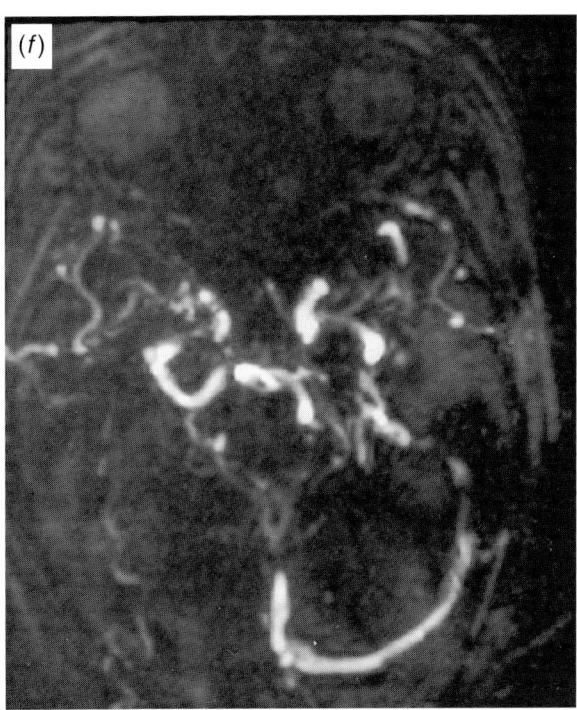

Fig. 6.8. (cont.)

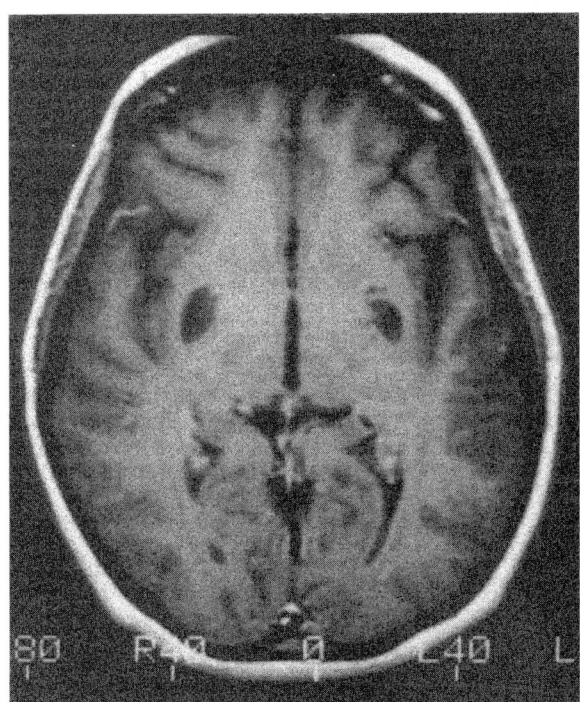

Fig. 6.9. Virchow–Robin (perivascular) spaces. T_1-weighted axial image shows symmetrical, large fluid filled ovoid spaces in the anterior perforated substance in close proximity to the anterior commissure.

appearance, both in mass effect and contrast enhancement pattern, while a tumour will be unchanged or slightly bigger.

Encephalitis/cerebritis

The clinical presentation will usually be significantly different, but the MRI appearances can be similar. The major difference is that inflammatory processes do not respect normal arterial territories. Herpes simplex encephalitis characteristically involves one or both temporal lobes (Fig. 6.10). The involvement is predominantly in the posterior cerebral artery supplied portion of the medial temporal lobe initially, but almost invariably has already involved the middle cerebral artery supplied lateral aspect by the time of first presentation. As the inflammation extends superiorly through the external capsule, the lentiform nucleus is almost always preserved, unlike middle cerebral artery territory infarcts.

The early cerebritis stage which precedes the development of cerebral abscess may manifest as an area of nonspecific non-enhancing edema, usually at the cortico-medullary junction. It is more

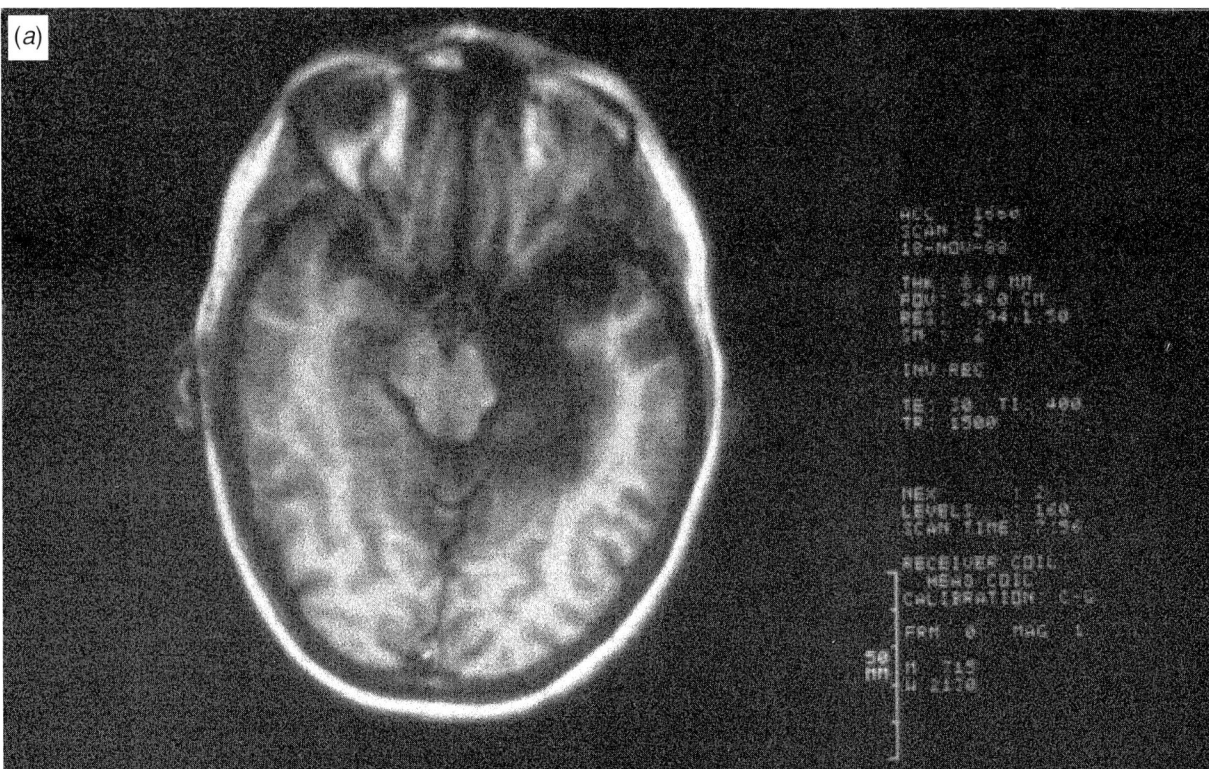
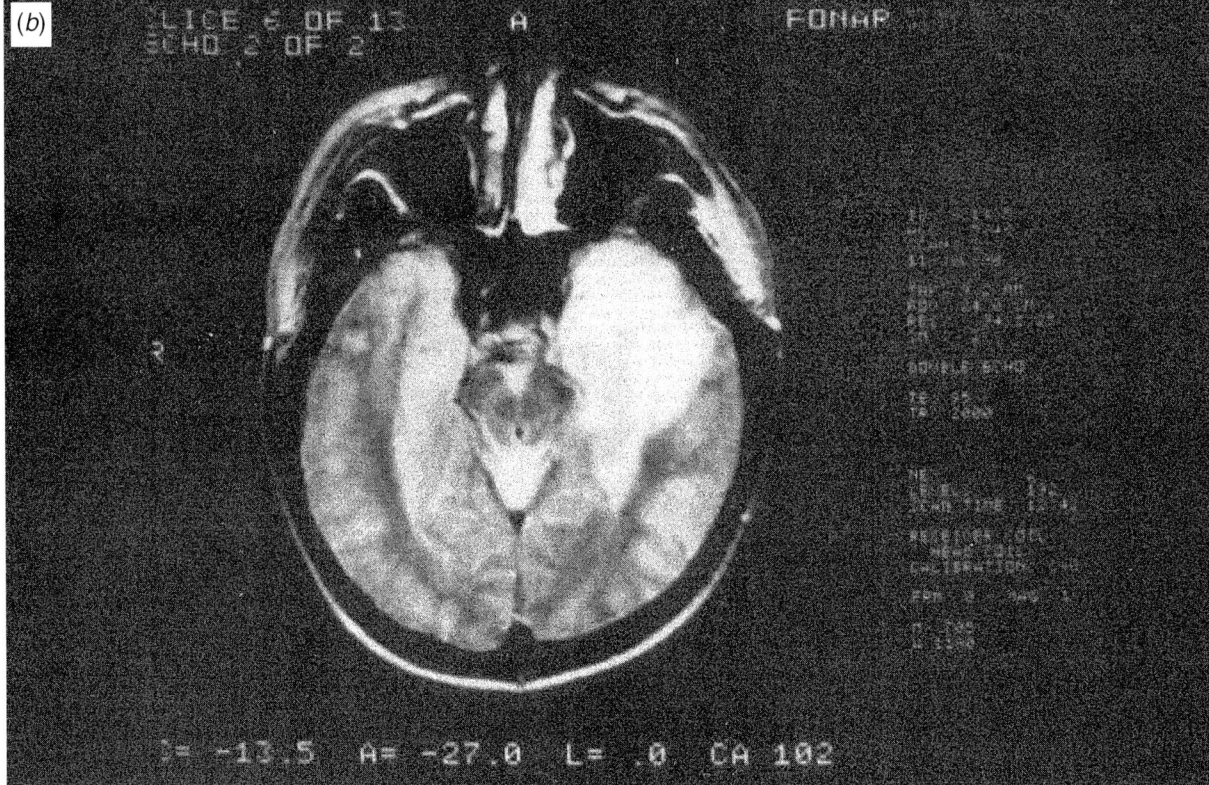

Fig. 6.10. Herpes simplex encephalitis. T_1-weighted (*a*) and T_2-weighted axial images, demonstrate abnormal signal and swelling in the anterior portion of the left temporal lobe and less marked changes in the medial portion of the right temporal lobe. Note that the left temporal lobe abnormality transgresses the left middle and posterior cerebral artery territory.

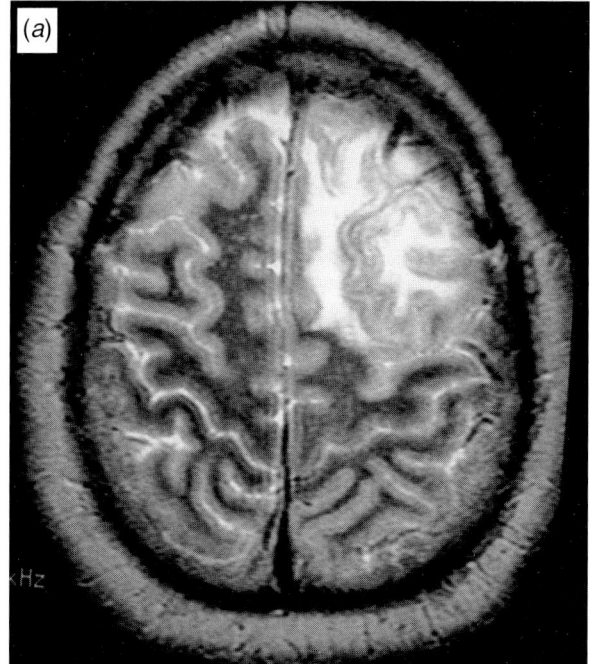 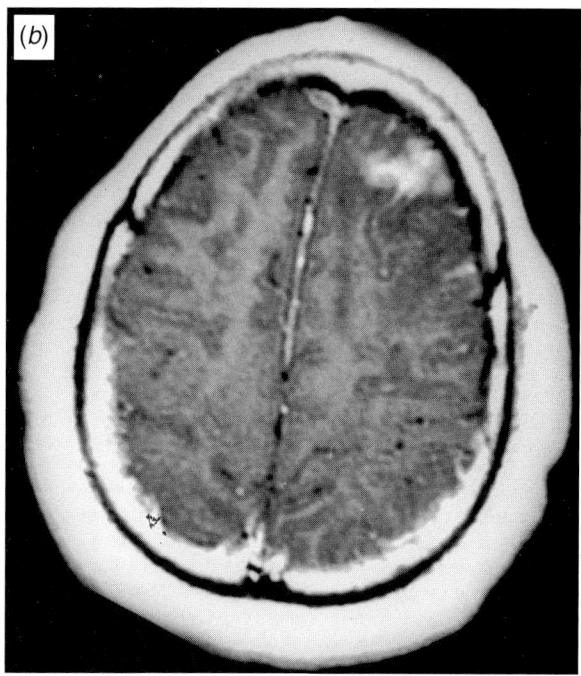

Fig. 6.11. Left frontal cerebritis. T_2-weighted scan (*a*) shows abnormal signal in left frontal lobe anteriorly with pattern of vasogenic edema in the underlying white matter. Note lesion crosses the left anterior and middle cerebral artery territories. Post-contrast T_1-weighted scan (b) shows patchy left frontal enhancement.

often associated with a vasogenic pattern of edema than are infarcts, but may have a patchy enhancement pattern before the development of a capsule and ring enhancement at about 2 weeks (Fig. 6.11). Once developed, the capsule will usually show evidence of signal voids on T_2-weighted scans, thought to be due to a combination of microhaemorrhages and free radicals.

Conclusion

Standard MRI sequences are extremely sensitive to the detection of acute, subacute and chronic infarcts. However, standard sequences are negative in the majority of infarcts (within the first 6–8 hours). Sensitivity is increased by the use of contrast enhancement and FLAIR, but accurate diagnosis of hyperacute infarction depends on the use of diffusion-weighted imaging. Standard MRA sequences add further valuable information regarding patency of major intracranial vessels.

REFERENCES

1 Noguchi K, Ogawa T, Inugami, A et al. Acute subarachnoid haemorrhage: MR imaging with fluid-attenuated inversion recovery pulse sequences. *Radiology* 1995; 196: 773–777.
2 Kamran S, Bates V, Bakshi R, Wright P, Kinkel W, Milatich R. Significance of hyperintense vessels on FLAIR MRI in acute stroke. *Neurology* 2000; 55: 265–269.
3 Toyoda K, Ida M, Fukuda K. Fluid-attenuated inversion recovery intraarterial signal: an early sign of hyperacute cerebral ischemia. *Am J Neuroradiol* 2001; 22: 1015–1016.
4 Pereira AC, Doyle VL, Clifton A, Howe FA, Griffiths JR, Brown MM. Case reports. The transient disappearance of cerebral infarction on T_2 weighted MRI. *Clin Radiol* 2000; 55: 725–727.
5 Elster AD, Moody DM. Early cerebral infarction; gadopentate dimeglumine enhancement. *Radiology* 1990; 177: 627–632.
6 Karonen JO, Partanen PL, Vanninen RL, Vainio PA, Aronen HJ. Evolution of MR contrast enhancement patterns during the first week after acute ischemic stroke. *Am J Neuroradiol* 2001; 22: 103–111.

7 Fellner FA, Felher C, Wufke, R et al. Fluoroscopically triggered contrast-enhanced 3D MR DSA and 3D time of flight turbo MRA of the carotid arteries: first clinical experiences in correlation with ultrasound, X-ray angiography and endarterectomy findings. *Magn Reson Imaging* 2000; 18: 575–585.

8 Patel MR, Kurtz KM, Klufas RA, et al. Preoperative assessment of the carotid bifurcation. Can magnetic resonance angiography and duplex ultrasonography replace contrast angiography? *Stroke* 1995; 26: 1753–1758.

9 Mathews VP, King JC, Elster AD, Hamilton CA. Cerebral infarction: effects of dose and magnetization transfer saturation at gadolinium-enhanced MR imaging. *Radiology* 1994; 190: 547–552.

10 Pendlebury ST, Lee MA, Blamire AM, Styles P, Matthews PM. Correlating magnetic resonance imaging markers of axonal injury and demyelination in motor impairment secondary to stroke and multiple sclerosis. *Magn Reson Imaging* 2000; 18: 369–378.

11 Patel MR, Edelman RR, Warach S. Detection of hyperacute primary intraparenchymal hemorrhage by magnetic resonance imaging. *Stroke* 1996; 27: 2321–2324.

12 Ayanzen RH, Bird CR, Keller PJ, McCully FJ, Theobald MR, Heiserman JE. Cerebral MR venography: normal anatomy and potential diagnostic pitfalls. *Am J Neuroradiol* 2000; 21: 74–78.

13 Provenzale JM, Joseph GJ, Barboriak DP. Dural sinus thrombosis: findings on CT and MR imaging and diagnostic pitfalls. *Am J Radiol* 1998; 170: 777–783.

14 Heier LA, Bauer CJ, Schwartz L, Zimmerman RD, Morgello S, Deck MD. Large Virchow-Robin spaces: MR-clinical correlation. *Am J Neuroradiol* 1989; 10: 929–936.

15 Bokura H, Kobayashi S, Yamaguchi S. Distinguishing silent lacunar infarction from enlarged Virchow-Robin spaces: a magnetic resonance imaging and pathological study. *J Neurol* 1998; 245: 116–122.

MR angiography of the head and neck: basic principles and clinical applications

Robert R. Edelman and Joel Meyer

Department of Radiology, Evanston Northwestern Healthcare
Northwestern University School of Medicine, 2650 Ridge Avenue, Evanston, IL 60201, USA

Since the first publication of a clinical magnetic resonance angiogram (MRA) in 1985,[1] there has been extensive growth in the vascular applications of magnetic resonance.[2] Although for many years a purely investigational tool, the technology and validation studies have progressed to the point that MRA has largely supplanted X-ray angiography (XRA) for evaluation of the extracranial carotid arteries, and is often an alternative to XRA for evaluation of the vertebral arteries and circle of Willis.

In this chapter, we will first review the basic principles of MRA, including time of flight and phase contrast techniques, and introduce the use of paramagnetic contrast agents for MRA. Advantages and pitfalls of MRA as compared with duplex sonography (DUS) and XRA will be addressed, and we will consider future directions for this rapidly advancing technology.

Basic principles of MRA

Unlike computed tomography (CT), which relies solely on the attenuation of X-ray photons to generate an image, MR uses a combination of magnetic fields and radiofrequency energy in order to produce images. The appearance of blood in an MR image depends on the intrinsic magnetic relaxation properties (T_1 and T_2), the oxygenation status and physical state of the blood (e.g. venous vs. arterial vs. hematoma), the direction, rate, and pulsatility of flow, as well as the presence of exogenously administered contrast agents. The variety of physical properties that can be manifested in an MR image can be a great advantage for distinguishing arteries and veins from stationary background tissue, and permits the measurement of flow (not possible by CT), but it also introduces ample sources for artefacts.

Blood has a long T_1 relaxation time (~ 1.2 s). The T_2 relaxation time is substantially longer for arterial blood (high oxyhemoglobin content), as compared with venous blood (high deoxyhemoglobin content). Without the confounding influence of flow, blood would appear dark (e.g. similar to muscle on T_1-weighted images) and bright on T_2-weighted images. However, flow has a profound effect on the signal intensity of blood so that the intrinsic relaxation properties of arterial and venous blood are not usually apparent, the exception being where flow is absent (i.e. stasis in a varix).

Time of flight

One class of MRA techniques is called 'time of flight'.[3] The term refers to the fact that the transit of blood from one position to another will alter the signal intensity from the spins, and enable its differentiation from stationary tissues. On spin-echo and fast spin-echo images, the time-of-flight effect causes rapidly flowing spins to appear dark (hence the terminology 'dark blood' technique). The reason is that the flowing spins wash out of the plane of section before the sequence of 90 and 180 degree pulses has been played out, so that the MR signal is lost. Additionally, extra radiofrequency pulses called 'saturation' pulses may be applied to the inflowing spins so as to further saturate and suppress their signal.[4] Alternatively, one can more effectively eliminate the signal from blood by using the dual inversion method.[5,6] Dark blood techniques are helpful for routine anatomic imaging and for direct imaging of the vessel wall and associated plaque or thrombus.[7,8]

For MRA, on the other hand, one is usually trying to render the flowing spins brighter than other tissues, so that one can apply a maximum intensity projection (MIP) algorithm to produce an angiogram-like picture.[9] In order to achieve this goal, a gradient-echo pulse sequence is applied. Unlike the spin-echo case, only a single radiofrequency pulse is used during each repetition of the sequence, so that the washout effects can be neglected. Typically, one uses a short repetition time (TR) so that scan times are minimized (of the order of a few seconds for 2D acquisitions and less than 30 seconds for 3D acquisitions). The combination of the short TR and a large excitation flip angle depresses the signal intensity of stationary tissues, as these spins do not have adequate time to recover their longitudal magnetization between sequence repetitions.

Conversely, rapidly flowing spins move into and out of the plane of section in such a short time period that they only experience one or a few radiofrequency pulses before they are replaced by fresh, fully magnetized spins. Thus, the flowing spins produce an intense signal that is readily differentiated from stationary tissue, particularly if the orientation of the blood vessel is nearly orthogonal to the plane of section. The data may be directly acquired as thin sections (2D) or as a thick slab that is subsequently reconstructed into thin sections (3D). In the case of 3D, the flow must be more rapid than in the 2D scenario since a thick slab, rather than thin slice, is imaged and the flowing spins have a greater distance to traverse before exiting. Thus, 3D time-of-flight MRA is reserved for situations where the expected flow velocities are high, such as the extracranial carotid arteries and Circle of Willis, whereas 2D time of flight would be greatly preferred where the velocities are lower, as for venography of the intracranial venous sinuses. Alternatively, one can use a multiple overlapping thin-slab 3D acquisition (MOTSA) (Fig. 7.1), which is less sensitive to signal loss from saturation and turbulence than 3D or 2D, respectively.[10]

Both 2D and 3D time-of-flight MRA are helpful for assessing the extracranial carotid bifurcation. The 2D technique generally yields good image quality for non-stenotic vessels and in slow flow situations (e.g. string sign). However, it is not as helpful for the circle of Willis. The 3D technique provides more accurate measurements of stenoses because of its lesser sensitivity to signal loss from turbulent flow and smaller voxels. In both cases, images are acquired over a small field of view in the axial orientation, so that only a relatively small portion of the carotids in the vicinity of the bifurcation is imaged. Thus, a tandem stenosis would be easily missed, as is also the case with duplex sonography.

Phase contrast

The pulse sequences used for MR imaging typically apply a pair of gradients of opposite polarity ('bipolar') along the frequency and slice-select directions. The net phase shift for stationary spins at the echo time (TE) is zero. However, moving spins accumulate a non-zero phase shift from the bipolar gradients; this velocity-dependent phase shift is the basis for phase contrast MRA. The phase shift can be used to quantify velocity on phase-contrast images.[11,12] Alternatively, the phase shift allows flowing blood to be displayed without any signal from the stationary tissues. This feature comes in handy when there are paramagnetic hemoglobin breakdown products or contrast-enhancing tissues in the vicinity of a blood vessel, as these structures would appear bright in a time of flight MRA. Two-dimensional (thick slice) phase-contrast MRA can be obtained in a matter of seconds, whereas 3D phase-contrast MRA more typically is acquired over several minutes.[13]

Phase-contrast MRA is sensitive to velocities over a range that is determined by the ratio of velocity to the user-selected velocity-encoding sensitivity (VENC). Ideally, a VENC is chosen that is slightly

MR angiography of the head and neck: basic principles and clinical applications

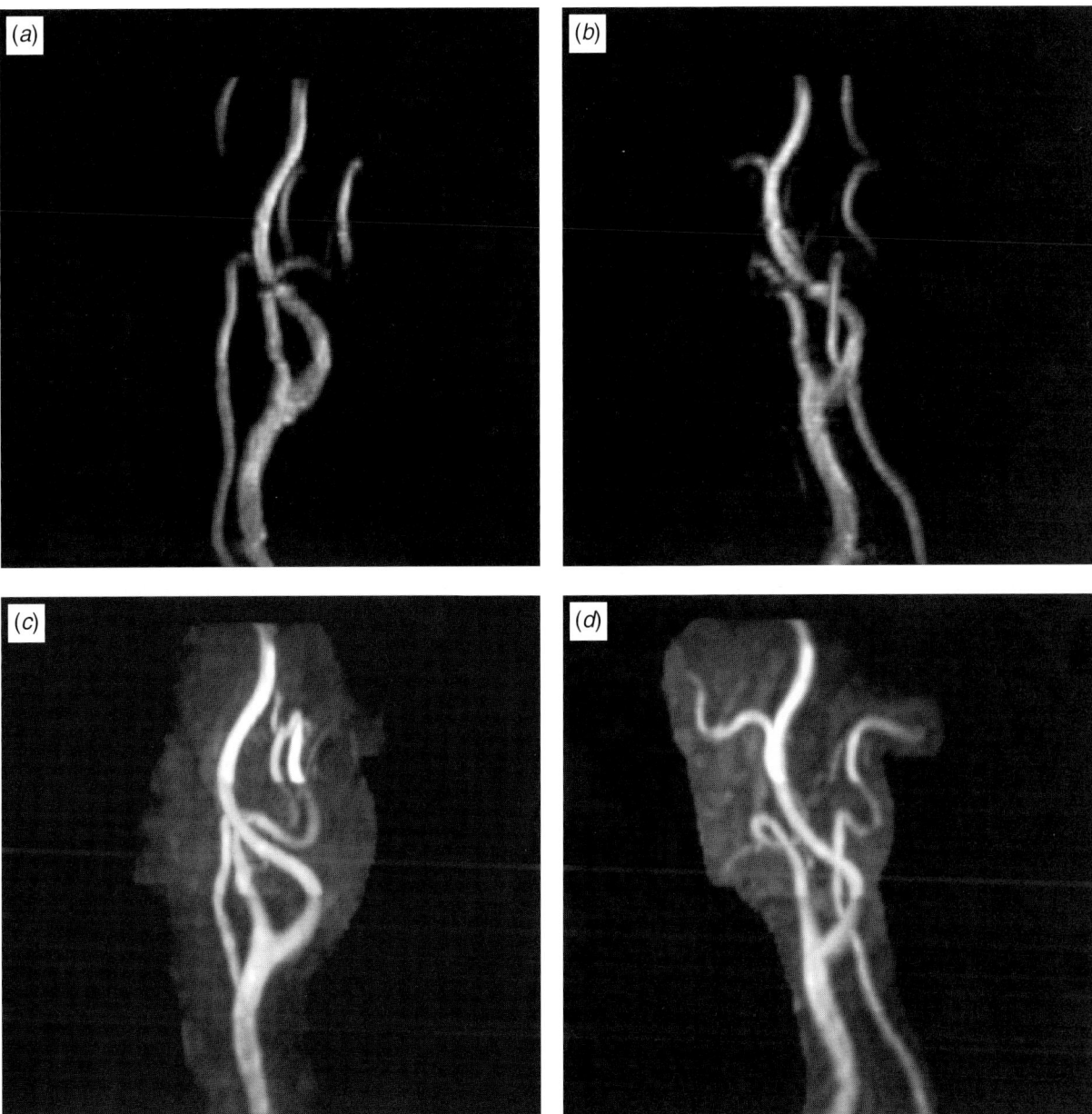

Fig. 7.1. Two-dimensional TOF v. MOTSA. (*a*), (*b*) Two-dimensional TOF MRA: targeted MIP projection of the left carotid and vertebral artery shows loss of normal signal of the left internal carotid artery several centimetres distal to the bifurcation. Similar loss of signal in the adjacent left external carotid artery favours swallowing artefact rather stenoses. (*c*), (*d*) MOTSA: targeted MIP projection of the left carotid bifurcation and verterbral artery confirms the presence of a swallowing artefact with normal appearance of both internal and external carotid arteries.

larger than the peak velocity. For instance, a VENC of 1 m/s might be chosen for an MRA of the abdominal aorta, whereas a VENC of 10 cm/s might be chosen for imaging of the intracerebral veins. If the VENC is too small, then the phase-contrast MRA will alias – blood flowing at high velocities will falsely appear to flow at lower velocities, or the signals may be lost due to dephasing. Conversely, if the VENC is too large, then the signal-to-noise ratio is diminished for the blood vessels.

There are several helpful clinical applications of phase-contrast MRA in the head and neck. Two-dimensional phase contrast can be used as a scout sequence for the carotid arteries, for rapid assessment of dural sinus patency and for the evaluation of collateral flow patterns. Three-dimensional phase-contrast MRA provides a lengthier but more complete depiction of the intracranial veins[14]. Phase-contrast MRA is effective even after the administration of a paramagnetic contrast agent; in fact, the vascular signal-to-noise ratio will benefit.

Contrast-enhanced MRA

Time-of-flight images can suffer from artefacts in the presence of slow flow or turbulence. The desire to eliminate such artefacts prompted the development of contrast-enhanced 3D techniques, which lessen the sensitivity to turbulence and slow flow.[15,16]

Paramagnetic contrast agents boost the signal intensity from blood by greatly shortening its T_1 relaxation time. For instance, during the first pass of a typical dose of gadolinium chelate (e.g. 0.1 mmol/kg or around 10–20 cc for an average-sized adult), the T_1 relaxation time of blood may be shortened by a factor of 10 or more. As a consequence, one can use a very short repetition time (TR, e.g. 5 ms) in order to acquire entire 3D data sets in much shorter times (e.g. 10–20 seconds) than with time-of-flight or phase contrast.

The benefits of using a contrast agent can be substantial. For instance, contrast-enhanced 3D MRA (CE 3DMRA) never suffers from saturation artefact, since the vessels appear bright by virtue of the effects of the contrast agent alone. Because the TE is so short (e.g. <2ms), CE 3DMRA is insensitive to signal loss from turbulent flow, an effect that artefactually enlarges stenoses in time-of-flight and phase-contrast MRA. The scan time is typically an order of magnitude shorter than with 3D time-of-flight and phase-contrast.

There are also drawbacks to the use of contrast agents. The need for a very short TR and TE may limit spatial resolution, so that the accuracy of measuring stenoses may be degraded. For instance, one typically needs at least 3 pixels to span a vessel in order to measure the diameter accurately. With current gradient technology, typical in-plane resolution for CE 3DMRA is of the order of 1 mm, which could not be adequate to measure a 2 mm stenosis of the internal carotid artery. Enhancement of background tissues can make it difficult to process the images into a MIP. This is particularly a problem for imaging of the carotid siphon due to rapid enhancement of the cavernous sinus, and as a result time of flight remains the preferred technique for MRA of the Circle of Willis. Another drawback is the cost of the contrast agent. However, the combination of shorter scan time allowing for higher patient throughput, the improved reliability and field of view as compared with time-of-flight, and better image quality may balance concerns about the additional cost.

Contrast agent dosage and timing

The typical dose of gadolinium chelate for extracranial carotid and vertebral studies is on the order of 0.1 mmol/kg delivered intravenously at a rate of approximately 2 cc/s, followed by 10 cc of saline administered at the same rate. The matrix and slice thickness should be selected such that the voxel dimensions are of the order of 1 mm or less. It is critical to time the start of the 3D data acquisition so that it is coincident with the arrival and filling of the target vessel with contrast medium. Several approaches have been used for this purpose. One can administer a 1–2 cc test bolus and image with a fast 2D sequence in order to time the arrival of contrast medium.[17] One can place a 'tracker' region within the vessel of interest and automatically detect the arrival of the contrast bolus.[18] A foolproof timing approach is to image with a rapid, fluoroscopic 2D acquisition and then trigger the 3D acquisition when the contrast medium is seen to arrive in the target vessel.

Technical considerations

The optimal technique used for CE 3DMRA depends on the particular hardware and software configurations of the MR system. For instance, MR systems with the newest gradient hardware can achieve TRs of the order of 4 ms or less, so that first-pass, high resolution studies of the extracranial carotid arteries can be acquired in the 15 s or less needed to avoid jugular venous enhancement. With further shortening of TR and a modest reduction in the number of phase-encodes, one can acquire multiphase MRA with a time resolution of 10 s or better, thereby eliminating the need to get the timing of the contrast bolus exactly right.[19] However, such rapid imaging may come at the expense of spatial resolution, which is needed for accurate measurement of carotid stenoses.[20] Moreover, older MR systems cannot provide such short TRs, in which case a different approach called 'elliptico-centric phase-encoding'[21] is helpful.

The concept underlying elliptico-centric phase-encoding is that the order in which the phase-encode gradients are played out will alter the appearance of the image in fundamental ways. Data acquired during the play-out of the weakest phase-encoding gradients (centre of k-space) determine the overall image contrast, whereas data acquired during the play-out of the stronger phase-encoding gradients (outer portions of k-space) determine spatial resolution. In a 3D sequence, two orthogonal phase-encoding gradients are played out (vs. one phase-encode gradient for a 2D sequence). If the two phase-encode gradients are played out in the usual linear order, then the image contrast is similar throughout the period of data acquisition. In the elliptico-centric scheme, the weakest phase-encodes are played out for both phase-encode directions at the start of the data acquisition, so that this early data determines the eventual tissue contrast of the MRA. For instance, if these early data are acquired during the first pass of contrast agent through the extracranial carotid arteries prior to enhancement of the jugular veins, then the jugular veins will not be visible in the MRA (Fig. 7.2). This is true even if the data acquisition is extended over a minute or longer. Thus, the benefit of elliptico-centric phase-encoding is that one can differentiate the arteries from veins even though one has a slower gradient system and must use a lengthier data acquisition. The longer data acquisition provides the opportunity to collect more data and therefore to obtain higher spatial resolution than would be possible during a first-pass study.

Comparison of time-of-flight and CE 3DMRA

Although the benefits of contrast enhancement are well recognized, published data do not yet fully support the replacement of time-of-flight techniques for carotid MRA. There are certain circumstances where CE 3DMRA is clearly advantageous (Fig. 7.3). For instance, because data can be acquired in a coronal or sagittal orientation spanning a large field of view, the method is preferred for studies that need to detect tandem stenoses involving the origin or siphon of the carotid artery. This is advantageously done in conjunction with a head and neck phased array coil, which spans the region from the aortic arch through the circle of Willis. The CE 3DMRA method is also preferred for patients with tortuous vessels, as well as for patients who might not hold still for the 5–10 minutes required for 3D time-of-flight MRA. Turbulence causes exaggeration of stenosis with time of flight or phase contrast methods, but is much less an issue with CE 3DMRA. On the other hand, the nominal spatial resolution for time-of-flight MRA is usually better than with CE 3DMRA, which in some circumstances improves the specificity of the stenosis measurement.

Clinical applications

Extracranial carotid and vertebral arteries

Stenotic disease

In 1991 the NASCET study showed that carotid endarterectomy gave superior outcomes to medical therapy for symptomatic patients with significant extracranial carotid stenosis.[22] A more recent study indicated that even asymptomatic patients may benefit from surgical therapy.[23] Although X-ray angiography was the gold standard for the NASCET study, it involves a small stroke risk of the order of 0.5–4%.[24] Consequently, there is a strong need for an accurate non-invasive test for extracranial carotid disease.

In a blinded study involving 176 carotid arteries, 3D TOF MRA had a sensitivity of 94%, a specificity of 85% and an accuracy of 88% for the identification of 70% to 99% stenosis; two-dimensional TOF MRA

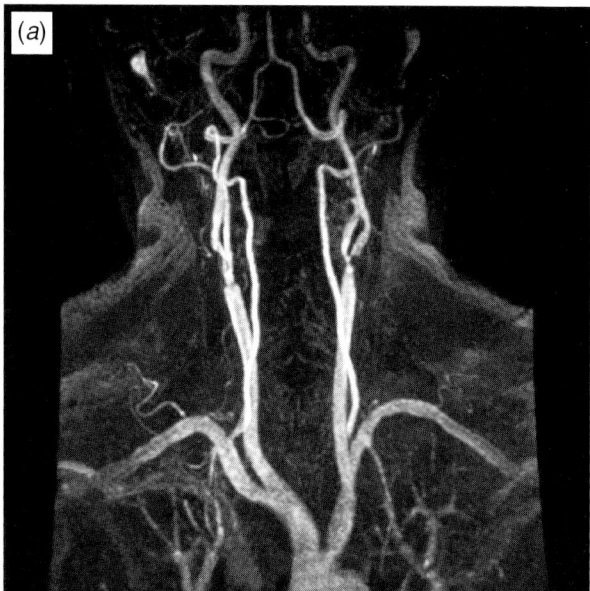
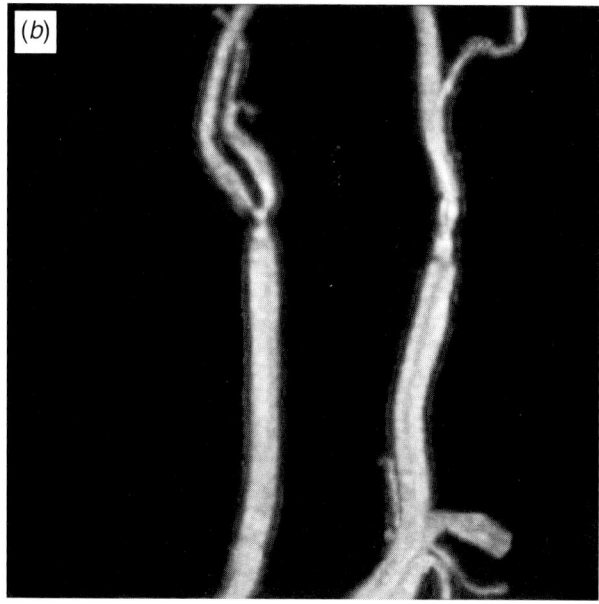
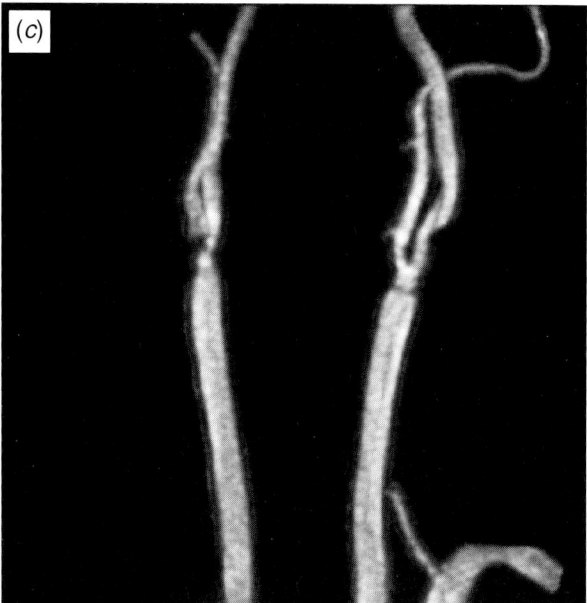

Fig. 7.2. Gadolinum-enhanced MRA with elliptic centric encoding: carotid stenosis. (*a*), (*b*), (*c*) AP view and multiple oblique projections show bilateral stenoses of the carotid arteries. On the left, there is high grade stenosis of the common and left internal carotid arteries. On the right, there is moderate stenosis of the common carotid artery bifurcation extending to involve the right internal carotid artery. Note the excellent visualization of the origins of the great vessels and the vertebral arteries.

had a sensitivity and specificity that were approximately 10% lower than those of three-dimensional TOF MRA.[25] Duplex sonography had a sensitivity of 94%, a specificity of 83%, and an accuracy of 86%. Combining data from three-dimensional TOF MRA and DU, allowing for CA only for disparate results, yielded a sensitivity of 100%, a specificity of 91%, and accuracy of 94% among concordant non-invasive tests, with CA required in 16% of arteries. The authors concluded that the combination of MRA and DUS can replace X-ray angiography in the majority of patients (Figs. 7.4, 7.5). The use of CE 3DMRA can eliminate the artefacts associated with time of flight MRA and also permit a much larger field of view that encompasses the carotid origins and siphons.[26] A recent study comparing CE 3DMRA, CTA, and digital subtraction angiography found that both MRA and CTA accurately depicted extracranial carotid stenoses, although the superior spatial resolution afforded by CTA made it easier to

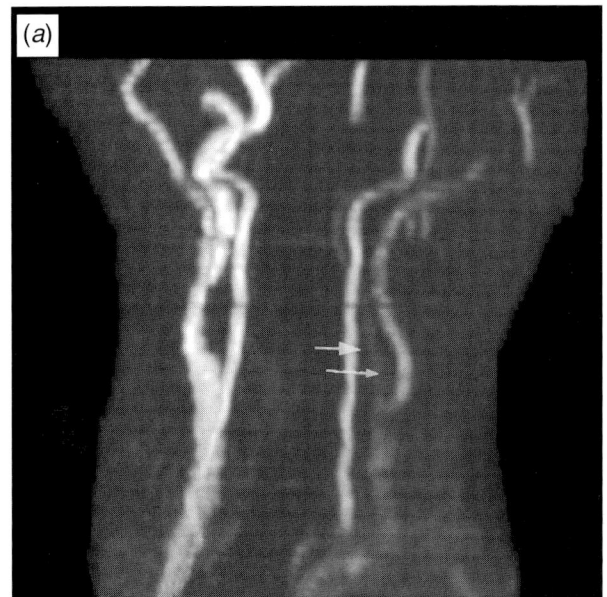
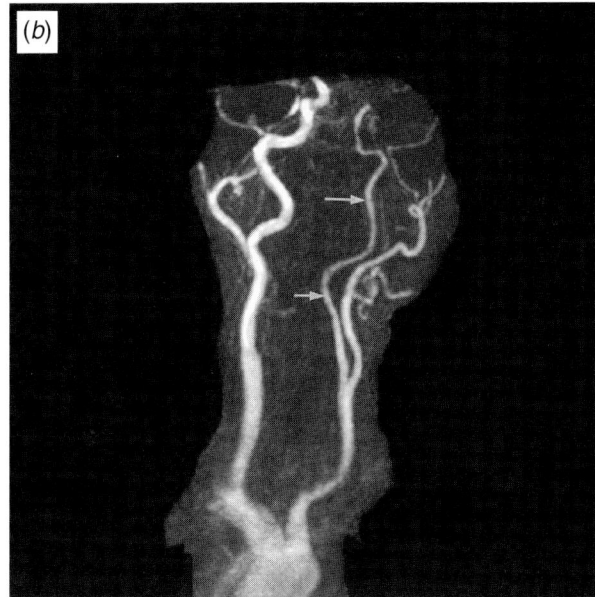
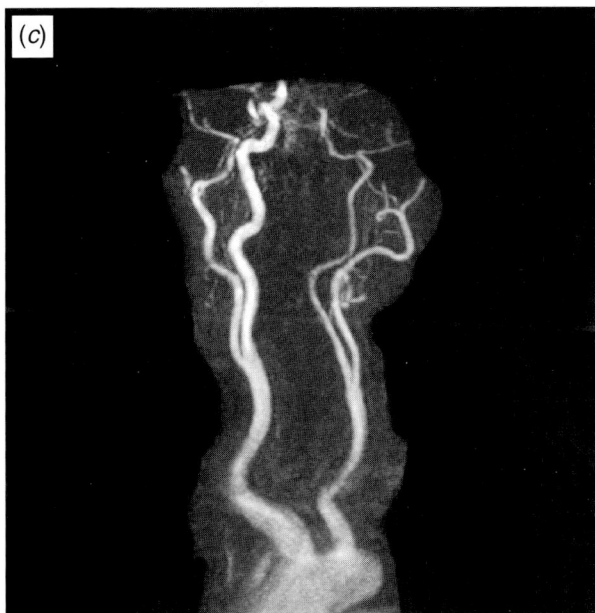

Fig. 7.3. Two-dimensional TOF vs. enhanced MRA: string sign. (a) Two-dimensional TOF demonstrates diminished flow within the left internal carotid artery (arrows). Note the decreased signal intensity of the left ICA vs. the right ICA. (b), (c) Enhanced MRA better demonstrates the abnormal left internal carotid through the level of the skull base (arrows). Note the irregular areas of narrowing involving the left pre-cavernous and cavernous internal carotid arteries.

detect ulcerations.[27] With ongoing improvements in spatial resolution, the performance of CE 3DMRA appears to match that of DSA.[28]

Flow measurement

By using 2D phase contrast angiography, particularly with cardiac-gated cine to depict flow over the entire cardiac cycle, one can measure flow velocities and flow rates in the extracranial carotid arteries as well as in other vessels. This method can be used in patients with extracranial carotid stenosis.[29,30] as well as lesions of the Circle of Willis.

Plaque

Magnetic resonance can be used not only to image the lumen of the vessel but the wall as well using dark blood imaging methods. MRI is highly accurate at measuring the carotid wall area[31] and T_2-weighted images can discriminate between the fibrous cap and lipid core of a plaque.[32]

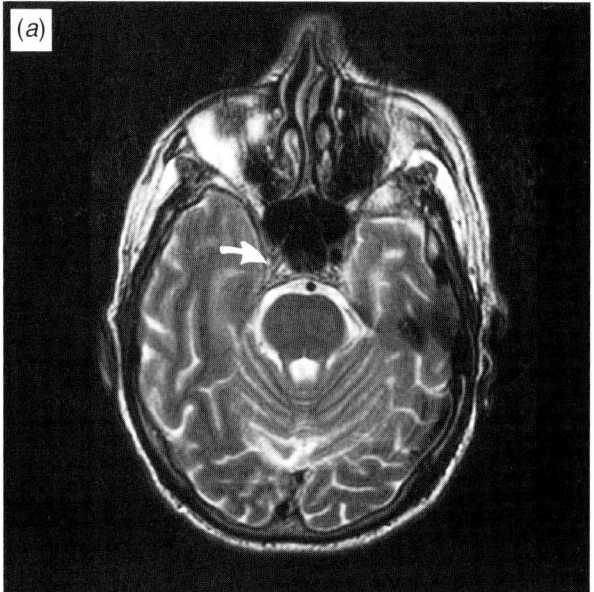
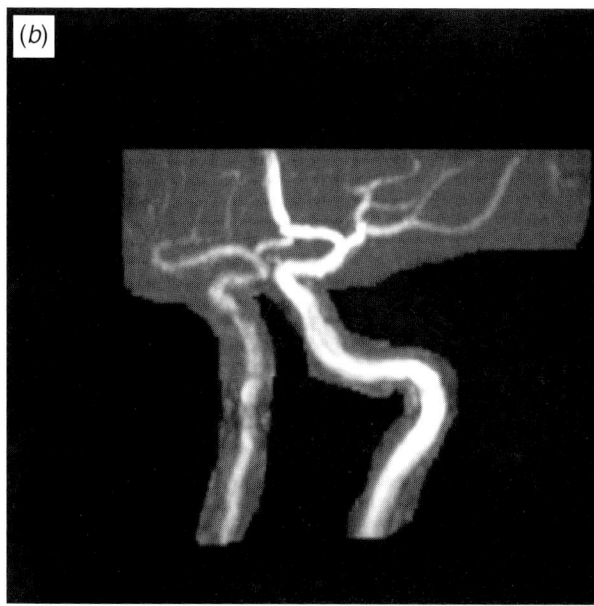
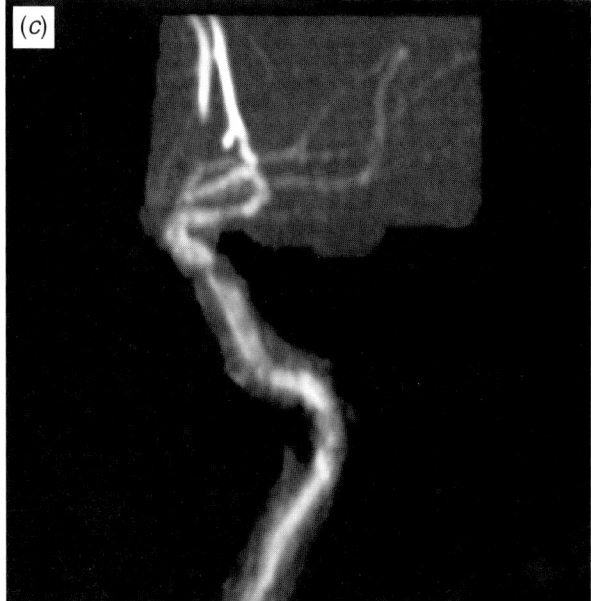

Fig. 7.4. Intracranial stenosis: right internal carotid artery. (*a*) Axial T_2-weighted MR shows absence of the normal flow void within the right internal carotid artery (curved arrow). (*b*) MIP projection of the anterior circulation demonstrates decreased signal intensity of the right internal carotid relative to the left internal carotid artery. (*c*) Targeted MIP of the right internal carotid artery confirms a high grade stenosis of the cavernous right internal carotid artery.

Dissection

Dissections of the extracranial portions of the carotid and vertebral arteries can be traumatic or spontaneous in origin. The combination of MRI and MRA is an accurate non-invasive means for the detection of carotid and vertebral dissections (Fig. 7.6).[33–37] Typically, MRI reveals a crescentic intramural hyperintensity on both T_1- and T_2-weighted images. MRA may reveal a smoothly tapered vessel or intimal flap, mural hematoma, and luminal irregularity similar to that demonstrated by X-ray angiography. One can also use MRA to serially follow the response to antiplatelet or anticoagulant therapy.[38] Most studies of MRA for carotid and vertebral dissection have relied on time of flight or phase contrast techniques. Consequently, patient motion, turbulence, or slow flow can cause an

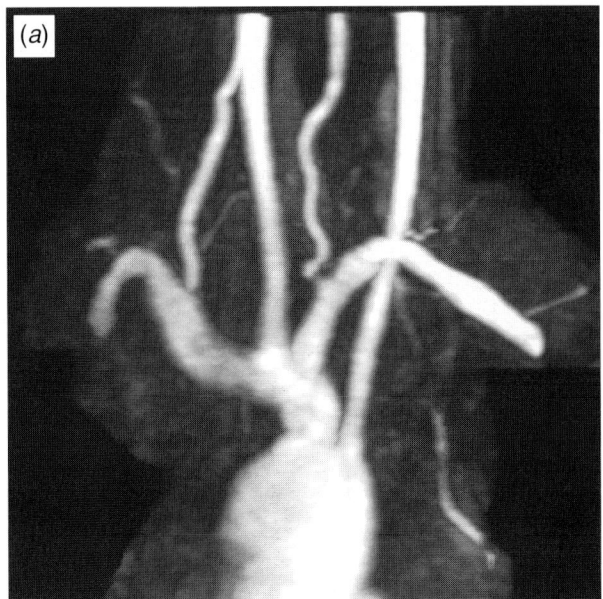
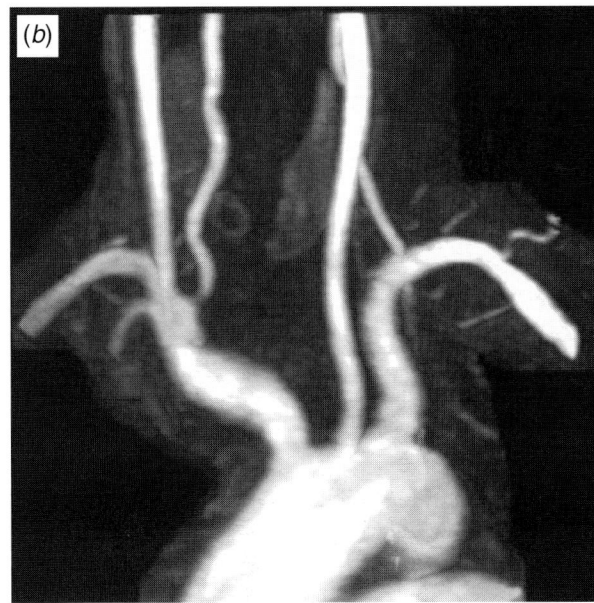
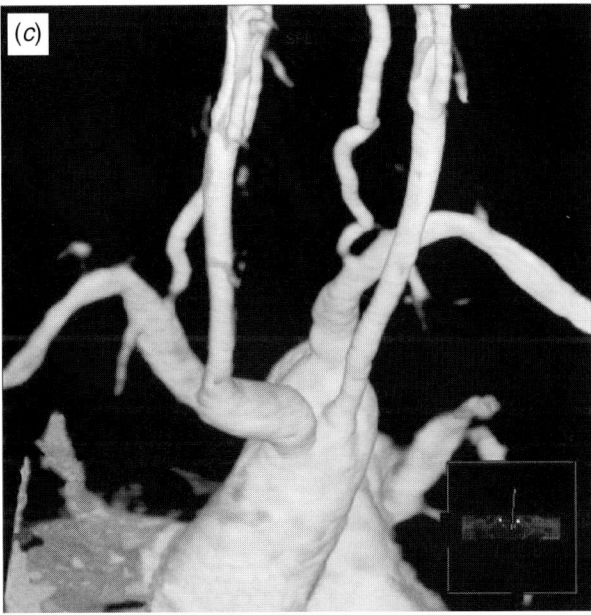

Fig. 7.5. Vertebral artery origin stenosis. (*a*), (*b*), (*c*) Enhanced MRA of the aortic arch and great vessels shows excellent visualisation of the vertebral artery origins with stenoses bilaterally. Volume rendered oblique projection better demonstrates the proximal vertebral lesions.

incomplete or erroneous interpretation. Given their smaller size and greater tortuousity, the accuracy is less for vertebral than carotid dissections. It is likely that CE 3DMRA will give more reliable results, but this is not yet verified in the published literature.

Circle of Willis

Stenotic disease

The incidence of intracranial arterial stenosis varies among ethnic groups. Whites tend to be afflicted more with extracranial carotid stenosis, whereas the intracranial circulation is affected more commonly in blacks, Hispanics, Japanese, and Chinese.[39] In setting of acute stroke, information about the status of the intracranial arteries is critical to determination of stroke subtype and associated prognosis, and helps to determine the choice to employ thrombolytic therapy.[40] Transcranial doppler, MRA,[41–43] and CTA are non-invasive approaches for evaluating intracranial

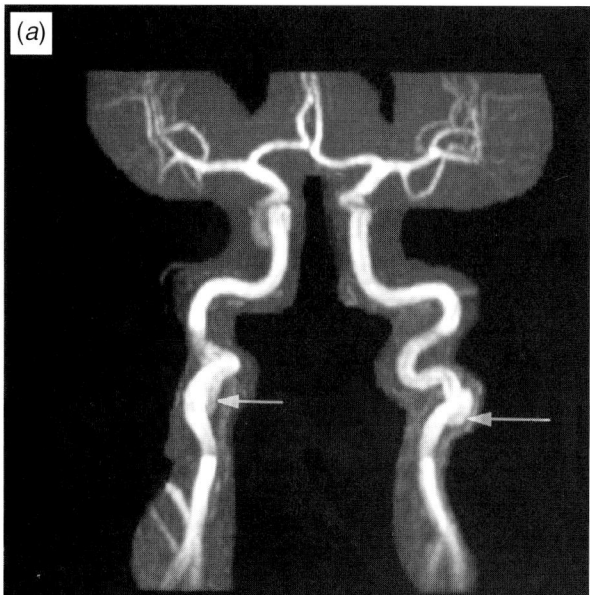
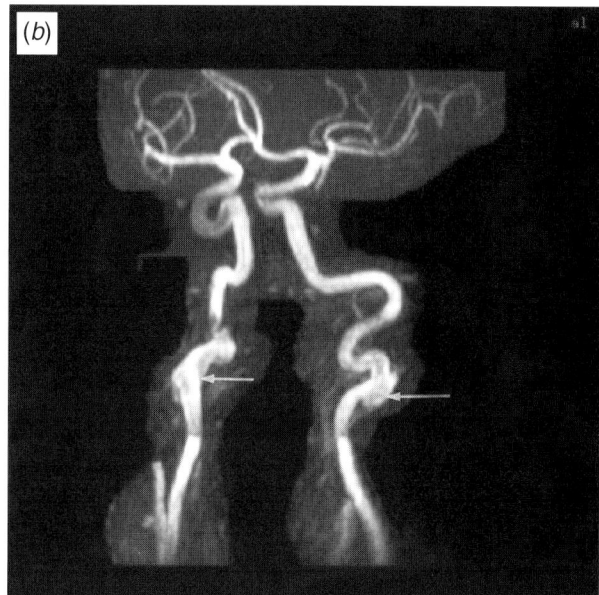
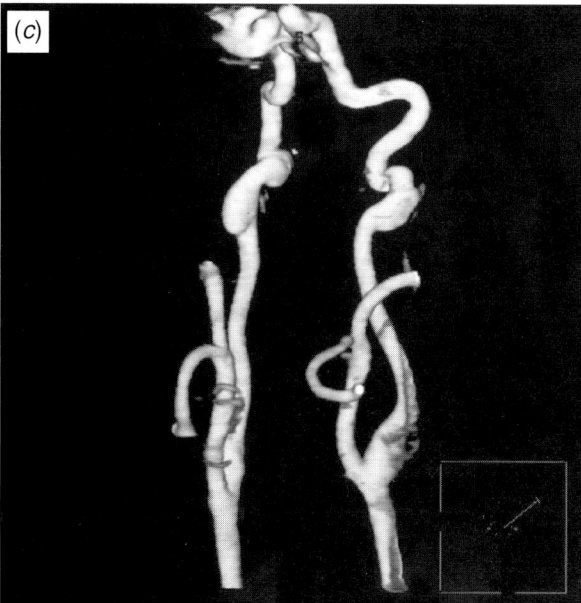

Fig. 7.6. Gadolinium-enhanced MRA with elliptic centric encoding: carotid dissection – bilateral pseudoaneurysms. (*a*), (*b*), (*c*) Oblique MIP projections demonstrate dilation of the cervical internal carotid arteries bilaterally consistent with pseudoaneurysms associated with bilateral carotid dissections (arrows). Volume rendered projections more clearly document the bilateral carotid pseudoaneurysms.

disease. Transcranial doppler is inexpensive and available at the bedside, but in some cases there is not an adequate temporal window. In one study, a total of 50 middle cerebral arteries in 25 patients with a history of ischemic stroke were studied with MRA and CTA.[44] Inter- and intraobserver variability was good and comparable to that achieved with duplex sonography for extracranial carotid stenosis, although MRA proved more reliable than CTA.

In another study, imaging with DWI and MRA within 24 hours of hospitalization substantially improved the accuracy of early ischemic stroke subtype diagnosis.[45] While useful for evaluation of the Circle of Willis,[46] time of flight MRA also has limitations. Whereas spatial resolution is adequate for the primary branches of the Circle of Willis, it is less so in the more distal, smaller branches and the level of diagnostic confidence diminishes.

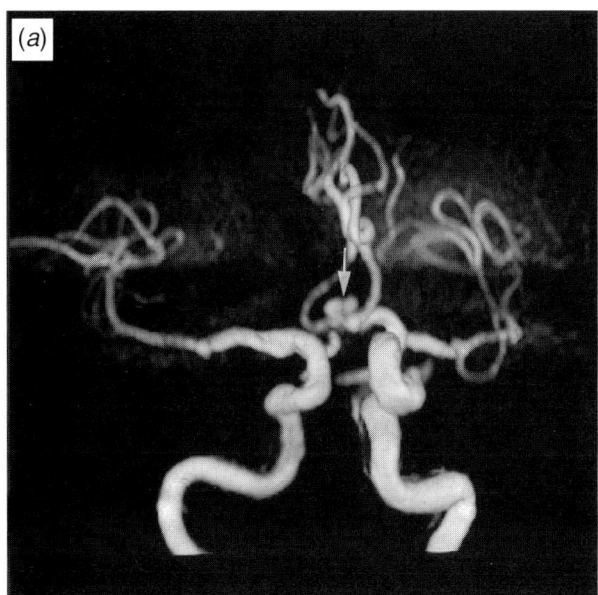 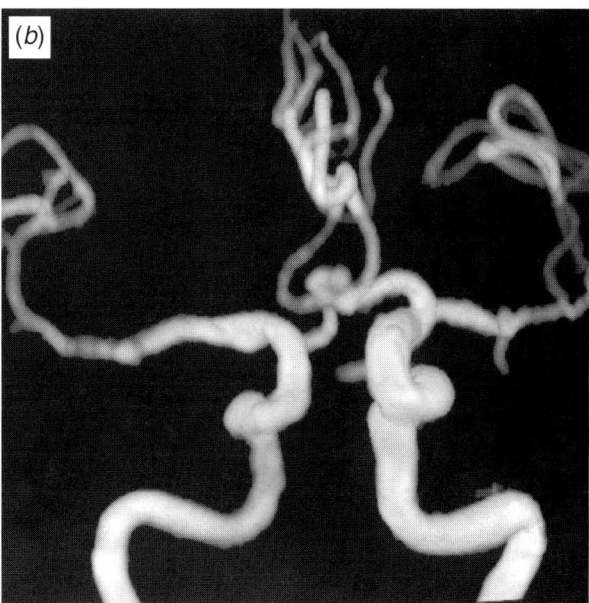

Fig. 7.7. Unruptured anterior communicating artery aneurysm. (*a*), (*b*) 73-year-old male with headache. MIP of the TOF MRA anterior circulation shows bilobed aneurysm of the anterior communicating complex. Note the hypoplastic right A1 segment. Volume rendering provides better appreciation of the relationship of the aneurysm to the anterior cerebral artery origins.

Collateral flow and function

Collateral flow patterns are readily shown by selective application of presaturation pulses over feeding vessels[47] or by phase contrast MRA. Phase contrast MRA has been applied to demonstrate collateral flow patterns in patients with internal carotid artery obstructions.[48,49] In patients with moyamoya, a progressive cerebrovascular occlusive disorder of unknown etiology, the diagnostic accuracy of MRA has been reported to be excellent, close to that of X-ray angiography.[50,51] Moreover, MRA can be used to assess vascular anatomy and hemodynamic response after surgical intervention.[52] MRA has also been used in conjunction with acetazolamide challenge to assess the vasoreactivity of the intracranial vessels for normal and stenotic vessels[53] and to show age-related decreases in cerebral blood flow.[54]

Aneurysm

Both MRA[55,56] and CTA have been reported to be accurate tests for intracranial aneurysms (Fig. 7.7), although the sensitivity diminishes greatly for smaller lesions. Despite an accuracy of the order of 90%, the reported sensitivities have ranged from 0.67 to nearly 1.[57–61] A prospective study involving 142 patients demonstrated an accuracy per patient of 0.87 at CTA and 0.85 at MRA.[62] The accuracy per aneurysm for the best observer was 0.73 at CTA and 0.67 at MRA. Interobserver agreement was good; however, the sensitivity for detection of aneurysms smaller than 5 mm was 0.57 for CTA and 0.35 for MRA compared with 0.94 and 0.86, respectively, for detection of aneurysms 5 mm or larger. The accuracy of both CTA and MRA was lower for detection of internal carotid artery aneurysms compared with that at other sites. Thus, MRA is not a complete replacement for X-ray angiography. The accuracy of MRA might be sufficient to screen patients who are at risk for intracranial aneurysms.[63] The cost–benefit of screening MRA is controversial. One study of screening MRA found aneurysms in 25 of 626 first-degree relatives of patients with history of subarachnoid bleed from ruptured intracranial aneurysms.[64] The authors state that 'Implementation of a screening program for the

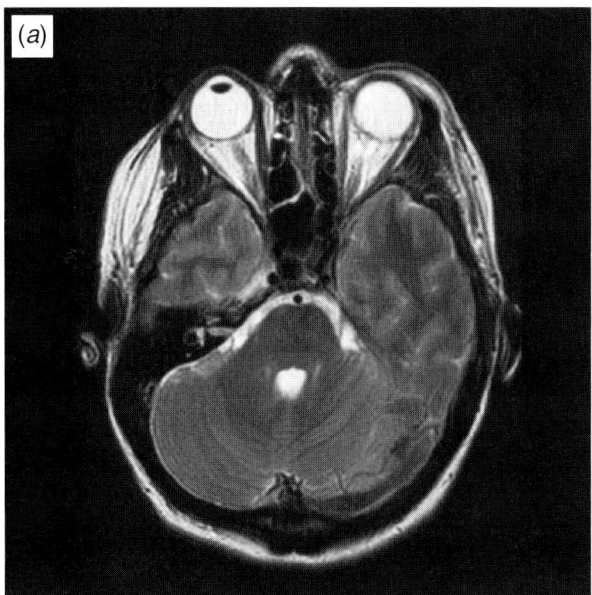
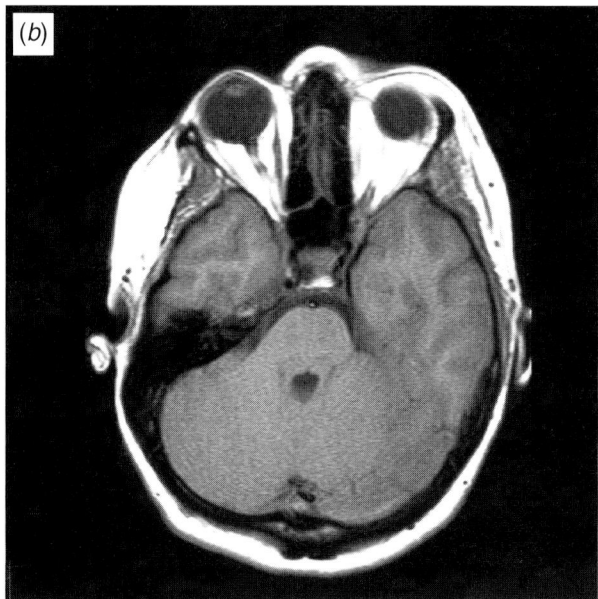
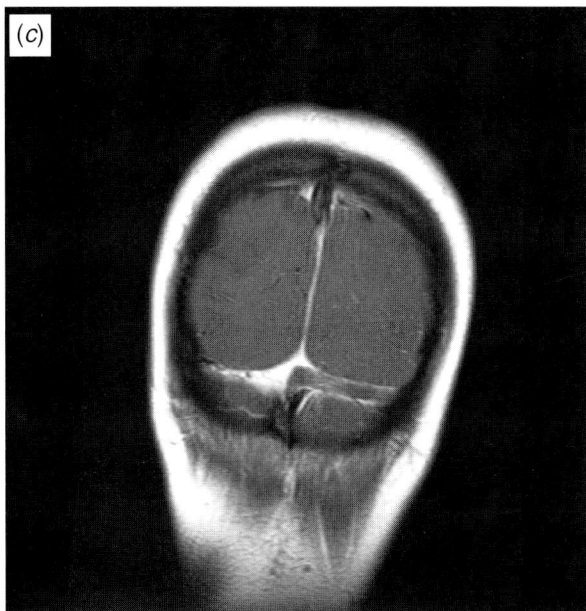

Fig. 7.8. MR venography 2D TOF: venous thrombosis. (*a*), (*b*), (*c*), (*d*), (*e*) Axial T_2-MR (*a*) imaging of the posterior fossa demonstrates low signal intensity involving the left transverse sinus mimicking a normal flow void. Axial T_1-weighted MR (*b*) of the transverse sinus show subtle increased signal that suggests recent sinus thrombosis. T_1-images with gadolinium (*c*), (*d*) document a large filling defect involving the left transverse sinus as well as collateral circulation along the left tentorium cerebellum. Two-dimensional TOF MR venography (*e*) shows no flow within the transverse sinuses bilaterally with collateral circulation noted on the right.

first-degree relatives of patients with sporadic subarachnoid hemorrhage does not seem warranted at this time, since the resulting slight increase in life expectancy does not offset the risk of postoperative sequelae.' Other studies favour the use of MRA.[65]

Vascular malformation

MRI depicts the nidus of a vascular malformation, whereas MRA depicts the feeding arteries and draining veins.[66–68] However, image quality is not sufficient to obviate the need for selective X-ray angiography prior to intervention. Contrast-enhanced 3D MRA should provide more complete evaluation. One study using real-time monitored auto-triggered elliptic centric-ordered MRA found it to be superior to TOF MRA for evaluation of intracranial AVMs, resulting in improved depiction of the components of an AVM, in particular the nidus and draining veins.[69] When compared with DSA, the authors reported that CE 3DMRA consis-

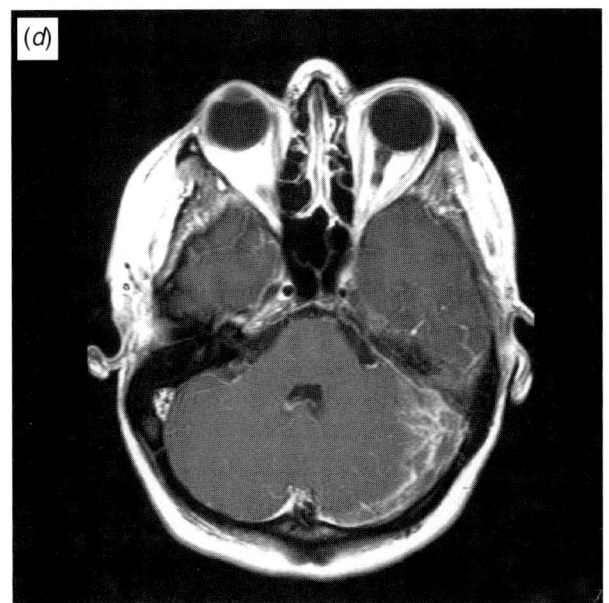 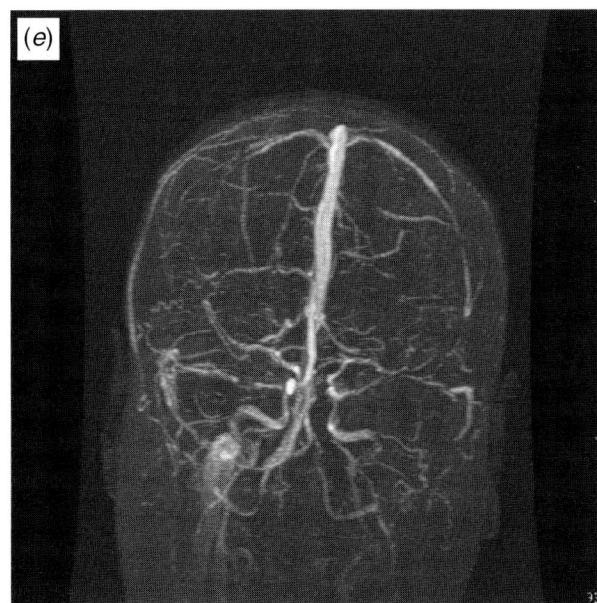

tently depicted AVM components and their orientation.

Intracranial veins

Patency of the dural sinuses and cerebral veins can be well assessed by any of several techniques, including 2D time of flight,[70] 3D phase contrast,[71–74] as well as CE 3D MRA (Fig. 7.8). The combination of MRI and MRA is ideal as it provides information about vessel patency as well as the signal characteristics and thus age of thrombus.[75]

Works in progress

Spiral imaging

Although spoiled gradient-echo pulse sequences such as FLASH (fast low angle shot) and MPSPGR (multiplanar spoiled gradient-echo) predominate for time of flight and CE 3D MRA, other pulse sequences may be helpful. For instance, spiral imaging is a method whereby two orthogonal gradients are oscillated to collect a series of echoes. The method is insensitive to flow-related dephasing so that vessels appear bright. However, excellent shimming of the main magnetic field is required to avoid blurring from off-resonance effects, which may be particularly difficult to achieve for neck applications.

Balanced steady-state free precession

Although available for many years, balanced steady-state free precession (SSFP) techniques have only come into their own with the availability of faster gradients and shorter TR/TE. Examples of SSFP include true FISP[76] and FIESTA. SSFP images show a contrast dependence on the T_2/T_1 ratio. Because of its long T_2 relaxation time, blood naturally appears bright with SSFP imaging. The technique enables the use of very short TR so that imaging is extremely rapid. Although SSFP acquisitions are relatively insensitive to the T_1 shortening effect of a contrast agent, one can sensitize the acquisition by means of an inversion prepulse for CE MRA. Drawbacks of SSFP include artefacts from off-resonance effects (improved through the use of very short TR) and the fact that other tissues, such as cerebrospinal fluid and fat, also appear bright.

Variants in K-space sampling

Since not all portions of k-space are equal with respect to tissue contrast, there are potential benefits to sampling the various portions of k-space at differing rates. This approach enables more rapid imaging during the first pass of a contrast agent. For instance, one might collect the outer portions of k-space less frequently than the central portions since the amplitudes of the latter are relatively insensitive to the effects of the contrast bolus and remain fairly constant. Examples of this approach include 'keyhole'[77] and 'TRICKS'.[78] By sampling the outer portions of k-space less frequently than usual, the scan time is substantially shortened providing the opportunity for rapid, multiphase imaging while maintaining spatial resolution.

Parallel imaging
The time and spatial resolution of neurovascular MRA studies can be greatly improved by the use of parallel imaging techniques.[79–81] Sample commercial nomenclature for parallel imaging methods includes 'SMASH', 'SENSE', and 'ASSET'. The basic idea of parallel imaging is that the individual elements of the phased array coil used to detect the MR signal have a sensitivity for the signal that depends on distance and orientation from the coil element. With the use of appropriate mathematical algorithms, this property can be used to extract phase-encode information in parallel to the phase-encode information acquired through the application of the magnetic field gradient. The net effect is that the scan time can be reduced by a factor up to the number of coil elements, or the spatial resolution can be improved by this factor. In practice, accelerations of 2–4 have been shown, and in principle much higher acceleration factors are feasible by the use of appropriately designed phased array coils. With the availability of parallel imaging, which is just beginning to come into clinical practice, the only real limit on speed and spatial resolution for MRA is the available signal-to-noise ratio, which will depend on magnetic field strength, contrast agent dosage and rate of infusion, as well as radiofrequency coil and patient-related factors.

Conclusions

In a relatively short period of time, MRA has come to occupy a valuable place in the diagnostic toolbox for neurovascular disorders. The technology is not entirely mature insofar as the pulse sequences and gradient hardware continue to improve. For instance, steady-state free precession and parallel imaging methods have not yet been extensively evaluated for neurovascular applications, but no doubt will improve the accuracy and speed of diagnosis. It is now generally accepted that MRA can replace X-ray angiography for the presurgical evaluation of the carotid endarterectomy candidate. There remain circumstances where X-ray angiography is still needed, such as in a patient who has a pacemaker or a potentially ferromagnetic intracranial aneurysm clip (MRI contraindicated), as well as in those patients who are unable to remain still long enough to acquire an artefact-free MRA study. X-ray angiography may be indicated as the arbitrating examination for the patient in whom the duplex sonogram and MRA yield strikingly divergent results. In addition to X-ray angiography, contrast-enhanced CTA using fast, multislice scanners can provide accurate depiction of the extra- and intracranial carotid arteries, and is advocated by some as a more reliable test than MRA. However, CT is relatively contraindicated in someone with significantly impaired renal function or allergy to iodinated contrast medium.

For the intracranial circulation, MRA is well accepted for imaging of the dural sinuses and larger intracranial veins, e.g. for the diagnosis of dural sinus thrombosis. Using phase contrast MRA one can easily depict patterns of collateral flow. Stenoses involving the proximal branches of the circle of Willis are well shown, although the accuracy declines as one attempts to image smaller, more distal vessels. MRA is reliable for detecting stenoses and occlusions involving the vertebrobasilar system, although the specificity will depend on the level of spatial resolution (as is also the case for the extracranial carotid arteries). Although MRI is invaluable for detecting vascular malformations and MRA can depict major feeding arteries and draining veins, it has not eliminated the need for X-ray angiography prior to embolization or surgical therapy.

We see that MRA has already had a major clinical impact despite the relative immaturity of the technology. No doubt the breadth and depth of clinical applicability will continue to expand as the technology moves forward.

REFERENCES

1. Wedeen VJ, Meuli RA, Edelman RR et al. Projective imaging of pulsatile flow with magnetic resonance. *Science* 1985; 230: 946–948.
2. Yucel EK, Anderson CM, Edelman RR et al. Magnetic resonance angiography: update on applications for extracranial arteries. *Circulation* 1999; 100: 2284.
3. Keller P. Time of flight magnetic resonance angiography. *Neuroimaging Clin N Am* 1992; 4: 639–656.
4. Felmlee JP, Ehman RL. Spatial presaturation: a method for suppressing flow artefacts and improving depiction of vascular anatomy in MR imaging. *Radiology* 1987; 164: 559–564.
5. Edelman RR, Chien D, Kim D. Fast selective black blood MR imaging. *Radiology* 1991; 181: 655–660.
6. Simonetti OP, Finn JP, White RD, Laub G, Henry DA. 'Black blood' T_2-weighted inversion-recovery MR imaging of the heart. *Radiology* 1996; 199: 49–57.
7. Demarco JK, Rutt BK, Clarke SE. Carotid plaque characterization by magnetic resonance imaging: review of the literature. *Top Magn Reson Imaging* 2001; 12: 205–217.
8. Edelman RR, Mattle HP, Wallner B et al. Extracranial carotid arteries: evaluation with 'black blood' MR angiography. *Radiology* 1990; 177: 45–50.
9. Laub G. Displays for MR angiography. *Magn Reson Med* 1990; 14: 222–229.
10. Blatter DD, Parker DL, Ahn SS et al. Cerebral MR angiography with multiple overlapping thin slab acquisition. *Radiology* 1992; 183: 379–389.
11. Dumoulin CL. Phase contrast MR angiography techniques. *Magn Reson Imaging Clin N Am* 1995; 3: 399–411.
12. Walker MF, Souza SP, Dumoulin CL. Quantitative flow measurement in phase contrast MR angiography. *J Comput Assist Tomogr* 1988; 12: 304–313.
13. Pernicone JR, Siebert JE, Potchen EJ, Pera A, Dumoulin CL, Souza SP. Three-dimensional phase-contrast MR angiography in the head and neck. *Am J Neuroradiol* 1990; 155: 457–466.
14. Tsuruda JS, Shimakawa A, Pelc NJ, Saloner D. Dural sinus occlusion: evaluation with phase-sensitive gradient-echo MR imaging. *Am J Neuroradiol* 1991; 12: 481–488.
15. Prince MR. Gadolinium-enhanced MR aortography. *Radiology* 1994; 191: 155–164.
16. Cloft HJ, Murphy KJ, Prince MR, Brunberg JA. 3D gadolinium-enhanced MR angiography of the carotid arteries. *Magn Reson Imaging* 1996; 14: 593–600.
17. Kim JK, Farb RI, Wright GA. Test bolus examination in the carotid artery at dynamic gadolinium-enhanced MR angiography. *Radiology* 1998; 206: 283–289.
18. Foo TKF, Saranathan M, Prince MR, Chenevert TL. Automated detection of bolus arrival and initiation of data acquisition in fast, three dimensional, gadolinium-enhanced MR angiography. *Radiology* 1997; 203: 275–280.
19. Levy RA, Makin JH. Three-dimensional contrast-enhanced MR angiography of the extracranial carotid arteries: two techniques. *Am J Neuroradiol* 1998; 19: 688–690.
20. Serfaty JM, Chirossel P, Chevallier JM. Accuracy of three-dimensional gadolinium-enhanced MR angiography in the assessment of extracranial carotid artery disease. *Am J Radiol* 2000; 175: 455–463.
21. Wilman AH, Riederer SJ. Performance of an elliptical spiral centric view order for signal enhancement and motion artefact suppression in breathhold three dimensional gradient echo imaging. *Magn Reson Med* 1997; 38: 793–802.
22. North American Symptomatic Carotid Endarterectomy Trial Collaborators. Beneficial effect of carotid endarterectomy in symptomatic patients with high-grade stenosis. *N Engl J Med* 1991; 325: 445–453.
23. Executive Committee for the Asymptomatic Carotid Atherosclerosis Study. Endarterectomy for asymptomatic carotid artery stenosis. *J Am Med Assoc* 1995; 273: 1421–1428.
24. Hankey GJ, Warlow CP, Sellar RJ. Cerebral angiographic risk in mild cerebrovascular disease. *Stroke* 1990; 21: 209–222.
25. Patel MR, Klufas RA, Kim D et al. Preoperative assessment of the carotid bifurcation: can magnetic resonance angiography and duplex ultrasonography replace contrast arteriography? *Stroke* 1995; 26: 1753–1758.
26. Remonda L, Heid O, Schroth G. Carotid artery stenosis, occlusion, and pseudo-occlusion: first-pass, gadolinium-enhanced, three-dimensional MR angiography – preliminary study. *Radiology* 1998; 209: 95–102.
27. Randoux B, Marro B, Koskas F et al. Carotid artery

stenosis: prospective comparison of CT, three-dimensional gadolinium-enhanced MR, and conventional angiography. *Radiology* 2001; 220: 179–185.
28 Huston J, Fain SB, Wald JT. Carotid artery: elliptic centric contrast-enhanced MR angiography compared with conventional angiography. *Radiology* 2001; 218: 138–143.
29 van Everdingen KJ, Klijn CJM, Kappelle LJ, Mali WPTM, van der Grond J. MRA flow quantification in patients with a symptomatic internal carotid artery occlusion. *Stroke* 1997; 28: 1595–1600.
30 Vanninen R, Koivisto K, Tulla H, Manninen H, Partanen K. Hemodynamic effects of carotid endarterectomy by magnetic resonance flow quantification. *Stroke* 1995; 26: 84–89.
31 Yuan C, Beach KW, Hillyer Smith L, Jr, Hatsukami TS. Measurement of atherosclerotic carotid plaque size in vivo using high resolution magnetic resonance imaging. *Circulation* 1998; 98: 2666–2671.
32 Toussaint JF, LaMuraglia GM, Southern JF, Fuster V, Kantor HL. Magnetic resonance images lipid, fibrous, calcified, hemorrhagic, and thrombotic components of human atherosclerosis in vivo. *Circulation* 1996; 94: 932–938.
33 Klufas RA, Hsu L, Barnes PD, Patel MR, Schwartz RB. Dissection of the carotid and vertebral arteries: imaging with MR angiography. *Am J Roentgenol* 1995; 164: 673–677.
34 Levy C, Laissy JP, Raveau V et al. Carotid and vertebral artery dissections: three-dimensional time-of-flight MR angiography and MR imaging versus conventional angiography. *Radiology* 1994; 190: 97–103.
35 Provenzale JM, Morgenlander JC, Gress D. Spontaneous vertebral dissection: clinical, conventional angiographic, CT, and MR findings. *J Comput Assist Tomogr* 1996; 20: 185–193.
36 Hoffman M, Sacco RL, Chan S, Mohr JP. Noninvasive detection of vertebral artery dissection. *Stroke* 1993; 24: 815–819.
37 Kitanaka C, Tanaka J, Kuwahara M, Teraoka A. Magnetic resonance imaging study of intracranial vertebrobasilar artery dissections. *Stroke* 1994; 25: 571–575.
38 Kasner SE, Hankins KK, Bratina P, Morgenstern LB. Magnetic resonance angiography demonstrates vascular healing of carotid and vertebral artery dissections. *Stroke* 1997; 28: 1993–1997.
39 Caplan LR, Gorelick PB, Hier DB. Race, sex and occlusive cerebrovascular diseases: a review. *Stroke* 1986; 17: 648–655.
40 Multicenter Acute Stroke Trial-Europe Study Group. Thrombolytic therapy with streptokinase in acute ischemic stroke. *N Engl J Med* 1996; 335: 145–150.
41 Rother J, Schwartz A, Wentz KU, Rautenberg W, Hennerici M. Middle cerebral artery stenosis: assessment by magnetic resonance angiography and transcranial Doppler ultrasound. *Cerebrovasc Dis* 1994; 4: 273–279.
42 Fujita N, Hirabuki N, Fujii K et al. MR imaging of middle cerebral artery stenosis and occlusion: value of MR angiography. *Am J Neuroradiol* 1994; 15: 335–341.
43 Korogi Y, Takahashi M, Mabuchi N et al. Intracranial vascular stenosis and occlusion: diagnostic accuracy of three-dimensional, Fourier transform, time-of-flight MR angiography. *Radiology* 1994; 193: 187–193.
44 Wong KS, Lam WWM, Liang E, Huang YN, Chan YL, Kay R. Variability of magnetic resonance angiography and computed tomography angiography in grading middle cerebral artery stenosis. *Stroke* 1996; 27: 1084–1087.
45 Lee LJ, Kidwell CS, Alger J, Starkman S, Saver JL. Impact on stroke subtype diagnosis of early diffusion-weighted magnetic resonance imaging and magnetic resonance angiography. *Stroke* 2000; 31: 1081.
46 Masaryk TJ, Modic MT, Ross JS et al. Intracranial circulation: preliminary clinical experience with three-dimensional volume MR angiography. *Radiology* 1989; 171: 793–799.
47 Edelman RR, Mattle HP, O'Reilly GV, Wentz KU, Cheng L, Zhao B. Magnetic resonance imaging of flow dynamics in the circle of Willis. *Stroke* 1990; 21: 56–65.
48 Miralles M, Dolz JL, Cotillas J et al. The role of the circle of Willis in carotid occlusion: assessment with phase contrast MR angiography and transcranial duplex. *Eur J Vasc Endovasc Surg* 1995; 10: 424–430.
49 Hartkamp MJ, van der Grond J, van Everdingen KJ, Hillen B, Mali WPTM. Circle of Willis collateral flow investigated by magnetic resonance angiography. *Stroke* 1999; 30: 2671.
50 Hasuo K, Mihara F, Matsushima T. MRI and MR angiography in moyamoya disease. *J Magn Reson Imaging* 1998; 8: 762–766.
51 Houkin K, Aoki T, Takahashi A, Abe H. Diagnosis of moyamoya disease with magnetic resonance angiography. *Stroke* 1994; 25: 2159–2164.
52 Yoon H-K, Shin H-J, Lee M, Byun HS, Na DG, Han BK. MR Angiography of moyamoya disease before and after encephaloduroarteriosynangiosis. *Am J Radiol* 2000; 174: 195–200.
53 Mandai K, Sueyoshi K, Fukunaga R et al. Evaluation of cerebral vasoreactivity by three-dimensional time-of-flight magnetic resonance angiography. *Stroke* 1994; 25: 1807–1811.

54. Buijs PC, Krabbe-Hartkamp MJ, Bakker CJ et al. Effect of age on cerebral blood flow: measurement with ungated two-dimensional phase-contrast MR angiography in 250 adults. *Radiology* 1998; 209: 667–674.
55. Ross JS, Masaryk TJ, Modic MT, Ruggieri PM, Haacke EM, Selman WR. Intracranial aneurysms: evaluation by MR angiography. *Am J Neuroradiol* 1990; 11: 449–455.
56. Schuierer G, Huk WJ, Laub G. Magnetic resonance angiography of intracranial aneurysms: comparison with intra-arterial digital subtraction angiography. *Neuroradiology* 1992; 35: 50–54.
57. Ogawa T, Okudera T, Noguchi K et al. Cerebral aneurysms: evaluation with three-dimensional CT angiography. *Am J Neuroradiol* 1996; 17: 447–454.
58. Preda L, Gaetani P, Rodriguez et al. Spiral CT angiography and surgical correlations in the evaluation of intracranial aneurysms. *Eur Radiol* 1998; 8: 739–745.
59. Huston J, III, Nichols D, Luetmer P et al. Blinded prospective evaluation of sensitivity of MR angiography to known intracranial aneurysms: importance of aneurysm size. *Am J Neuroradiol* 1994; 15: 1607–1614.
60. Aprile I. Evaluation of cerebral aneurysms with MR-angiography. *Riv Neuroradiol* 1996; 9: 541–550.
61. White PM, Wardlaw JM, Easton V. Can noninvasive imaging accurately depict intracranial aneurysms? A systematic review. *Radiology* 2000; 217: 361–370.
62. White PM, Teasdale EM, Wardlaw JM, Easton V. Intracranial aneurysms: CT angiography and MR angiography for detection – prospective blinded comparison in a large patient cohort. *Radiology* 2001; 219: 739–749.
63. Raaymakers TW, Buys PC, Verbeeten Jr B et al. MR angiography as a screening tool for intracranial aneurysms: feasibility, test characteristics, and interobserver agreement. *Am J Radiol* 1999; 173: 1469–1475.
64. The Magnetic Resonance Angiography in Relatives of Patients with Subarachnoid Hemorrhage Study Group. Risks and benefits of screening for intracranial aneurysms in first-degree relatives of patients with sporadic subarachnoid hemorrhage. [see comments]. *N Engl J Med* 1999; 341: 1344–1350.
65. Brown BM, Soldevilla F. MR angiography and surgery for unruptured familial intracranial aneurysms in persons with a family history of cerebral aneurysms. *Am J Radiol* 1999; 173: 133–138.
66. Edelman RR, Wentz KU, Mattle HP et al. Intracerebral arteriovenous malformations: evaluation with selective MR angiography and venography. *Radiology* 1989; 173: 831–837.
67. Marchal G, Bosmans H, Van Fraeyenhoven L et al. Intracranial vascular lesions: optimization and clinical evaluation of three-dimensional time-of-flight MR angiography. *Radiology* 1990; 175: 443–448.
68. Kauczor HU, Engenhart R, Layer G et al. 3D TOF MR angiography of cerebral arteriovenous malformations after radiosurgery. *J Comput Assist Tomogr* 1993; 17: 184–190.
69. Farb RL, McGregor C, Kim JK et al. Intracranial arteriovenous malformations: real-time auto-triggered elliptic centric-ordered 3D gadolinium-enhanced MR angiography – initial assessment. *Radiology* 2001; 220: 244–251.
70. Mattle HP, Wentz KU, Edelman RR et al. Cerebral venography with MR. *Radiology* 1991; 178:453–458.
71. Liauw L, van Buchem MA, Spilt A et al. MR angiography of the intracranial venous system. *Radiology* 2000; 214: 678–682.
72. Tsuruda J, Saloner D, Normal D. Artefacts associated with MR neuroangiography. *Am J Neuroradiol* 1992; 13: 1411–1422.
73. Medlock MR, Olivero WC, Hanigan WC, Wright RM, Winek SJ. Children with cerebral venous thrombosis diagnosed with magnetic resonance imaging and magnetic resonance angiography. *Neurosurgery* 1991; 31: 870–876.
74. Vogl TJ, Bergman C, Villringer A, Einhaupl K, Lissner J, Felix R. Dural sinus thrombosis: value of venous MR angiography for the diagnosis and follow-up. *Radiology* 1994; 162: 1191–1198.
75. Isensee C, Reul J, Thron A. Magnetic resonance imaging of thrombosed dural sinuses. *Stroke* 1994; 25: 29–34.
76. Carr JC, Simonetti O, Bundy J et al. Angiography of the heart with segmented true fast imaging with steady-state precision. *Radiology* 2001; 219: 828–834.
77. van Vaals JJ, Brummer ME, Dixon WT et al. 'Keyhole' method for accelerating imaging of contrast agent uptake. *J Magn Reson Imaging* 1993; 3: 671–675.
78. Korosec FR, Frayne R, Grist TM, Minstretta CA. Time-resolved contrast-enhanced 3D MR angiography. *Magn Reson Med* 1996; 36: 588–595.
79. Sodickson DK, Manning WJ. Simultaneous acquisition of spatial harmonics (SMASH): fast imaging with radiofrequency coil arrays. *Magn Reson Med* 1997; 38: 591–603.
80. Sodickson DK, McKenzie CA, Li W, Wolff S, Manning WJ, Edelman RR. Contrast-enhanced 3D MR angiography with simultaneous acquisition of spatial harmonics: A pilot study. *Radiology* 2000; 217: 284–289.
81. Weiger M, Pruessmann KP, Kassner A et al. Contrast-enhanced 3D MRA using SENSE. *J Magn Reson Imaging* 2000; 12: 671–677.

Stroke MRI in intracranial hemorrhage

Peter D Schellinger,[1] Olav Jansen[2] and Werner Hacke[1]

[1]Department of Neurology, University of Heidelberg, Germany
[2]Department of Neuroradiology, University of Kiel, Germany

Introduction

Non-traumatic intracranial hemorrhage (ICH) accounts for 10–15% of all strokes, but up to 25% of more severe strokes.[1,2] The etiology of ICH in the vast majority of patients is arterial hypertension (63.5%), followed by coagulopathies (15%) and vessel malformations (8.5%), and less frequently amyloid angiopathy, vasculitis, intoxications, cavernoma, or cerebral venous thrombosis.[3] In the hyperacute emergency assessment (< 6–12 h) computed tomography (CT) is the diagnostic standard and modality of choice to differentiate between hyperacute ICH and ischemic stroke.[4–6] In general, MRI at this stage is considered to be of little value for the diagnosis of intracerebral or subarachnoidal hemorrhage, and many authors claim that the sensitivity of MRI for detecting hyperacute ICH is poor.[7–10] Throughout the chapter we arbitrarily defined hyperacute as (< 12 h), acute (12 h to 7 d), subacute (7 d to 3 mo) and chronic (> 3 mo) stages. While hyperacute ICH is hyperdense on acute CT scans with progressing time and hematoma degradation, there is a loss of density and the ICH may appear isodense or hypodense. MRI is far superior to CT in the subacute and chronic stages especially with regard to concomitant or underlying pathology.[11] In a study of 129 patients with ICH Steinbrich et al. found sensitivities of 46% (MRI) and 93% (CT) in the hyperacute and acute stage but 97% (MRI) and 58% (CT) in the subacute and 93% (MRI) and 17% (CT) in the chronic stage.[12] Also, petechial bleeding, discrete foci of contusion and evidence of residues from ICH were only demonstrated by MRI. This chapter will cover the MRI signatures of ICH in all stages, but with a focus on the differential diagnosis in hyperacute stroke patients, where stroke MRI becomes more and more important for guiding therapy in ischemic stroke patients. It will briefly deal with subarachnoid hemorrhage (SAH), and discuss future prospects such as the detection of perihemorrhagic pathological processes, which may contribute to the morbidity of ICH.

MRI signatures of acute, subacute and chronic ICH

Gomori and Grossman had already described in the mid-1980s the stage-dependent signal intensity of ICH in different MRI sequences in experimental[13] as well as clincial situations.[14–17] The ability to detect acute hemorrhage by MRI is related to the oxygen saturation of hemoglobin and its degradation. As a hematoma ages, the hemoglobin passes through several forms (oxyhemoglobin, deoxyhemoglobin, and methemoglobin) prior to red cell lysis and breakdown into ferritin and hemosiderin. The T_2 relaxation rate varies quadratically with the concentration of deoxyhemoglobin.[13] Acute hematomas are characterized by central hypointensity on T_2-weighted images (T_2–WI) whereas they appear isointense on conventional T_1–WI. Methemoglobin formation leads to T_1-shortening and therefore to a centripetal hyperintensity on T_1–WI, which also changes

Table 8.1. Signal characteristics of ICH

Sequence	Hyperacute (< 12 h)	Acute (12 h–7 d)	Subacute (7 d–3 m)	Chronic (> 3 m)
T_1–WI Spin echo	Isointense	Isointense to Hyperintense	Hyperintense	Cystic defect
T_2–WI Spin echo	Hyperintense	Hypointense	Hypointense	Hypointense scar
FLAIR	Hyperintense rim, Hypointense core	Signal loss	Signal loss	Hypointense scar
DWI	Hyperintense rim, Hypointense core	Hypointense/ Signal loss	Signal loss	Hypointense scar
T_2*–WI (PWI)	Signal loss	Signal loss	Signal loss	Hypointense scar

T_2–WI causing a hyperintense signal. This may allow approximate classification of the stage of the ICH. In late subacute and chronic ICH, a hypointense rim caused by the paramagnetic effect of hemosiderin demarcates the border zone of the hematoma, which is better seen on T_2–WI than on T_1–WI. Hyperacute ICH presents as a non-specific hyperintensity on T_2–WI and cannot be seen on T_1–WI unless there is a substantial mass effect. An excellent overview about this can be found in Osborn, *Diagnostic Neuroradiology*.[18] New sequences, which are more susceptible to paramagnetic effects of deoxyhemoglobin, however, may detect hyperacute ICH (see below). Due to the complexity of ICH appearance in different sequences at different stages (see Table 8.1) as opposed to CT, there is a considerable amount of discomfort among clinicians and radiologists with regard to the role of MRI especially in the evaluation of hyperacute stroke. Besides differentiation between ischemia and hemorrhage, MRI may provide information with regard to the etiology of ICH. Basal ganglia hemorrhage in combination with older microbleeds or vascular leukencephalopathy implies a hypertensive etiology of ICH as do lobar hematomas in the elderly.[19] Multiple cortical ICH in the elderly may suggest an amyloid angiopathy.[20] In young patients, additional information from MRA may detect aneurysms, arteriovenous malformations, vasculitis like changes, such as multiple intracranial stenoses, or cerebral venous thrombosis and thus may make an invasive conventional angiography unnecessary.[21,22]

MRI in hyperacute ICH

Hyperacute stroke demands the differentiation between ischemic stroke and intracranial hemorrhage from the radiologist, which is impossible by clinical means.[6,23] It also demands a generalized diagnostic workup, where the important pathophysiologic aspects of hyperacute ischemic stroke can be investigated: (i) where and how large is the actual area of irreversible ischemic brain damage? (ii) how old is the infarction? (iii) is there tissue at risk of infarction that is potentially salvageable and how much tissue is at risk? (iv) is there a vessel occlusion and where is it? (5) is an ICH or another underlying, nonischemic disease present? The advent of new MRI techniques such as perfusion- (PWI) and diffusion- (DWI) weighted imaging has revolutionized diagnostic imaging in ischemic stroke.[24,25] DWI may delineate infarcted brain tissue in less than 1 h after symptom onset, probably within minutes,[26] although there is cumulating evidence that in the very early stage of stroke there may be reversible DWI changes.[27,28] while PWI defines the area of cerebral hypoperfusion. Several studies have reported early findings of stroke MRI within the first 6 to 12 hours, demonstrating the feasibility and practicality of this method in the setting of acute stroke and thrombolytic therapy.[25,29–35] In essence, the presence of a vessel occlusion by MRA is associated with a PWI/DWI mismatch, the stroke MRI setting that defines the ideal candidate for thrombolysis.[33,36] As already stated, the diagnosis of ICH is still the domain of CT rather MRI. The need to perform both, CT for exclusion of ICH and stroke MRI to guide therapeutic efforts, is time-consuming ('time is brain'), medicoeconomically questionable, and also inefficient.[37,38] Therefore, characteristic MRI features of hyperacute ICH especially on newer sequences should be described and utilized.

Many authors claim that the sensitivity of MRI for detecting hyperacute ICH is poor.[7,10] The appearance of intracranial hemorrhage on magnetic resonance (MR) imaging depends primarily on the age of the hematoma and the type of MR contrast (i.e. T_1- or T_2-weighted). Immediately after ICH there are intact red blood cells with intracellular oxyhemoglobin within a protein and fluid-rich serum.[12] Oxyhemoglobin is diamagnetic and does not cause any susceptibility effects.[18] The key substrate for early MRI visualization of hemorrhage is deoxyhemoglobin, a blood degradation product with paramagnetic properties due to unpaired electrons. As long as the deoxyhemoglobin is intracellular within the erythrocytes during the very first hour(s) after ICH onset, it does not cause rapid dephasing of proton spins in T_2–WI or in T_2*–WI thus not allowing for a signal loss within the first 12 hours.[12,39] However, the paramagnetic deoxyhemoglobin changes the local magnetic field gradient and this subsequently may lead to a dephasing of stationary or passing protons inside and in the vicinity of the ICH.[11] The short T_2 observed when deoxyhemoglobin forms is enhanced on higher-field-strength systems and on gradient-echo images and is reduced with 'fast spin-echo' MR techniques.[10]

There are only few publications which report a high diagnostic accuracy of MRI for ICH within a time window of 6 hours or less after symptom onset.[40–43] Patel et al. were the first to demonstrate early MRI changes in susceptibility-weighted T_2*–WI within 5 hours in six patients with acute ICH.[41] These authors, however, did not use a standardized MRI protocol and did not perform a volumetric comparative analysis of CT and MRI.

Our group compared CT and stroke MRI findings in nine patients with acute ICH in a randomized stroke imaging protocol (CT, DWI, PWI with T_2*–W source images, T_2–WI, FLAIR images, MRA); all patients received CT and MRI within a 3 to 6 h time window.[42] ICH was unambiguously identified on the basis of all stroke MRI sequences. Volumetric analysis showed a good raw correlation of hematoma volumes in all MRI images compared to CT. As already reported by Rosen et al., images obtained with sequences with a high sensitivity for susceptibility effects (T_2*-WI, FLAIR) generally overestimate the actual hematoma size in comparison to the lesion volume assessed on CT.[44] Hematoma volumes on DWI (median and mean difference 3.97%/−4.36%, SD $\sigma = 37.42\%$) followed by FLAIR (median and mean difference −2.91%/−6.25%, SD $\sigma = 28.39\%$) corresponded best with lesion size on CT. Conventional T_2–WI substantially underestimated (median and mean difference 17.24% / 12.98%, SD $\sigma = 34.46\%$) and T_2*-WI substantially overestimated (median and mean difference −17.94% / −18.86%, SD $\sigma = −24.45\%$) the hematoma size. The typical appearance of ICH on the MRI images was a heterogeneous focus of high and low signal intensities. With increasing susceptibility weight, the central area of hypointensity became more pronounced. The T_2*-WI showed no or few areas of hyperintensity, or merely a faint ring around a central core of signal loss. Figures 8.1 and 8.2 illustrate the appearance of a larger and a smaller hyperacute ICH on CT and MRI in two representative patients; these findings were common to all nine patients.

Linfante et al. successfully investigated 5 hyperacute ICH-patients with MRI between 23 minutes and 2 hours from symptom onset.[43] They report a characteristic signal- and evolution pattern of hyperacute ICH, dividing the lesion into three parts. In the very first minutes after symptom onset, the centre of the lesion appears heterogeneous on all images (T_2-WI, T_2*-WI, T_1-WI), which is due to a local predominance of oxyhemoglobin. The periphery of the hematoma is hypointense on susceptibility-weighted images more than on T_2-WI and shows a progressive enlargement over the next minutes and first hours. This is due to a progressive centripetal increase in concentration of deoxyhemoglobin. There is a surrounding rim, which appears hyperintense on T_2-WI and T_2*-WI but hypointense on T_1-WI and represents perifocal vasogenic edema. While both authors[42,43] suggest that stroke MRI is

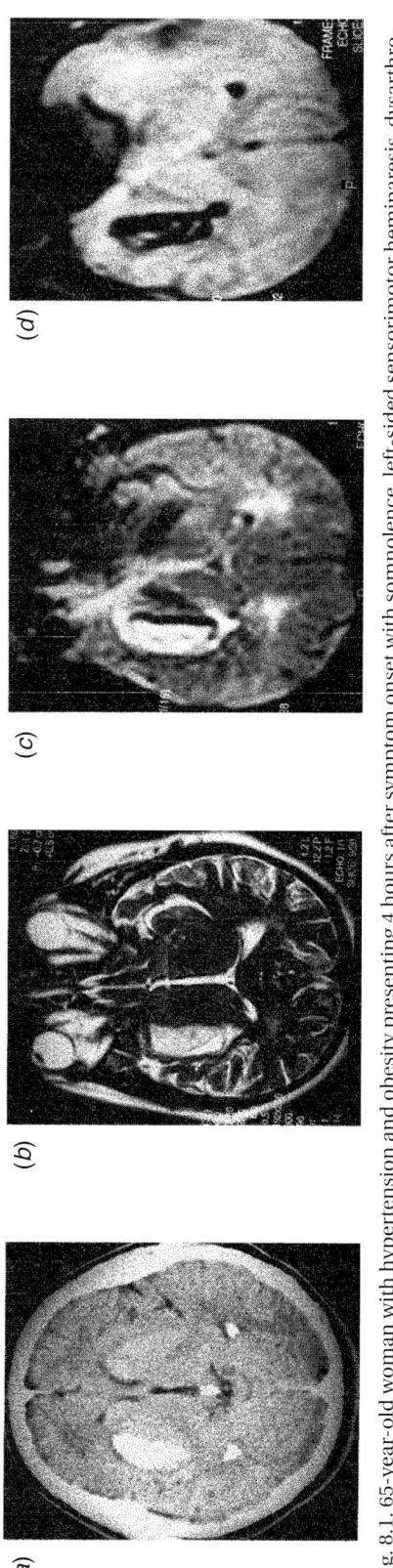

Fig. 8.1. 65-year-old woman with hypertension and obesity presenting 4 hours after symptom onset with somnolence, left-sided sensorimotor hemiparesis, dysarthrophonia, and hemineglect to the left. CT 1½ h and MRI 3¾ h after symptom onset: (a) initial CT shows an ICH located in the right external capsule, (b) T_2-WI shows the same hyperintense lesion. (c) FLAIR and (d) DWI revealed an irregular hyperintense right putaminal lesion with a hypointense core more prominent on the strongly susceptibility-weighted and strongest on T_2^*-weighted images.

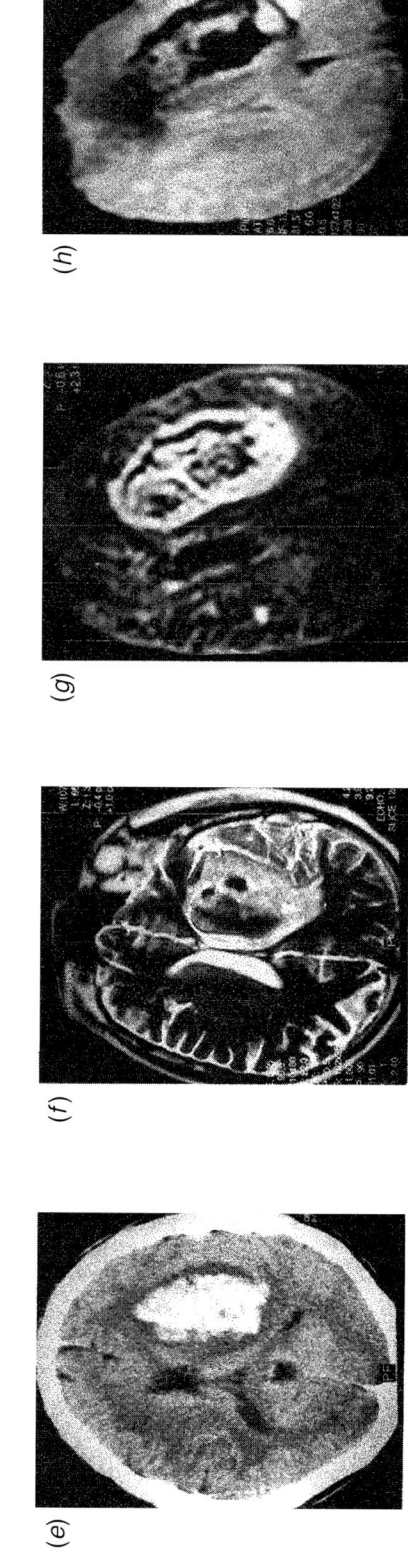

Fig. 8.1 cont. 40-year-old man with untreated arterial hypertension suffering from severe headache, dense right-sided paresis, severe non-fluent aphasia, and forced gaze deviation to the left. CT 2 h and MRI 3 h after symptom onset: (e) initial CT shows a left putaminal ICH and (f–h) T_2–WI an irregular hyperintense putaminal lesion on the left DWI, FLAIR, and T_2^*-weighted PWI source images show an increasing area of signal loss within the core of the left-sided hematoma with a heterogeneous appearance caused by small amounts of deoxyhemoglobin.

Stroke MRI in intracranial hemorrhage 107

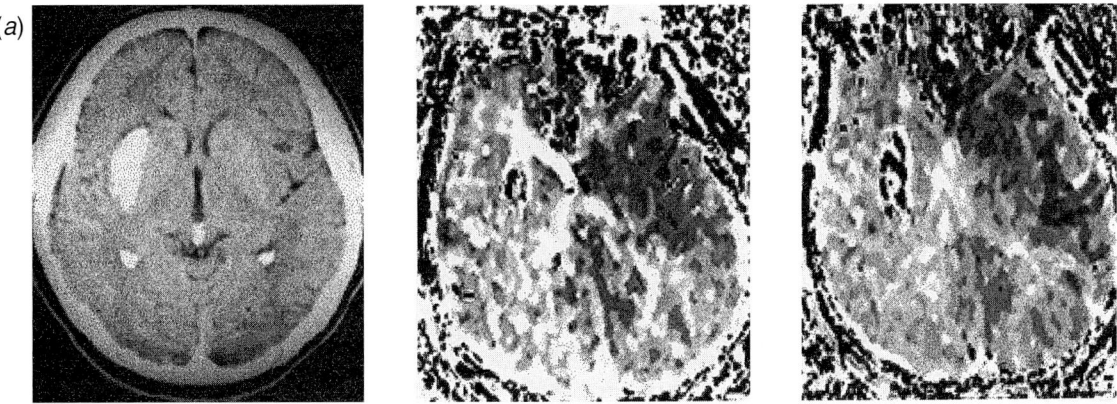

Fig. 8.2. 65-year-old patient with left-sided hemiplegia. Baseline CT shows an external capsule ICH 4 h after symptom onset (left). Perfusion-weighted images (PWI, MTT-maps) show a large perfusion deficit (hyperintensity) of the complete right hemisphere (middle and right).

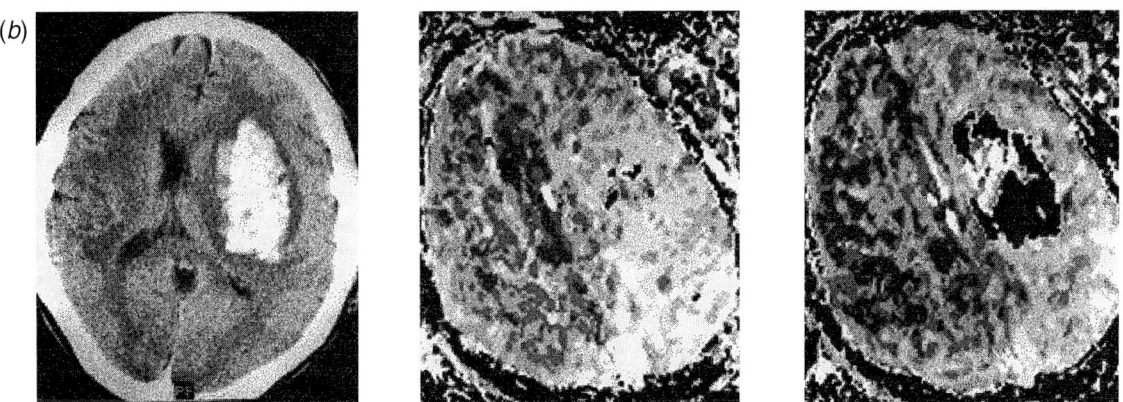

41-year-old patient with right-sided hemiplegia and aphasia. Baseline CT shows a large basal ganglia ICH 3 h after symptom onset (left). Perfusion-weighted images (PWI, MTT-maps) show a large perfusion deficit (hyperintensity) of the complete left hemisphere (middle and right).

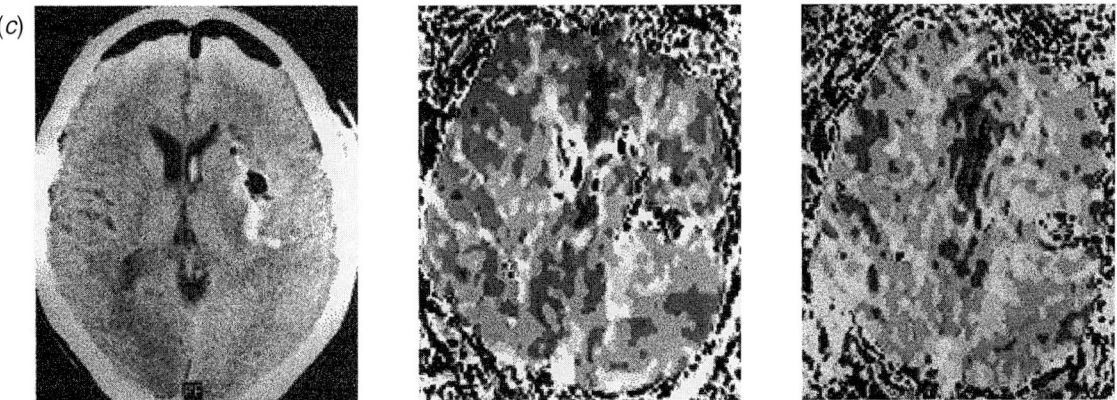

Same patient as middle row 24 h after symptom onset. Surgical removal of the hematoma as seen on the postsurgical CT (left). Normalization of perfusion disturbance on the left hemisphere according to PWI (middle and right) with small artefacts in the former ICH cavity due to susceptibility (T_2^*) effects.

diagnostic in the evaluation of hyperacute ICH, they conclude consistently that the randomized and prospective acquisition of a larger group with blinded evaluation is needed to confirm these preliminary observations.

These results support the hypothesis that small amounts of deoxyhemoglobin are present within the very first minutes after onset of ICH and detectable by susceptibility-weighted MRI sequences. Figure 8.1 suggests that T_2^*–WI are suited best for the diagnosis of ICH, which holds true for the qualitative detection also of relatively small hematomas without mass effect. Further information such as the presence of space occupying edema, midline shift, and ventricular hemorrhage is best derived from conventional T_2–WI. In addition to the standardized stroke protocol, postcontrast T_1–WI scans may be obtained after PWI if another primary disease is suspected (e.g. apoplectic glioma or metastases). Multicentre trials to acquire larger patient numbers are currently under way. Patients should be randomized for the sequence of CT and MRI to avoid a negative selection bias for CT, if both modalities are to be compared with regard to sensitivity and specifity.

MRI in subarachnoid hemorrhage

CT is also the (imaging) standard of care for the diagnosis of acute subarachnoid hemorrhage[45,46] with a sensitivity of 85–100%. The CT-based diagnosis of SAH may be difficult in the posterior fossa due to bone artefacts as well as with small amounts of blood. In the subacute stage the sensitivity of CT for SAH diminishes substantially with sensitivities of 50% after 1 week, 30% after 2 weeks and ≈0% at 3 weeks[45] necessitating the diagnostic gold standard in SAH, i.e. lumbar puncture. There currently is only scarce information about the sensitivity of stroke MRI for SAH. Initial assumptions that MRI may also be suitable in the diagnosis of acute SAH were derived from in vitro studies.[47,48] In subacute SAH (5 days to 2 weeks) MRI with fluid attenuated inversion recovery (FLAIR) sequences and proton density (PD) weighted images is clearly superior to CT (sensitivity 100% vs. 45%).[49] Some investigators reported that MRI may also be effective in the diagnosis of acute SAH.[50–54] Conventional T_1–WI and T_2–WI were shown to be ineffective in the diagnosis of acute SAH with sensitivities of 35–50%.[55] This may, in part, be due to the fact that the rules, which apply for intracerebral degradation of ICH may not be valid for SAH due to a higher oxygen partial pressure in cerebrospinal fluid (CSF)[17] and that the formation of blood clots which also causes T_2-shortening is impaired.[9] The paramagnetic susceptibility effect, which may be utilized to detect intracerebral hemorrhage is not suitable for the detection of SAH as the latter frequently is localized in the vicinity of the cranial vault or skull base, thus areas which are prone to artifacts. A rise in CSF-protein concentration leads to a T_1-shortening and therefore signal intensity increase, which is seen better on PD–WI than T_1–WI,[50,56] an observation contradicted by other authors.[57,58] The detection of SAH may be improved by using PD–WI with shorter repetition times (TR) to visualize the T_1-effect.[59] FLAIR sequences have been reported to be suitable for the diagnosis of not only subacute but also acute SAH.[48,49,52,54,60] The latter studies have all been performed with low field scanners (≤0.5 tesla), however, with increasing field strengths and faster FLAIR sequences (usually 10 to 15 min, TURBO–FLAIR ≈3 to 6 min) there also are more pulsation artefacts, which may impair their sensitivity for SAH. Wiesmann et al. recently reported a very high sensitivity (100%) for the combined use of PD–WI and FLAIR images in 19 patients.[59,60] Artefacts, which were seen in one-third of their patients could be determined as such by the combined use of PD–WI and FLAIR images, all PD and FLAIR studies were negative in ten control patients. Also many newer MRI sequences such as MRA, DWI and PWI be useful to detect early complications of SAH such as vasospasm and spreading depression.[61] Further studies aimed at the diagnostic reach of stroke MRI in acute SAH are worthwhile.

Future prospects of stroke MRI in ICH

Even in the new millenium there is still controversy with regard to which patients should receive best medical treatment and whom should surgery performed on.[62,63] In general, patients with mild symptoms and small ICH, severe symptoms and large ICH as well as deep grey matter ICH are not operated, because surgery does not affect the natural disease course and may even lead to complications and deterioration in patients with mild symptoms or basal ganglia hemorrhage.[64] Conversely, young patients with a low comorbidity, moderately sized right hemispheric ICH, moderate clinical symptoms at presentation with a rapid deterioration are likely to profit from hematoma evacuation, especially when microsurgical techniques are applied.[65] There are inconsistent data with regard to the pathological processes in the vicinity of the ICH and their contribution to acute and chronic clinical deficit. Some authors postulate the presence of perihemorrhagic ischemic lesions (animal experimental data) whether caused by toxic effects, apoptosis or reduction of cerebral blood flow,[66,67] others deny this.[68] Also in clinical studies evidence has been provided for[69,70] and against[71] the presence of ischemic perihemorrhagic areas. Results of the studies by Videen et al., however, suggest that oligemia may be reactive to ICH and represent a reduced metabolic oxygen rate with a constant oxygen extraction fraction rather than being pathologic oligemia or ischemia.[70] A small pilot study utilized a stroke MRI protocol with T_2–WI, FLAIR, DWI, PWI and MRA to evaluate ICH.[42] There were perihemorrhagic perfusion deficits according to PWI in all nine patients, and large deficits in three of nine patients, while there were no manifest ischemic infarcts according to DWI (Fig. 8.2).[72] However, whether this was due to raised intracranial pressure, local compression of the middle cerebral artery, diaschisis, toxic effects of blood products or other mechanisms cannot be answered at this point. Further animal studies and a prospective clinical study, which may shed more light on the pathophysiological, clinical and prognostic relevance of a perihemorrhagic zone of cerebral impairment are currently under way.

Conclusion

In hyperacute stroke, it is of utmost importance that diagnostic efforts are as specific and time efficacious as possible, especially with the time constraints imposed by acute therapies for ischemic stroke such as thrombolytic therapy. MRI stroke protocols including DWI, PWI and susceptibility weighted images are very promising with regard to the characterization of acute stroke patients and the identification of patients suitable for specific therapy. Surprisingly, though, MRI is still not generally considered to be the primary and only diagnostic tool in hyperacute stroke patients, as there is doubt regarding the ability to detect hyperacute ICH. While a larger number of patients would be useful to confirm these findings, preliminary results suggest that stroke MRI with T_2*–WI is as sensitive as CT in the diagnosis of ICH and that there are characteristic features of hyperacute intracerebral hemorrhage on MRI. Also, the combination of PD–WI and FLAIR images may reliably differentiate acute and subacute SAH from ICH and ischemic strokes. In addition to that, SAH usually presents with a different clinical picture than do ICH and ischemic stroke, unless there is a substantial intracerebral hemorrhage accompanying primary SAH, which then is apparent on T_2*–WI. The initial and exclusive use of stroke MRI therefore is feasible, cost-effective and time saving. In conclusion, stroke MRI may be the diagnostic tool of choice not only for patients with subacute and chronic ICH and SAH but also in the initial assessment of patients with hyperacute ischemic or hemorrhagic stroke as well as hyperacute SAH.

REFERENCES

1 WHO Task Force. Stroke – 1989. Recommendations on stroke prevention, diagnosis, and therapy. Report of the WHO Task Force on Stroke and other Cerebrovascular Disorders. *Stroke* 1989; 20: 1407–1431.
2 Jorgensen HS, Nakayama H, Raaschou HO, Olsen TS. Intracerebral hemorrhage versus infarction: stroke severity, risk factors, and prognosis. *Ann Neurol* 1995; 38: 45–50.
3 Rosenow F, Hojer C, Meyer-Lohmann C et al. Spontaneous intracerebral hemorrhage. Prognostic factors in 896 cases. *Acta Neurol Scand* 1997; 96: 174–182.

4. Higer HP, Pedrosa P, Schaeben W, Bielke G, Meindl S. Intracranial hemorrhage in MRT. *Radiology* 1989; 29: 297–302.

5. Jansen O, Heiland S, Schellinger P. Neuroradiological diagnosis in acute ischemic stroke. Value of modern techniques. *Nervenarzt* 1998; 69: 465–471.

6. Hacke W, Stingele R, Steiner T, Schuchardt V, Schwab S. Critical care of acute ischemic stroke. *Intens Care Med* 1995; 21: 856–862.

7. Hayman LA, Taber KH, Ford JJ, Bryan RN. Mechanisms of MR signal alteration by acute intracerebral blood: old concepts and new theories. *Am J Neuroradiol.* 1991; 12: 899–907.

8. Hayman LA, Pagani JJ, Kirkpatrick JB, Hinck VC. Pathophysiology of acute intracerebral and subarachnoid hemorrhage: applications to MR imaging. *Am J Radiol* 1989; 153: 135–139.

9. Weingarten K, Zimmerman RD, Cahill PT, Deck MD. Detection of acute intracerebral hemorrhage on MR imaging: ineffectiveness of prolonged interecho interval pulse sequences. *Am J Neuroradiol* 1991; 12: 475–479.

10. Bradley WG, Jr. MR appearance of hemorrhage in the brain. *Radiology* 1993; 189: 15–26.

11. Felber S, Auer A, Wolf C et al. MRI characteristics of spontaneous intracerebral hemorrhage. *Radiology* 1999; 39: 838–846.

12. Steinbrich W, Gross-Fengels W, Krestin GP, Heindel W, Schreier G. Intracranial hemorrhages in the magnetic resonance tomogram. Studies on sensitivity, on the development of hematomas and on the determination of the cause of the hemorrhage. *Rofo Fortschr Geb Rontgenstr Neuen Bildgeb Verfahr* 1990; 152: 534–543.

13. Gomori JM, Grossman RI, Yu-Ip C, Asakura T. NMR relaxation times of blood: dependence on field strength, oxidation state, and cell integrity. *J Comput Assist Tomogr* 1987; 11: 684–690.

14. Gomori JM, Grossman RI, Goldberg HI, Zimmerman RA, Bilaniuk LT. Intracranial hematomas: imaging by high-field MR. *Radiology* 1985; 157: 87–93.

15. Gomori JM, Grossman RI. Mechanisms responsible for the MR appearance and evolution of intracranial hemorrhage. *Radiographics* 1988; 8: 427–440.

16. Grossman RI, Gomori JM, Goldberg HI et al. MR imaging of hemorrhagic conditions of the head and neck. *Radiographics* 1988; 8: 441–454.

17. Grossman RI, Kemp SS, Ip CY et al. Importance of oxygenation in the appearance of acute subarachnoid hemorrhage on high field magnetic resonance imaging. *Acta Radiol Suppl.* 1986; 369: 56–58.

18. Osborn AG. Intracranial hemorrhage. In: Osborn AG, ed *Diagnostic Neuroradiology*. Mosby: Year Book Inc; 1994: 154–198.

19. Fazekas F, Kleinert R, Roob G, Kleinert G et al. Histopathologic analysis of foci of signal loss on gradient-echo T_2*-weighted MR images in patients with spontaneous intracerebral hemorrhage: evidence of microangiopathy-related microbleeds. *Am J Neuroradiol* 1999; 20: 637–642.

20. Hagen T. Intracerebral hemorrhage in the context of amyloid angiopathy. *Radiology* 1999; 39: 847–854.

21. Ruiz-Sandoval JL, Cantu C, Barinagarrementeria F. Intracerebral hemorrhage in young people: analysis of risk factors, location, causes, and prognosis. *Stroke* 1999; 30: 537–541.

22. Jansen O, Knauth M, Sartor K. Advances in clinical neuroradiology. *Akt Neurologie* 1999; 26: 1–7.

23. Hacke W, Steiner T, Schwab S. Critical management of the acute stroke: medical and surgical therapy. In: Batjer HH, Caplan LR, Freiberg L, Greenlee RG, Jr., Kopitnik TH, Jr. and Young WL, eds *Cerebrovascular Disease*. Hagerstown: Lippincott-Raven; 1996: 523–533.

24. Warach S, Boska M, Welch KM. Pitfalls and potential of clinical diffusion-weighted MR imaging in acute stroke. *Stroke* 1997; 28: 481–482.

25. Barber PA, Darby DG, Desmond PM et al. Prediction of stroke outcome with echoplanar perfusion- and diffusion-weighted MRI. *Neurology* 1998; 51: 418–426.

26. Conturo TE, McKinstry RC, Aronovitz JA, Neil JJ. Diffusion MRI: precision, accuracy and flow effects. *NMR Biomed* 1995; 8: 307–332.

27. Kidwell CS, Alger JR, Di Salle F et al. Diffusion MRI in patients with transient ischemic attacks. *Stroke* 1999; 30: 1174–1180.

28. Kidwell CS, Saver JL, Mattiello J et al. Thrombolytic reversal of acute human cerebral ischemic injury shown by diffusion/perfusion magnetic resonance imaging. *Ann Neurol* 2000; 47: 462–469.

29. Tong DC, Yenari MA, Albers GW, O'Brien M, Marks MP, Moseley ME. Correlation of perfusion- and diffusion-weighted MRI with NIHSS score in acute (<6.5 hour) ischemic stroke. *Neurology* 1998; 50: 864–870.

30. Jansen O, Schellinger PD, Fiebach JB, Hacke W, Sartor K. Early recanalization in acute ischemic stroke saves tissue at risk defined by MRI. *Lancet* 1999; 353: 2036–2037.

31. Baird AE, Warach S. Imaging developing brain infarction. *Curr Opin Neurol* 1999; 12: 65–71.

32. Beaulieu C, de Crespigny A, Tong DC, Moseley ME, Albers GW, Marks MP. Longitudinal magnetic resonance imaging study of perfusion and diffusion in stroke: evolution of lesion volume and correlation with clinical outcome. *Ann Neurol* 1999; 46: 568–578.
33. Schellinger PD, Jansen O, Fiebach JB et al. Monitoring intravenous recombinant tissue plasminogen activator thrombolysis for acute ischemic stroke with diffusion and perfusion MRI. *Stroke* 2000; 31: 1318–1328.
34. Schellinger PD, Jansen O, Fiebach JB et al. Feasibility and practicality of MR imaging of stroke in the management of hyperacute cerebral ischemia. *Am J Neuroradiol* 2000; 21: 1184–1189.
35. Schellinger PD, Fiebach JB, Jansen O et al. Stroke magnetic resonance imaging within 6 hours after onset of hyperacute cerebral ischemia. *Ann Neurol* 2001; 49: 460–469.
36. Rordorf G, Koroshetz WJ, Copen WA et al. Regional ischemia and ischemic injury in patients with acute middle cerebral artery stroke as defined by early diffusion-weighted and perfusion-weighted MRI. *Stroke* 1998; 29: 939–943.
37. Powers WJ, Zivin J. Magnetic resonance imaging in acute stroke: not ready for prime time. *Neurology* 1998; 50: 842–843.
38. Powers WJ. Testing a test: a report card for DWI in acute stroke. *Neurology* 2000; 54: 1549–1551.
39. Mattle HP, Edelman RR, Schroth G, O'Reilly GV. In: *Spontaneous and Traumatic Hemorrhage in Clinical and Magnetic Resonance Imaging, Vol. 1*. 2nd ed. Philadelphia, PA: W B Saunders Co; 1996: 652–702.
40. Ebisu T, Tanaka C, Umeda M, et al. Hemorrhagic and nonhemorrhagic stroke: diagnosis with diffusion-weighted and T_2-weighted echo-planar MR imaging. *Radiology* 1997; 203: 823–828.
41. Patel MR, Edelman RR, Warach S. Detection of hyperacute primary intraparenchymal hemorrhage by magnetic resonance imaging. *Stroke* 1996; 27: 2321–2324.
42. Schellinger PD, Jansen O, Fiebach JB, Hacke W, Sartor K. A standardized MRI stroke protocol: comparison with CT in hyperacute intracerebral hemorrhage. *Stroke* 1999; 30: 765–768.
43. Linfante I, Llinas RH, Caplan LR, Warach S. MRI features of intracerebral hemorrhage within 2 hours from symptom onset. *Stroke* 1999; 30: 2263–2267.
44. Rosen BR, Belliveau JW, Chien D. Perfusion imaging by nuclear magnetic resonance. *Magn Reson Q* 1989; 5: 263–281.
45. van Gijn J, van Dongen KJ. The time course of aneurysmal haemorrhage on computed tomograms. *Neuroradiology* 1982; 23: 153–156.
46. Scotti G, Ethier R, Melancon D, Terbrugge K, Tchang S. Computed tomography in the evaluation of intracranial aneurysms and subarachnoid hemorrhage. *Radiology* 1977; 123: 85–90.
47. Chakeres DW, Bryan RN. Acute subarachnoid hemorrhage: in vitro comparison of magnetic resonance and computed tomography. *Am J Neuroradiol* 1986; 7: 223–228.
48. Melhem ER, Jara H, Eustace S. Fluid-attenuated inversion recovery MR imaging: identification of protein concentration thresholds for CSF hyperintensity. *Am J Roentgenol* 1997; 169: 859–862.
49. Noguchi K, Ogawa T, Seto H et al. Subacute and chronic subarachnoid hemorrhage: diagnosis with fluid-attenuated inversion-recovery MR imaging. *Radiology* 1997; 203: 257–262.
50. Jenkins A, Hadley DM, Teasdale GM, Condon B, Macpherson P, Patterson J. Magnetic resonance imaging of acute subarachnoid hemorrhage. *J Neurosurg* 1988; 68: 731–736.
51. Matsumura K, Matsuda M, Handa J, Todo G. Magnetic resonance imaging with aneurysmal subarachnoid hemorrhage: comparison with computed tomography scan. *Surg Neurol.* 1990; 34: 71–78.
52. Noguchi K, Ogawa T, Inugami A et al. Acute subarachnoid hemorrhage: MR imaging with fluid-attenuated inversion recovery pulse sequences. *Radiology* 1995; 196: 773–777.
53. Chrysikopoulos H, Papanikolaou N, Pappas J et al. Acute subarachnoid haemorrhage: detection with magnetic resonance imaging. *Br J Radiol* 1996; 69: 601–609.
54. Noguchi K, Seto H, Kamisaki Y, Tomizawa G, Toyoshima S, Watanabe N. Comparison of fluid-attenuated inversion-recovery MR imaging with CT in a simulated model of acute subarachnoid hemorrhage. *Am J Neuroradiol* 2000; 21: 923–927.
55. Ogawa T, Inugami A, Shimosegawa E et al. Subarachnoid hemorrhage: evaluation with MR imaging. *Radiology* 1993; 186(2): 345–351.
56. Satoh S, Kadoya S. Magnetic resonance imaging of subarachnoid hemorrhage. *Neuroradiology* 1988; 30: 361–366.
57. Atlas SW. MR imaging is highly sensitive for acute subarachnoid hemorrhage . . . not! *Radiology* 1993; 186(2): 319–322; discussion 323.
58. Atlas SW, Thulborn KR. MR Detection of hyperacute parenchymal hemorrhage of the brain. *Am J Neuroradiol* 1998; 19: 1471–1477.

59 Wiesmann M, Mayer TE, Medele R, Bruckmann H. Diagnosis of acute subarachnoid hemorrhage at 1.5 Tesla using proton-density weighted FSE and MRI sequences. *Radiology* 1999; 39: 860–865.

60 Noguchi K, Ogawa T, Inugami A, Toyoshima H, Okudera T, Uemura K. MR of acute subarachnoid hemorrhage: a preliminary report of fluid-attenuated inversion-recovery pulse sequences. *Am J Neuroradiol* 1994; 15: 1940–1943.

61 Busch E, Beaulieu C, de Crespigny A, Moseley ME. Diffusion MR imaging during acute subarachnoid hemorrhage in rats. *Stroke* 1998; 29: 2155–2161.

62 Kanno T, Nagata J, Nonomura K et al. New approaches in the treatment of hypertensive intracerebral hemorrhage. *Stroke* 1993; 24: 196–100.

63 Morgenstern LB, Frankowski RF, Shedden P, Pasteur W, Grotta JC. Surgical treatment for intracerebral hemorrhage (STICH). *Stroke* 1998; 51: 1359–1363.

64 Fernandes HM, Gregson B, Siddique S, Mendelow AD. Surgery in intracerebral hemorrhage : the uncertainty continues. *Stroke* 2000; 31: 2511–2516.

65 Auer LM, Deinsberger W, Niederkorn K et al. Endoscopic surgery versus medical treatment for spontaneous intracerebral hematoma: a randomized study. *J Neurosurg* 1989; 70: 530–535.

66 Bullock R, Brock Utne J, van Dellen J, Blake G. Intracerebral hemorrhage in a primate model: effect on regional cerebral blood flow. *Surg Neurol* 1988; 29: 101–107.

67 Deinsberger W, Vogel J, Fuchs C, Auer LM, Kuschinsky W, Boker DK. Fibrinolysis and aspiration of experimental intracerebral hematoma reduces the volume of ischemic brain in rats. *Neurol Res* 1999; 21: 517–523.

68 Mun Bryce S, Kroh FO, White J, Rosenberg GA. Brain lactate and pH dissociation in edema: 1H- and 31P-NMR in collagenase-induced hemorrhage in rats. *Am J Physiol* 1993; 265: R697–R702.

69 Dethy S, Goldman S, Blecic S, Luxen A, Levivier M, Hildebrand J. Carbon-11-methionine and fluorine-18–FDG PET study in brain hematoma. *J Nucl Med* 1994; 35: 1162–1166.

70 Videen TO, Dunford-Shore JE, Diringer MN, Powers WJ. Correction for partial volume effects in regional blood flow measurements adjacent to hematomas in humans with intracerebral hemorrhage: implementation and validation. *J Comput Assist Tomogr* 1999; 23: 248–256.

71 Hirano T, Read SJ, Abbott DF et al. No evidence of hypoxic tissue on 18F-fluoromisonidazole PET after intracerebral hemorrhage. *Neurology* 1999; 53: 2179–2182.

72 Schellinger PD, Fiebach JB, Jansen O, Hacke W. Penumbra Nachweis bei Hirnblutungen mit multimodaler MRT. *Akt Neurol* 1998; 25: 150.

Using diffusion–perfusion MRI in animal models for drug development

Marc Fisher

Department of Neurology, University of Massachusetts, Medical School, Worcester, MA, USA

Introduction

The development of therapies for acute ischemic stroke is a difficult venture with many potential pitfalls. Currently, the only approved therapy for acute ischemic stroke is intravenous tissue plasminogen activator (t-PA) given within 3 hours of stroke onset. The approval of rt-PA stemmed from the National Institutes of Neurological Disorders and Stroke (NINDS) trials that demonstrated a significant treatment effect with rt-PA on several different types of 90-day outcome measures and global assessment of these measures.[1] Two other acute stroke therapy trials yielded statistically significant positive effects on the prespecified primary outcome measures. In the Stroke Therapy Ancrod Trial (STAT), ancrod, a defrinogenating agent, initiated within 3 hours of stroke onset improved outcome, but not as favorably as rt-PA given within the same time window.[2] Another ancrod trial with a 6-hour window to the initiation of treatment was stopped and the drug has not been approved by regulatory agencies. The other positive acute stroke trial was the PROACT 2 trial that evaluated the thrombolytic agent, proUrokinase, within 6 hours of stroke onset in a group of relatively severe stroke patients with angiographically confirmed middle cerebral artery occlusion.[3] The trial only included 180 patients and did not lead to regulatory approval. There have been a large number of other acute stroke therapy trials, both phase 2 and phase 3 trials that have not achieved a favourable outcome.[4] These non-successful trials have engendered a careful reassessment of the development plan, both preclinical and clinical, used to bring the drugs in question to advanced evaluation.

Preclinical evaluation of purported acute stroke therapies plays a vital role in the drug development process. A cogent argument would be that a drug not demonstrating efficacy in animal stroke models is very unlikely to show efficacy in humans. Conversely, treatment effects in animal stroke models certainly do not guarantee success in clinical trials. For both thrombolytic and neuroprotective drugs, the 'gold standard' for detecting treatment efficacy in animal models remains effects on ischemic lesion volume evaluated postmortem by histological methods.[5] The goal of acute stroke therapy is to salvage ischemic brain tissue and prevent progression to infarction. The salvage of ischemic tissue is then presumed to be associated with improved neurological and functional outcome. Animal stroke models and their use in evaluating treatment effects of potential acute stroke therapies are prone to many difficulties.[6] Experiments must be performed in a blinded–randomized manner with careful attention to the measurement and maintenance of physiological variables. A dose–response relationship between drug treatment effects and lesion volume should be defined, as well as the relationship of dose to side effects. The survival time of animals after dosing should be extended for days or even weeks after initial success with shorter survival to ensure that the treatment effect is not transient.[6] Lastly, drugs are typically initially evaluated in rodent stroke models, but consideration of further testing in gyrencephalic species closer to humans should be entertained for novel, first in class drugs. In addition to determining effects on ischemic lesion volume, it has been recommended that effects on behavioural and functional outcome be evaluated to more closely reproduce the likely outcomes to be used in clinical trials.[7] The important role of animal stroke models for screening of potentially effective drugs for acute ischemic stroke is clear and the main treatment effect to be assessed in animals will likely remain reduction of acute and/or subacute infarct volume.

Proceeding from animal evaluation of novel acute stroke therapies to clinical development is a major step that requires a substantial investment of time, money and other resources by the drug's developer, e.g. a pharmaceutical or biotechnology company. Clinical trials require a large sample size to be adequately powered to detect treatment effects on the traditional neurological, functional and handicap measures used to determine treatment effects.[8] The sample size employed in most phase 2 trials is insufficient to detect even substantial trends of treatment efficacy and decisions about proceeding to phase 3 trials are largely based on safety data and intuition. Recently, it has been proposed that diffusion–perfusion MRI might help to bridge the gap between preclinical evaluation and advanced clinical trials.[9] For a neuroprotective drug, an effect on ischemic lesion growth on a baseline diffusion MRI to a day 30–90 T_2 scan might confirm an effect on ischemic lesion evolution in vivo and potentially be predictive of salutary effects on clinical outcome in a phase 3 trial.[10] For a thrombolytic drug, demonstrating reperfusion effects on perfusion imaging in a phase 2 trial would reassure participants and sponsors that the agent restores blood flow and the appropriate dose to be used in the phase 3 trial.[11] Diffusion–perfusion MRI can be used in animal models to evaluate the same parameters as those to be assessed in phase 2 and 3 clinical trials, providing a link between preclinical and clinical drug development. The two MRI techniques have been used extensively in animal stroke models and more recently in clinical stroke trials.

Diffusion–perfusion MRI in animal stroke models

Diffusion MRI (DWI) is an imaging technique that allows for the rapid and easy identification of regions of focal brain ischemia in animal stroke models (Fig. 9.1, see colour plate section). With DWI, ischemic lesions can be detected within minutes of stroke onset and the evolution of the ischemic lesion can be followed both temporally and spatially.[12] With serial DWI imaging, the pattern of lesion growth can be assessed, e.g. the spread of the ischemic lesion from the basal ganglia to the cortex. Information about the severity of the ischemic lesion can also be derived because absolute values of the apparent diffusion coefficient (ADC) can be determined. The precise derivation of low ADC values in focal ischemic brain injury remains uncertain, but the most likely explanation is the development of cytotoxic edema secondary to high-energy metabolism failure.[13] This energy failure leads to loss of ion homeostasis and an influx of extracellular water into the cell, i.e. cytotoxic edema. It appears that lower ADC values are associated with a greater degree of ischemic injury and less chance for reversibility with an appropriate and timely intervention. Rats have been the species most widely studied in DWI animal stroke studies and these experiments have provided much valuable information about stroke pathophysiology and temporal characteristics.

DWI animal stroke studies are providing information about the development of secondary lesions after successful reperfusion, so-called reperfusion injury. With early reperfusion, either with a thrombolytic drug or by mechanical reperfusion, several laboratories have demonstrated that initially detected ADC abnormalities can be reversed.[14,15] However, a few hours later secondary declines in ADC values are observed, occurring initially in regions where the initial ADC declines were most severe (Fig. 9.2, see colour plate section). By 12 hours after reperfusion, the secondary DWI lesion volumes are approximately 50% of the volume observed prior to reperfusion.[16] This lesion volume continues to increase, becoming almost the same as the volume observed during occlusion by 24

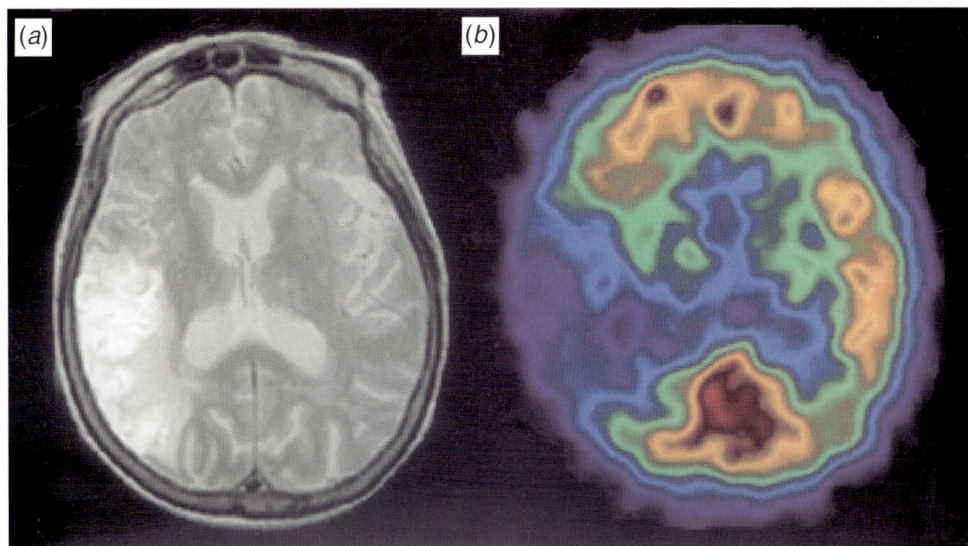

Fig. 2.4. Perfusion SPECT delineates regions of hypoperfusion. (a) T_2-weighted imaging (T_2-WI) and (b) single photon emission computed tomography (SPECT) in a patient imaged at 97 days. A hyperintense region of infarction is visible in the right middle cerebral artery territory on T_2-WI with a corresponding region of hypoperfusion on SPECT.

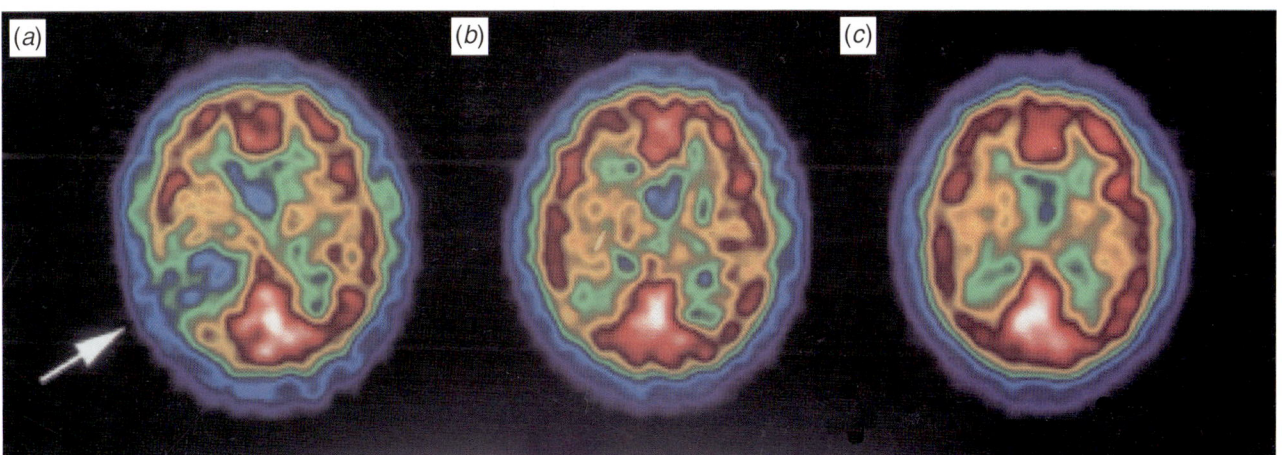

Fig. 2.5. Serial single photon emission computed tomography (SPECT) studies can show spontaneous and therapy-induced perfusion changes over time. (a) ^{99}Tc-HMPAO SPECT studies at 3.5 hours showing right middle cerebral artery territory hypoperfusion (arrow). (b) At 100 hours the hypoperfusion deficit has largely resolved, consistent with early reperfusion. (c) At 99 days the early reperfusion has been maintained. Thus the early reperfusion was into tissue that had not yet infarcted (nutritional reperfusion).

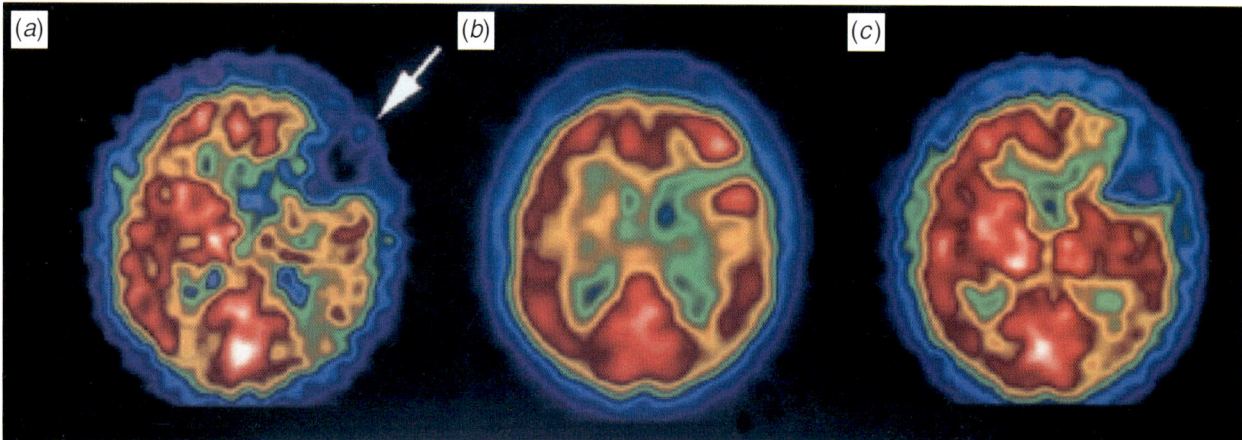

Fig. 2.6. Perfusion SPECT is unable to identify hypoperfused but potentially viable tissue of the ischemic penumbra. (*a*) ^{99}Tc-HMPAO SPECT studies at 10.5 hours showing a region of left frontal hypoperfusion deficit (arrow). (*b*) At 30 hours, the hypoperfusion deficit has largely resolved, consistent with early reperfusion. (*c*) At 95 days, the hypoperfusion deficit has reappeared. Thus, the early reperfusion was not maintained at outcome and can therefore be presumed to have been non-nutritional to the ischemic tissues.

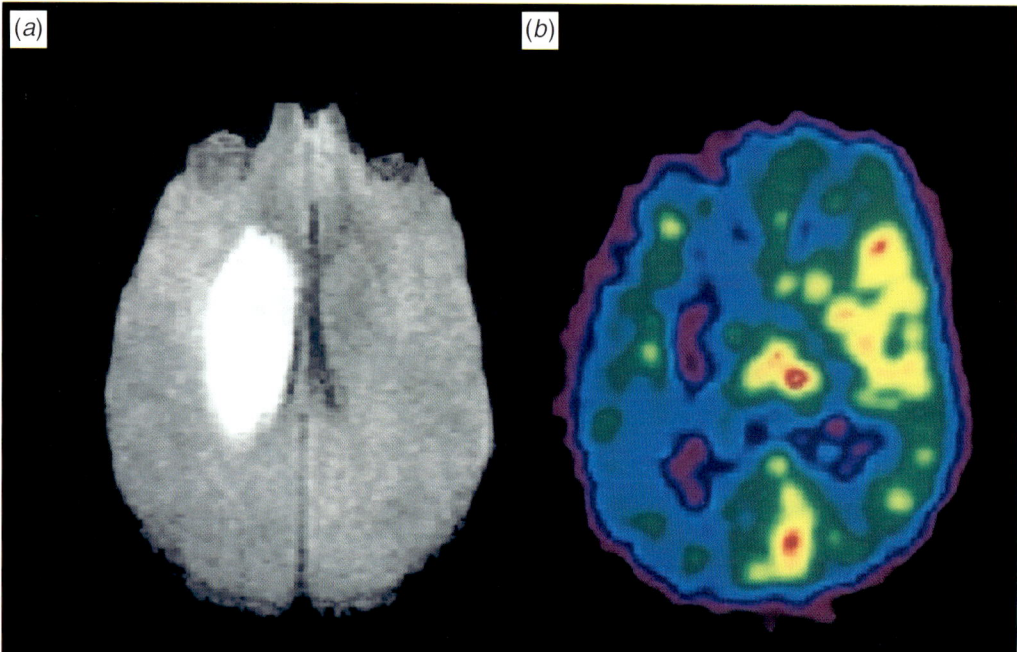

Fig. 2.7. Positron emission tomography (PET) and diffusion-weighted images (DWI) obtained at 3 days after stroke onset demonstrates a moderate right striatocapsular infarct on DWI with surrounding hypoperfusion on $H_2^{15}O$ cerebral blood flow PET. (Images provided by Drs JSR Markus and P Wright, Austin and Repatriation Medical Centre, Heidelberg, Australia.)

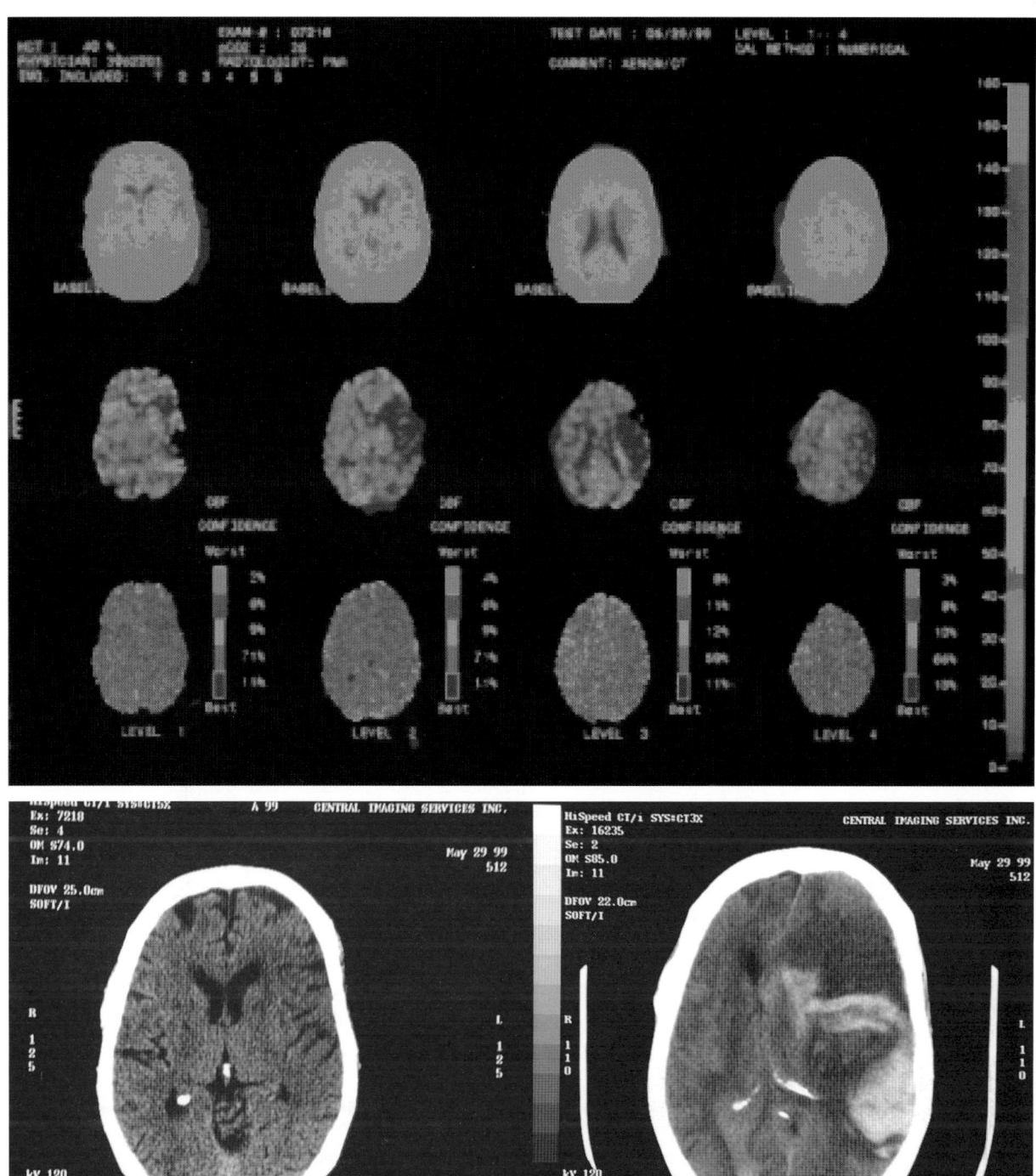

Fig. 4.1. The pretreatment XeCT CBF study with the pretreatment and post-treatment CT in a case of severe hypoperfusion with a median T-qCBF in the left MCA territory of 9.6 ml/100 g per min and a F-qCBF of 6.1 ml/100 g per min treated with combined i.v. t-PA and i.a. t-PA which resulted in symptomatic hemorrhagic conversion and death.

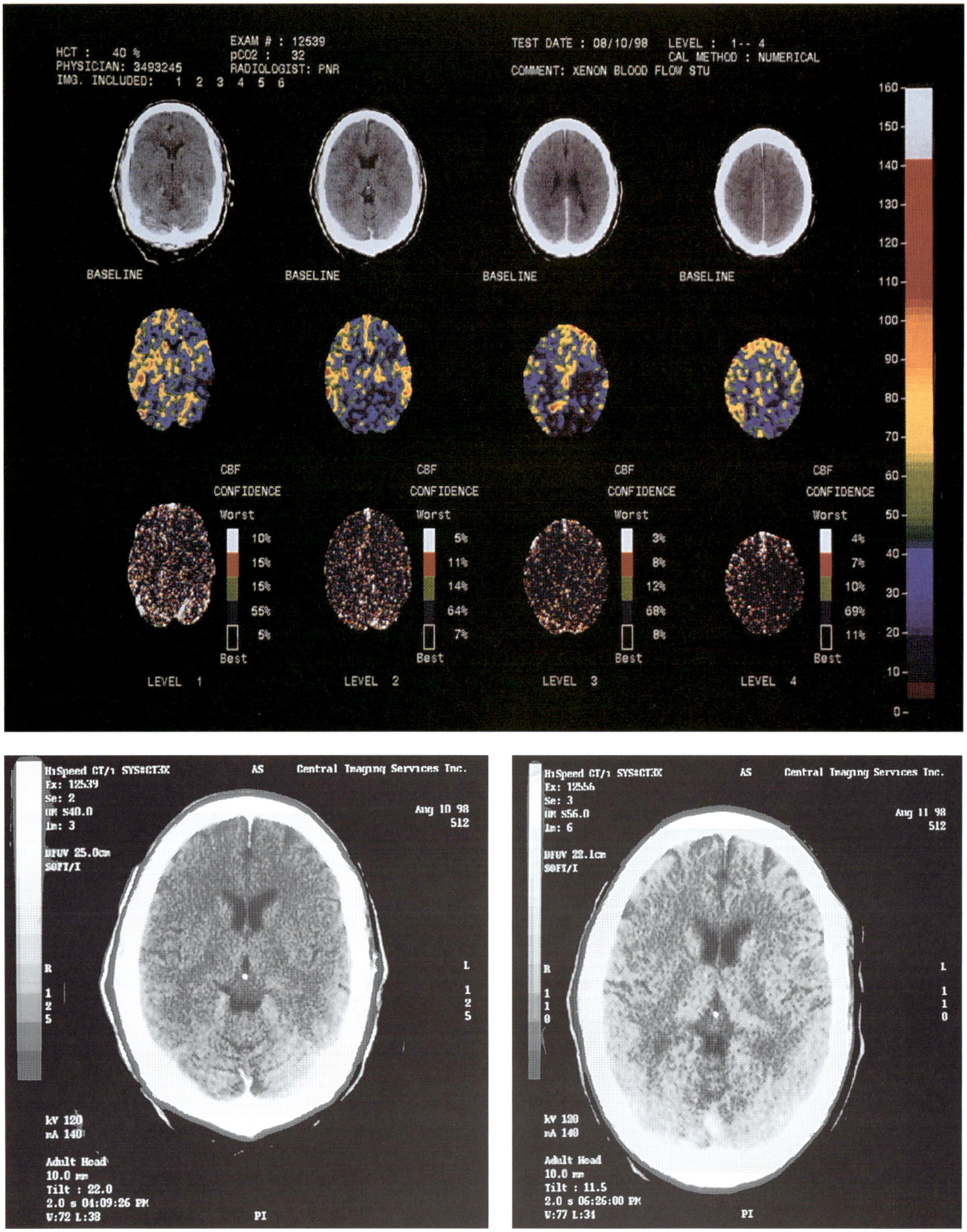

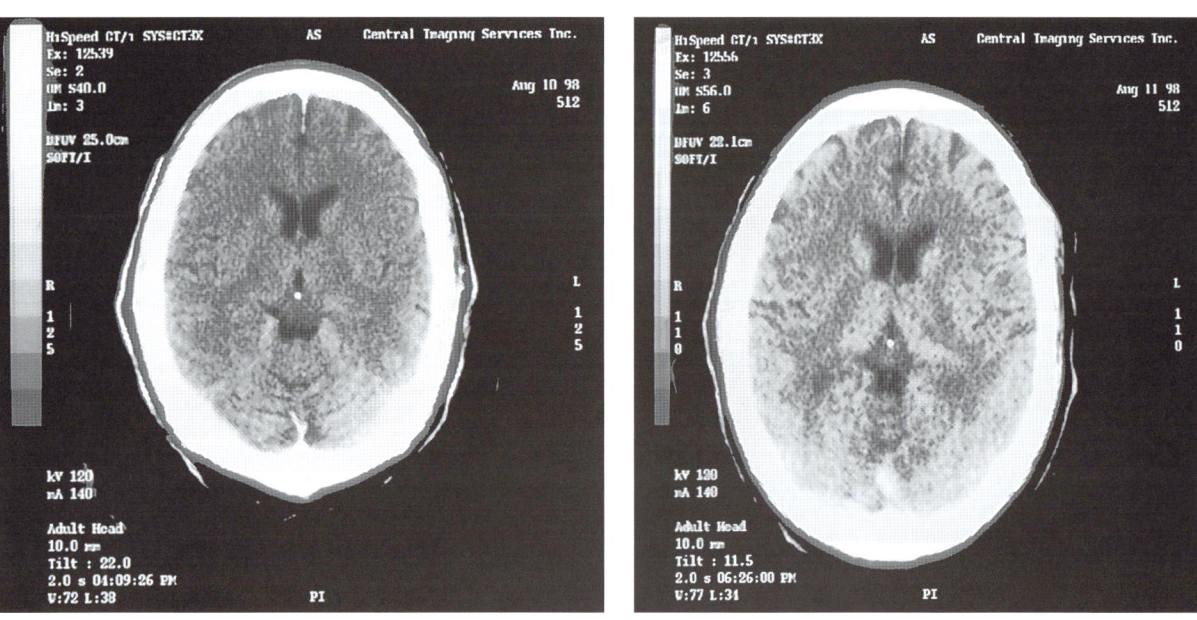

Fig. 4.2. The pretreatment XeCT CBF study with pretreatment and post-treatment CT in a case of mild hypoperfusion with a median T-qCBF in the left MCA territory of 39.4 ml/100 g per min and a F-qCBF of 30.7 ml/100g per min treated with i.v. t-PA (Modified Rankin at discharge equalled 0–1; no or minimal disability.)

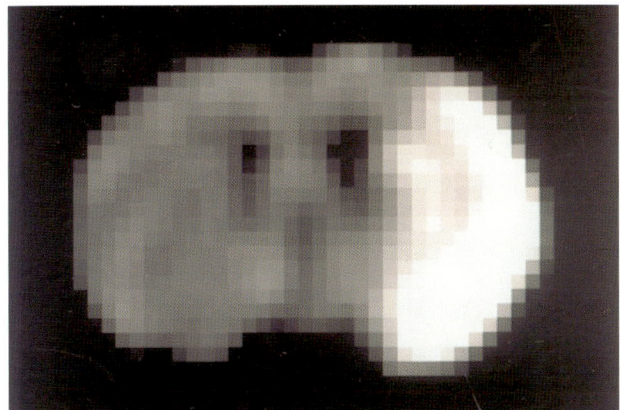

Fig. 9.1. A diffusion MRI in a rat 30 minutes after the onset of focal brain ischemia induced by the suture occlusion method. A large region of hyperintensity is seen in the left middle cerebral artery territory.

Fig. 9.2. During temporary focal ischemia, reduced apparent diffusion coefficient values are seen in the left middle cerebral artery territory (left panel). These revert to normal 90 minutes after reperfusion (centre panel) but secondary declines are seen 12 hours later (right panel).

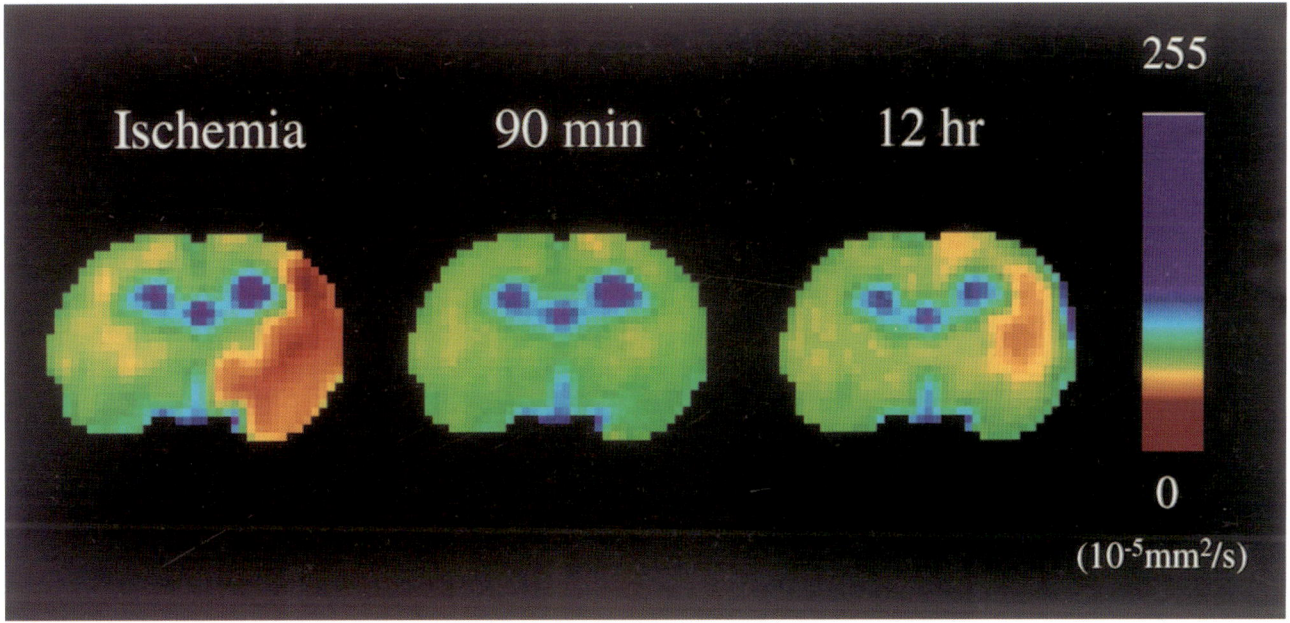

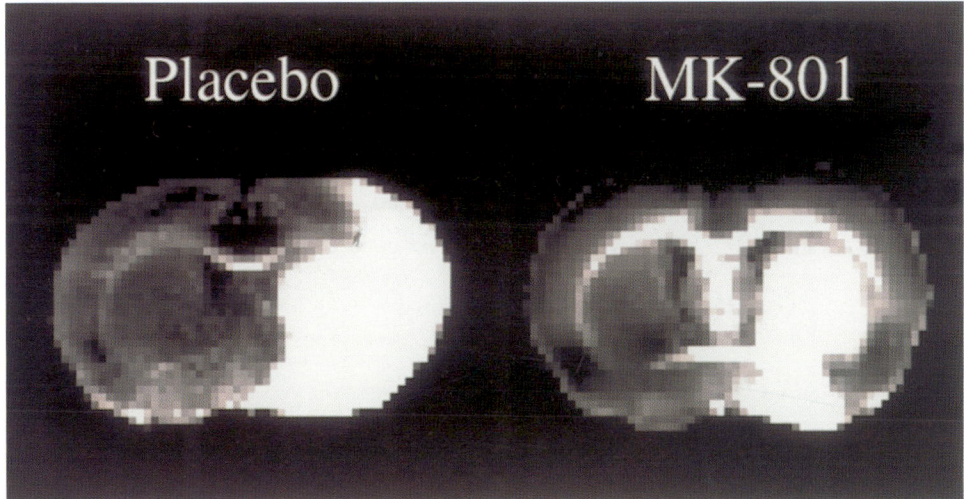

Fig. 9.3. Diffusion MRI studies from an animal treated with MK-801 and placebo showing a smaller region of hyperintensity in the treated animal.

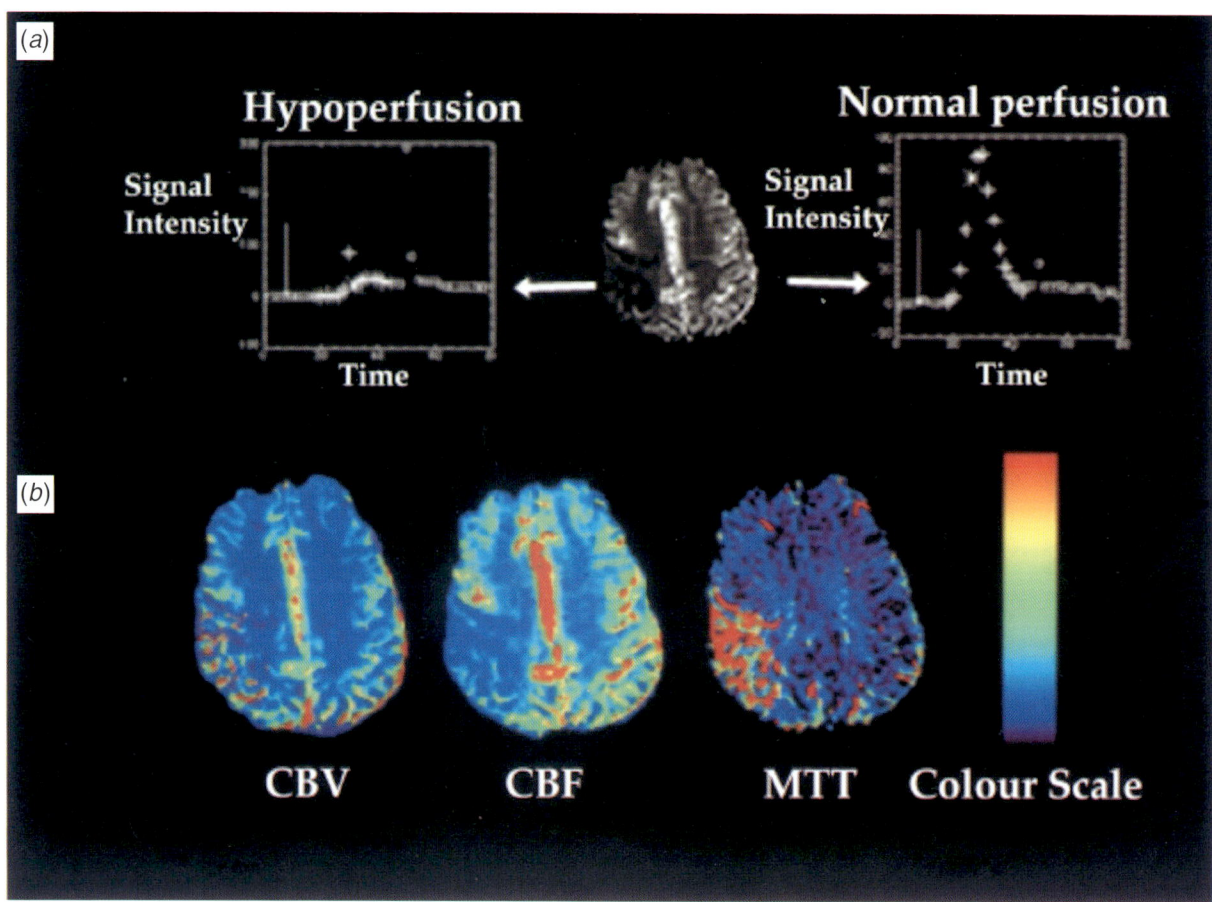

Fig. 14.3. (*a*) Perfusion-weighted imaging. Comparison of signal intensity vs. time curves during injection of Gd-DTPA in hypoperfused (left) and normally perfused tissue (right). Note that there is little reduction in signal intensity as the contrast bolus passes through the hypoperfused region. (*b*) Colour PWI maps generated from the same patient. Note reduced CBF and prolonged MTT in the inferior division of the right MCA.

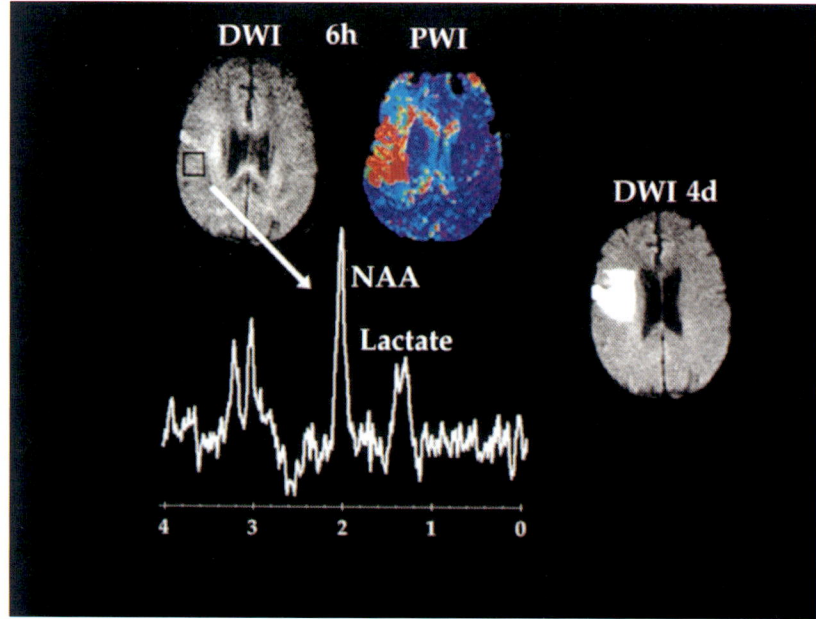

Fig. 14.13. MRS of the penumbra. Single voxel placed in the region of PWI > DWI mismatch at 6 hours after stroke onset shows intact NAA but lactate is present indicating ischemia despite no diffusion lesion being visible. This region consequently progressed to infarction (DWI at 4 days after stroke onset on right).

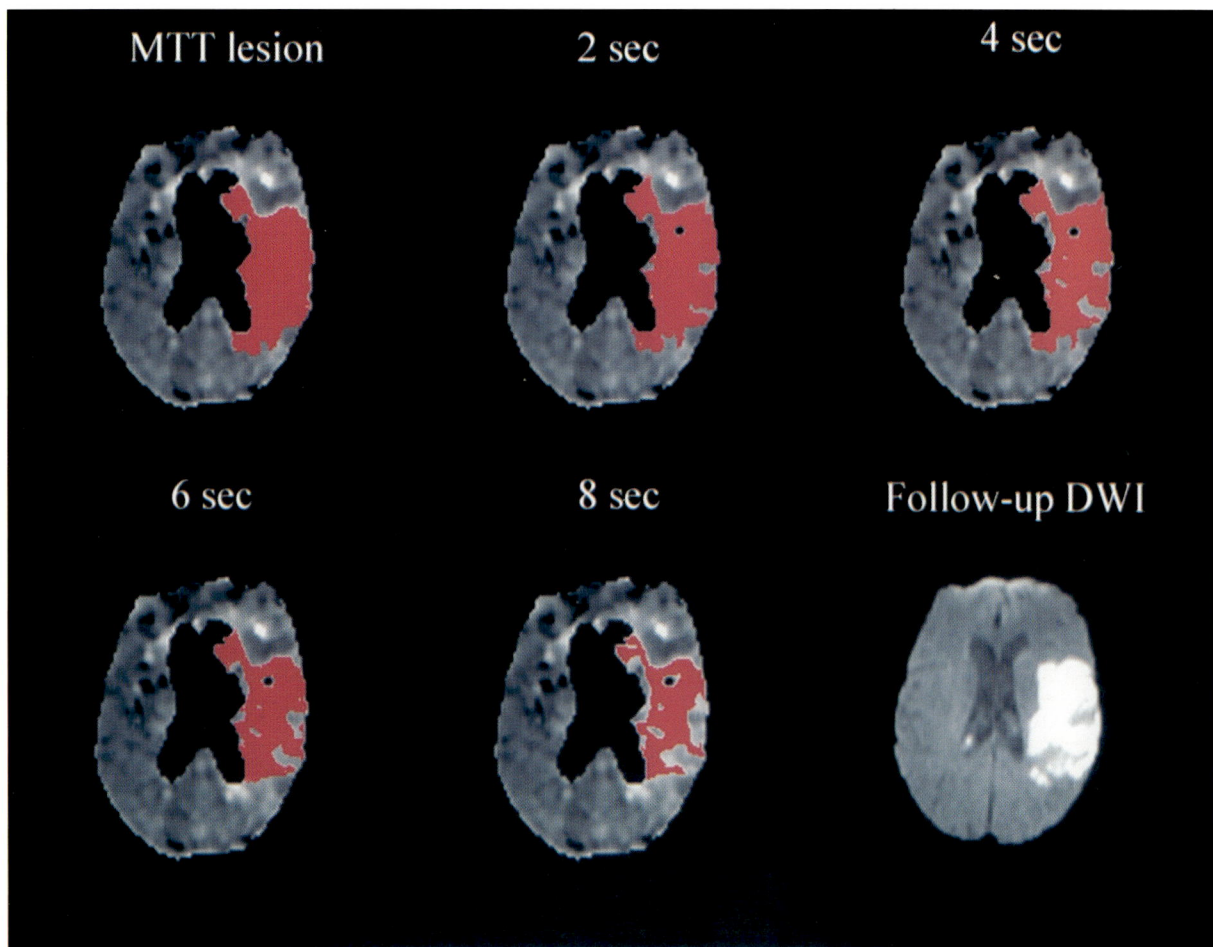

Fig. 16.2. A graded analysis of the MTT lesion may distinguish tissue at risk of infarction from hypoperfused tissue that is not at risk of infarction. Both the manually outlined MTT lesion and the MTT lesion with an increase of 2 s compared to the contralateral side overestimate the final infarct volume.

Fig. 19.1. (opposite) FMRI statistical parametric map and time course MR signal intensity analysis of a touch discrimination study in a recovered stroke patient. The FMRI data was obtained during a controlled touch discrimination experiment performed by the right 'sensory recovered' hand, 6 months poststroke. The study was conducted on a 1.5 Tesla Siemens Vision MR scanner. In (a)–(c), two axial brain slices including the primary somatosensory cortex (SI, top slice) and secondary somatosensory cortex (SII, bottom slice) are shown. (a) Statistical parametric map t-test analysis (SPM) of raw functional data (unthresholded). (b) SPM of significant sites of functional activation shown on the 1.5 tesla echoplanar images at $p_{uncorrected} < 0.005$. (c) SPM overlaid on anatomical images obtained at the same session. Activation is evident in the hand region of the left postcentral gyrus (SI; lesioned hemisphere) and left Sylvian fissure (SII), as would be expected based on findings from healthy volunteers. (d) Signal intensity time course shown in the large graph relates to a selected voxel of statistically significant activation, as indicated in the image to the left. The relative MR signal intensity (y-axis; yellow lines) is shown over time (x-axis; number of whole brain acquisitions, 1 per 10 seconds). The red blocks depict the task conditions (sensory stimulation) alternating with rest in this blocked trial paradigm. Signal intensity is higher during the touch discrimination epochs and changes of approximately 5% are evident between task and rest conditions. Time course analysis of the selected voxel may also be interpreted relative to that of surrounding voxels as shown

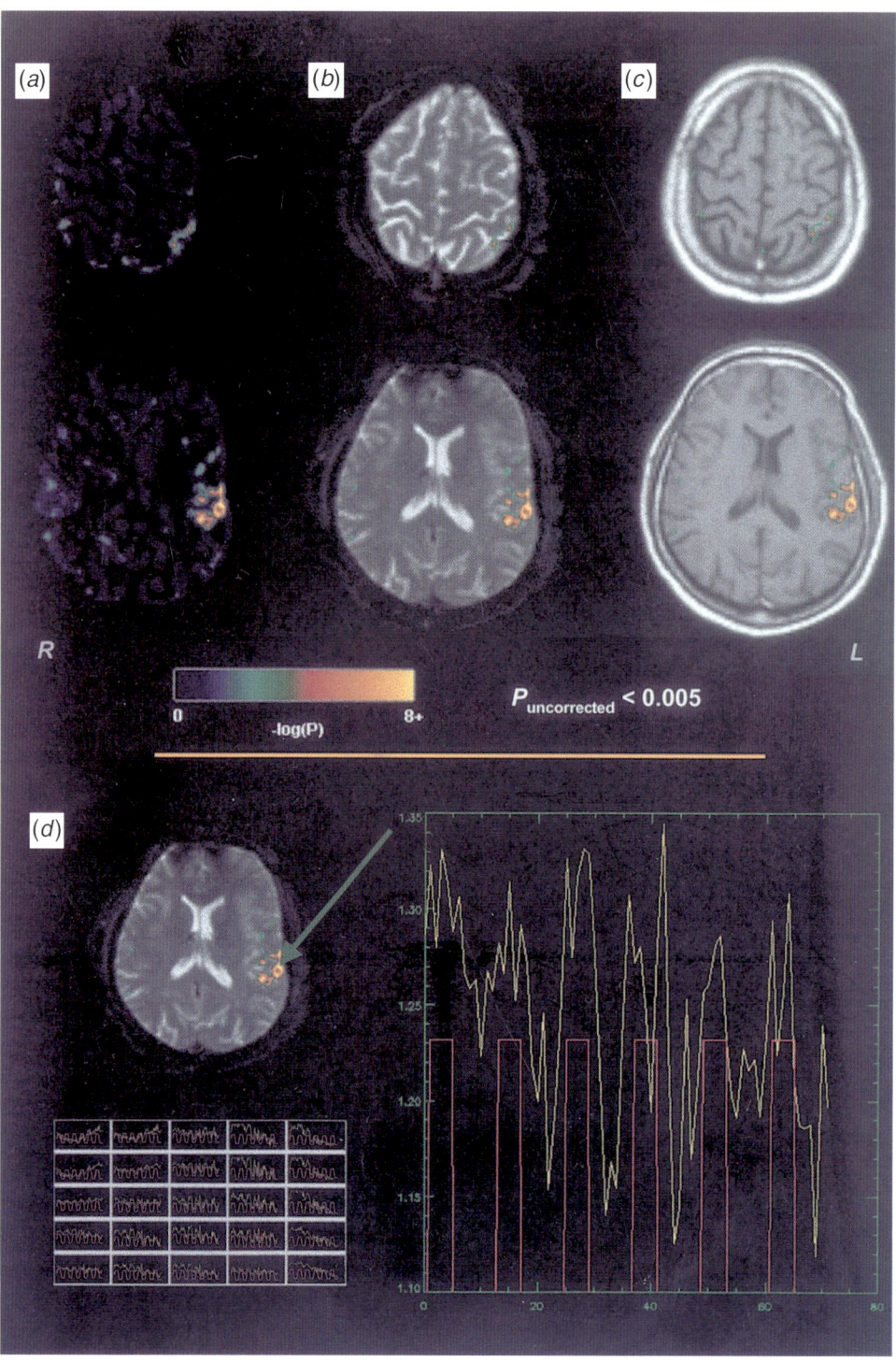

in the montage of graphs (bottom left). The large graph corresponds to the centre graph of this montage. (Figure produced by Carey. Study conducted by Carey, Abbott, Jackson, Syngeniotis and Donnan at the National Stroke Research Institute and Brain Research Institute (BRI), Melbourne, Australia. MR imaging was conducted with the assistance of the Radiology Department at Monash Medical Centre. Image analysis performed using iBrain® software, developed at the BRI.)

hours after reperfusion and this late secondary ischemic lesion is highly correlated with the histologically confirmed infarct volume. The secondary ADC decline observed after reperfusion might in part represent reperfusion injury, but the situation may be more complex. A recent histology study demonstrated that ischemic regions where ADC values had returned to normal still have neuronal and glial cell abnormalities that tend to worsen over time.[17] This observation implies that a normal DWI study after reperfusion does not necessarily indicate tissue normalization, although late secondary deterioration appears to occur even without complete reperfusion related ADC recovery. The mechanisms for the secondary ADC declines and tissue injury are not clearly established, but likely contributors are secondary energy failure, mitochondrial respiratory function deterioration and apoptosis. Secondary ADC declines is not limited to animal studies. The UCLA group has seen such secondary ADC declines in approximately half of their patients after successful intra-arterial thrombolysis.[18] The clinical significance of these secondary ADC declines remains to be firmly established, but a worse clinical outcome is likely when this occurs.

Perfusion MRI (PWI) is the other MRI modality that has been widely applied in animal stroke models. The two techniques used to acquire PWI are the bolus-tracking method and the arterial spin-labelling technique.[19] Bolus-tracking PWI is much more commonly used and requires the injection of a contrast agent that has susceptibility effects, impairing the acquisition of T_2^*-signal. Multiple, repetitive images are obtained over a 30-second time interval to generate a signal intensity curve. This signal intensity curve can then be used to obtain a number of perfusion-related parameters including the mean transit time, cerebral blood volume and an estimate of the cerebral blood flow.[20] With accurate determination of the arterial input function and deconvolution techniques, more precise measurements of cerebral blood flow can be obtained. In clinical practice or animal studies, perfusion maps based upon the mean transit time or time to peak of the signal intensity curve are commonly employed. These PWI maps can be used to document reduced perfusion in the ischemic region, the severity of the perfusion abnormality and the return of adequate perfusion with mechanical or thrombolytic intervention in an animal model or stroke patient.

Combining information from PWI with DWI provides a powerful tool for the study of acute ischemic stroke in animal models. PWI changes can be related to ADC declines to study the relationship between the severity of perfusion changes to the development and severity of tissue injury. Using the two MRI parameters together can provide insights about the existence or lack of an ischemic penumbra. An estimate of the ischemic penumbra would be hypoperfused tissue on PWI that is not yet abnormal on DWI.[21] This region is the so-called 'diffusion–perfusion mismatch' and the presence of a DWI–PWI mismatch is being used currently in clinical stroke trials to enrich patient selection for enrolment. The hypothesis being that mismatch patients are those likely to still have an ischemic penumbra and a better chance to respond to therapeutic intervention. In a preliminary animal study of the DWI–PWI mismatch, it was observed that with the permanent suture occlusion model the mismatch was no longer significantly different by 90 minutes after occlusion and that it had essentially disappeared by 120 minutes.[22] There was a significant mismatch at 30 and 60 minutes after occlusion. In another group of animals who were mechanically reperfused after 60 minutes of temporary occlusion, the ischemic lesion volume on DWI did not increase after reperfusion. This observation supports the concept that the hypoperfused region with normal ADC values can be salvaged with timely reperfusion. The DWI–PWI mismatch is likely only a rough approximation of the ischemic penumbra because some of the abnormal region on DWI can be reversed and infarction prevented. A more precise definition of the ischemic penumbra on DWI–PWI will likely require determination of absolute ADC, cerebral blood flow and perhaps other MRI parameters. These determinations will come from successful treatment experiments initially in animal stroke models and later in stroke patients.

Preclinical evaluation of new stroke therapies

Animal stroke models are used to assess in vivo therapeutic responses of novel pharmaceuticals to determine if the agents have activity in focal brain ischemia. A large variety of stroke models are used to evaluate therapy in several different animal species. None of the animal stroke models precisely reproduce the clinical conditions associated with ischemic stroke. Therefore, relating experiences with these animal stroke models to human stroke requires an extrapolation and extension of the results. The typical paradigm employed for the development of neuroprotective stroke drugs is to develop a molecule targeted at one or more aspects of the cascade of ischemic injury. The drug is then screened for obvious toxicology problems such as blood pressure lowering effects, effects on body–brain temperature, cancer inducing effects and other major side effects. Non-toxic agents are then applied to rodent models of focal brain ischemia and the recommended initial experiments usually are performed in a rat permanent ischemia model with a short period of poststroke survival (24–48 hours). Currently, the most commonly used rat stroke model is the suture occlusion model that can be used for both permanent and temporary occlusion experiments.[23] Dose ranging is then preformed around the initially effective dose to define the minimally effective and maximally tolerated dose. The endpoint of these investigations is infarct size as determined by histological evaluation. Functional and behavioural endpoints should also be evaluated, especially as the length of survival is extended to determine if initial treatment effects are maintained over an extended time period. The time to initiation of treatment is another important variable that should be assessed in the animal models. Drugs that are only effective when given before or shortly after stroke onset are not attractive candidates for clinical development for practical and financial reasons. A short time window will make clinical trial design difficult and a short time window for initiation of therapy will only have a small market, if proven to be successful. Drugs that are shown to be effective with a reasonable time window in rats should then be evaluated in higher species such as cats and/or primates. Determining effectiveness in higher species with a time window to initiation of treatment 1–2 hours or longer after stroke onset will likely provide more reassurance of drug activity than relying solely on rodent data. Experiments employing cats and especially primates are difficult, time consuming and expensive to perform. The data derived are very likely to be worth the effort because they will provide important clues as to how best to proceed with clinical development of the drug. However, the leap from animal studies that focus on infarct size and to some extent behavioural measures to clinical trials that use neurological and/or functional handicap measures remains problematic. Using diffusion–perfusion MRI in animal stroke models and clinical drug development may help to bridge the gap.

Using diffusion–perfusion MRI in animals to assess therapy

The ability of diffusion–perfusion MRI to rapidly evaluate stroke in vivo provides a powerful tool to assess the effects of neuroprotective and thrombolytic therapies in animal stroke models. Much more experience with diffusion MRI to assess effects of neuroprotectants is currently available. The first report using diffusion MRI to evaluate the sodium–calcium channel modulator, RS-87476, appeared in 1991, demonstrating that an in vivo treatment effect could be detected.[24] Subsequently, reduction of ischemic lesion size in vivo on diffusion MRI with the NMDA antagonist, Cerestat, was observed in both temporary and permanent rat focal ischemia models.[25] The treatment effect observed during the 3 hours of imaging and drug infusion was somewhat larger than the reduction of infarct size observed histologically. This observation was then used to model what the likely optimal infusion time of Cerestat should have been to maintain maximal neuroprotective benefits. Other neuroprotective drugs have also been evaluated with diffusion MRI with the detection of significant in vivo treatment effects that were confirmed by delayed histological confirmation of infarct size reductions (Fig. 9.3, see colour plate section). Another important piece of information that can be obtained with the use of diffusion MRI to evaluate neuroprotective therapeutic effects is the time course of activity. Two groups evaluated the glycine antagonist, ZD9379, and an interesting and unexpected delayed treatment effect was observed. When therapy with ZD9379 was initiated 30 minutes after permanent middle cerebral artery occlusion with the suture model, Takano et al. did not observe any obvious difference in lesion volume between the treated and placebo groups until 3.5 hours after occlusion when a trend towards a smaller ischemic lesion volume was seen in the ZD9379 group (Fig. 9.4).[26] The diffusion imaging ceased at that time point, but at 24 hours after stroke onset the treated group had a 43% smaller ischemic lesion volume by histological analysis. This experiment suggested a delayed treatment effect with ZD9379 that would not have been appreciated with analysis of delayed, histological infarct size alone. Interestingly, the delayed tissue salvage occurred primarily in the border zone between the middle and anterior cerebral arteries, a region of modest blood flow decline thought to represent a portion of the ischemic penumbra in the suture occlusion model. In a second reported treatment experiment with ZD9379, Qiu et al. initiated treatment immediately after stroke onset and imaged for 6 hours with diffusion MRI.[27] No significant difference of ischemic lesion size was detected at 2.5 hours after stroke onset, but at 6 hours ischemic lesion size was 41% smaller in the ZD9379 group. This experiment with a longer imaging time window supports the implications of the first experiment that ZD9379 had a delayed treatment effect and was able to reverse initially abnormal ADC regions.

PWI has been used to evaluate reperfusion effects of both mechanical reperfusion and thrombolytic therapy. The suture occlusion model is amenable to reperfusion experiments by withdrawal of the suture and this can be accomplished in the MRI unit to allow for rapid and continuous assessment. PWI can be used to confirm successful suture withdrawal and to quantify the percentage of initially hypoperfused tissue that is subsequently ade-

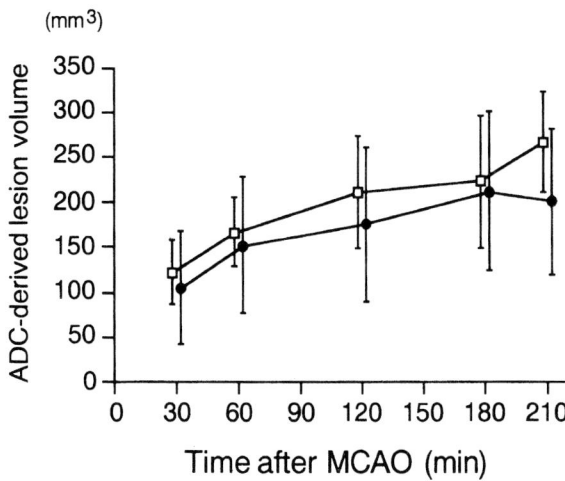

Fig. 9.4. Ischemic lesion volumes are similar in the placebo and ZD9379 groups for the first 3 hours after stroke onset. At 3.5 hours the volume in the treated group (closed circles) begins to diverge from the volume in the placebo group (open squares)(reproduced with permission, *Stroke* 1997; 28: 1255–1263).

quately reperfused. Combining PWI with DWI allows for assessment of the effects of reperfusion on ischemic lesion size. Several groups have reported that mechanical reperfusion by withdrawal of the suture occluder 30–60 minutes after stroke onset is associated with a marked reduction in the hypoperfused zone and shrinkage of the ischemic region on DWI.[15,28] Withdrawal of the suture occluder 90 minutes or later after stroke onset is typically associated with adequate reperfusion on PWI, but little or no reduction of the ischemic lesion on DWI.

Several reports have appeared concerning the use of PWI and DWI to assess thrombolytic therapy in animal stroke models. Jiang et al. evaluated rt-PA in a rat embolic stroke model.[14] Initiating treatment with rt-PA 1 hour after embolization was associated with significant reduction in the hypoperfused region on PWI and an improvement in the extent of the ischemic lesion determined by a combination of DWI and T_2 findings. Treatment effects of ProUrokinase were evaluated by another group in a rat embolic model.[29] Pro-urokinase was given either intravenously or intra-arterially beginning 30 minutes after embolization. Frequent PWI and DWI

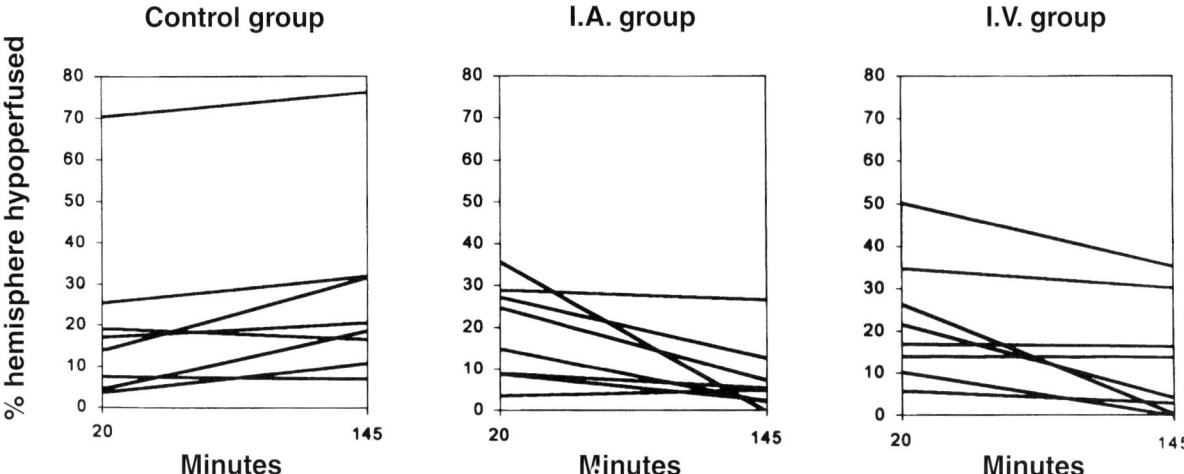

Fig. 9.5. The percentage of the ischemic hemisphere that is hypoperfused declined in most animals treated with intra-arterial (I.A.) or intravenous (I.V.) pro-urokinase (reproduced with permission, *Neurology* 1998; 50: 870–875).

studies were performed to evaluate the effects of treatment on brain perfusion and ischemic lesion growth. In comparison to the vehicle group, both pro-urokinase treatment approaches were observed to significantly improve perfusion and to maintain the ischemic lesion at the same size as before treatment began (Fig. 9.5). In the vehicle group, a significant increase of ischemic lesion size on DWI occurred over time, and the postmortem ischemic lesion size was significantly larger in this group at 24 hours than in the two pro-urokinase groups. Combining PWI and DWI in temporary occlusion models evaluating neuroprotective drugs may also be useful. A treatment experiment with an endothelin antagonist in a 90-minute temporary occlusion experiment demonstrated an interesting result. The 24-hour infarct volume demonstrated by histology was significantly smaller in the treated group as compared to the placebo group.[30] Interestingly, PWI disclosed that only 60% of the animals adequately reperfused after withdrawal of the suture occluder and it was these successfully reperfused animals that demonstrated a neuroprotective effect. This result suggested that the endothelin antagonist would not be effective in permanently occluded animals and, indeed, a subsequent experiment with a permanent occlusion model did not demonstrate a significant reduction of ischemic lesion size. Without the combination of PWI and DWI, the true efficacy of the drug would not have been realized in the temporary occlusion experiment. The power of using both PWI and DWI in animal treatment is thus apparent.

Conclusions

The limited success so far in the development of acute stroke therapies strongly suggests that new approaches to the drug development process will be necessary to enhance the likelihood of finding effective therapies in the future. Diffusion–perfusion MRI in animal stroke models should be valuable in this process for a number of reasons. These MRI techniques provide important information about in vivo drug activity that can help to confirm the site of action, time window of treatment effect and appropriate duration of therapy. The experience in animals can then be directly transferred to early clinical trials where the same endpoints can be evaluated, confirming or refuting the preclinical results in stroke patients. The use of diffusion–perfusion MRI both in preclinical testing and in clinical development of acute stroke therapies will likely continue to expand, especially once the MRI modalities provide support for the approval of a new acute stroke therapy. Additionally, their utility will also increase as we move into the multi-therapy era of acute stroke therapy when combinations of neuroprotective and thrombolytic therapy are employed together to maximize outcome.

REFERENCES

1. The National Institute of Neurological Disorders and Stroke rt-PA Stroke Study Group. Tissue plasminogen activator for acute ischemic stroke. *N Engl J Med* 1995; 333: 1581–1587.
2. Sherman DG, Atkinson RP, Chippendale T et al. for the STAT participants. Intravenous ancrod treatment for acute ischemic stroke. *J Am Med Assoc* 2000; 283: 2395–2403.
3. Furlan AJ, Higashida R, Wechsler L et al. for the PROACT Investigators. Intra-arterial prourokinase for acute ischemic stroke. The PROACT-II Study. *J Am Med Assoc* 1999; 282: 2003–2011.
4. Fisher M, Schaebitz W. An overview of acute stroke therapy. *Arch Neurol* 2000; 160: 3196–4006.
5. Li F, Irie K, Anwer U, Fisher M. Delayed triphenyltetrazolium chloride staining remains useful for evaluating cerebral infarct volume in a rat stroke model. *J Cereb Blood Flow Metab* 1997; 12: 1132–1135.
6. Stroke Therapy Academic Industry Roundtable. Recommendations for standards regarding preclinical neuroprotective and restorative therapies. *Stroke* 1999; 30: 2752–2758.
7. Marshall JWB, Duffin KJ, Green AR, Ridley RM. NXY-059, a free radical-trapping agent substantially lessens the functional disability resulting from cerebral ischemia in a primate species. *Stroke* 2001; 32: 190–198.
8. Davis SM. Endpoints and statistical concerns. In Fisher M, ed., *Stroke Therapy*, Butterworth-Heinemann, Boston, 2000.
9. Neumann-Haefelin T, Moseley ME, Albers GW et al. New magnetic resonance imaging methods for cerebrovascular disease: Emerging clinical applications. *Ann Neurol* 2000; 31: 559–570.
10. Warach S, Pettigrew LC, Dashe JF et al. Effect of citicoline on ischemic lesions as measured by diffusion-weighted MRI. *Ann Neurol* 2000; 48: 713–772.
11. Schellinger FD, Jansen O, Fiebach JB et al. Monitoring intravenous recombinant tissue plasminogen activator thrombolysis for acute ischemic stroke with diffusion and perfusion MRI. *Stroke* 2000; 31: 1318–1328.
12. Reith W, Hasegowa Y, Latour LL et al. Multislice diffusion mapping for 3–D evolution of cerebral ischemia in a rat stroke model. *Neurology* 1995; 45: 172–177.
13. Latour LL, Svoboda K, Mitra PP, Sotak CH. Time-dependent diffusion of water in biological model system. *Proc Natl Acad Sci USA* 1994; 91: 1229–1233.
14. Jeans Q, Zhang RL, Zhang ZB et al. Diffusion, T2, and perfusion-weighted magnetic resonance imaging of middle cerebral artery embolic stroke and recombinant tissue plasminogen activator intervention in the rat. *J Cereb Blood Flow Metab* 1998; 18: 758–767.
15. Li F, Haw S, Tatlisumak T et al. Reversal of acute apparent diffusion coefficient abnormalities and delayed neuronal death following transient focal cerebral ischemia in rats. *Ann Neurol* 1999; 46: 333–342.
16. Li F, Liu KF, Silva MD et al. Secondary decline in apparent diffusion coefficient and neurological outcome after a short period of focal brain ischemia in rats. *Ann Neurol* 2000; 48: 236–244.
17. Li F, Liu KF, Silva MD et al. Acute normalization of the apparent diffusion coefficient of water is not associated with reversal of astrocytic swelling and neuronal shrinkage. *Am J Neuroradiol* 2002; 23: 180–188.
18. Kidwell CS, Saver JL, Mattiello J et al. Thrombolytic reversal of acute human cerebral ischemic injury shown by diffusion/ perfusion magnetic resonance imaging. *Ann Neurol* 2000; 47: 462–469.
19. Rosen BR, Belliveau JW, Vevea JM, Brady TJ. Perfusion imaging with NMR contrast agents. *Magn Reson Med* 1990; 14: 249–265.
20. Sorensen AG, Copen WA, Ostergaard L et al. Hyperacute stroke: simultaneous measurement of relative cerebral blood volume, relative cerebral blood flow, and mean tissue transit time. *Radiology* 1999; 212: 519–527.
21. Neuman-Hacflin T, Wittsack H-J, Wenerski F et al. Diffusion and perfusion-weighted MRI: The DWI/PWI mismatch region in acute stroke. *Stroke* 1999; 30: 1591–1597.
22. Omae T, Silva M, Mayzel O et al. Temporal evolution of diffusion-perfusion mismatch in a rat stroke model. *Stroke* 2001; 32: 352.
23. Laing RJ, Jablonski J, Laing RW. Middle cerebral artery occlusion in the rat. Which method works best? *Stroke* 1993; 294–298.
24. Kucharczyk KJ, Mintorovitch J, Moseley ME et al. Ischemic brain damage: reduction by sodium–calcium ion channel modulator RS-87476. *Radiology* 1991; 179: 221–227.

25 Minematsu K, Fisher M, Li L et al. Effects of a novel NMDA antagonist on experimental stroke rapidly and quantitatively assessed by diffusion-weighted MRI. *Neurology* 1993; 42: 397–403.

26 Takano K, Tatlisumak T, Formato J et al. A glycine site antagonist attenuates infarct size in experimental focal ischemia: postmortem and diffusion mapping studies. *Stroke* 1997; 28: 1255–1263.

27 Qiu H, Hedlund CW, Gewalt SL, Benveniste H, Bare TM, Johnson GA. Progression of a focal ischemic lesion in a rat brain during treatment with a novel glycine NMDA antagonist. *JMRI* 1997; 7: 793–744.

28 Muller TB, Haraldseth D, Jones RA et al. Combined perfusion and diffusion-weighted magnetic resonance imaging in a rat model of reversible middle cerebral artery occlusion. *Stroke* 1995; 26: 451–458.

29 Takano K, Carano RAD, Tatlisumak T et al. The efficacy of intraarterial and intravenous Prourokinase in an embolic stroke model evaluated by diffusion–perfusion magnetic resonance imaging. *Neurology* 1998; 50: 870–875.

30 Tatlisumak T, Carano RAD, Takano K, Opgenorth TJ, Sotak CH, Fisher M. A novel endothelin antagonist, A-127722, attenuates ischemic lesion size in rats with temporary middle cerebral artery occlusion. *Stroke* 1998; 29: 850–858.

Localization of stroke syndromes using diffusion-weighted MR imaging (DWI)

Max Wintermark,[1] Marc Reichhart,[2] Reto Meuli[1] and Julien Bogousslavsky[2]

[1]Department of Diagnostic and Interventional Radiology and
[2]Department of Neurology, University Hospital (CHUV), 1011 Lausanne, Switzerland

Introduction

DWI is an MR imaging technique in which microscopic water motion is responsible for the contrast within the image.[1-5] DWI has assumed the role of a valuable imaging technique because it provides information that is not available on standard T_1- and T_2-weighted MR images. By showing hyperacute brain ischemia within minutes after stroke onset, diffusion-weighted imaging has gained importance in the assessment of stroke, whereas CT or T_2-weighted MR images become positive only after several, usually 5 or 6 hours after stroke onset. In a rodent model, sensitivity of diffusion-weighted imaging in the detection of acute infarction has amounted to 60% within 50 minutes and 100% within 2 hours after symptomatology onset.[6-12]

Clinical representations of DWI results

Diffusion of water molecules alters conventional T_1- and T_2-weighted MR imaging, because it induces a signal dephasing and a signal loss. On the other hand, through adequate MR sequences, this signal loss can be turned into a specific information, which constitutes the basis of DWI. Enhancement of the DWI signal is afforded by adding a bipolar gradient, which consists of two sequential pulses superimposed to the classical 90°–180° spin echo sequence. The first gradient pulse is applied between the 90° and the 180° pulses. Motion during and after this gradient pulse induces dephasing of the transverse magnetization of the static and mobile molecules. Both the 180° pulse and the second gradient pulse, which is the same size as the first but opposite in sign, rephase the stationary spins, but not the mobile molecules, thus resulting in substantial signal loss.[2-5]

Clinical practice uses different representations of the results of DWI data processing: diffusion-weighted images, DWI trace and ADC maps, which are all equivalent.

Diffusion of bipolar gradient pulses used to outline diffusion properties of matter is typically applied in one direction at a time. Because of anisotropic effects, data obtained in using a one-direction diffusion gradient only can give misleading information. Application of a diffusion gradient perpendicular (rather than parallel) to the orientation of a white matter tract results in a lower ADC measurement. If this particularity can be used in myelin fibre tractography, it may also be confusing and thus result in diagnostic pitfalls in the detection and delineation of cerebral ischemia. This is the reason why bipolar gradient pulses are usually applied along at least three orthogonal sampling directions, and the diffusion coefficients thus sampled allow for calculation of a DWI-trace, which represents the average of diffusion-weighted images in all three directions:

$$S = \left(S_0 \times e^{-\frac{TE}{T_2}} \right) \times e^{-b \times D}$$

in which the first term in brackets represents the 'T_2 shine-through effect', D the diffusion coefficient and *b* a factor describing the strength of bipolar gradient pulses. On a DWI trace, the anisotropy and orientation of myelin fibres are completely removed. Such images show small contrast between white and grey matter and, as discussed later, the diffusion coefficient of white matter is decreased in acute stroke to approximately the same extent as that of grey matter.[13–15]

The DWI trace is not solely the result of diffusion characteristics but also of the T_2 decay: some investigators have called this phenomenon the 'T_2 shine-through effect'.[16] One can get rid of this 'T_2 shine-through effect' through computing isotropic or directionally averaged diffusion coefficient (ADC) (Fig. 10.3). Admitting a single water compartment due to fast exchange across cell membranes, and thus a monoexponential decay in voxels, the ADC map can be calculated from at least two b values, typically 500 and 1000 $[s/mm^2]$. The ADC map shows relative signal intensities only due to differences in tissue diffusion.[14,16]

On ADC maps, tissues have an appearance opposite to that seen on the DWI trace, reflecting the negative exponent in the equation relating signal intensity to the ADC. Thus, CSF is hyperintense on ADC maps, whereas on a DWI trace, CSF is hypointense. On diffusion-weighted images, lesions with restricted water diffusion are hyperintense while they are hypointense on ADC maps.[14]

Information carried by a DWI trace and ADC maps are complementary. The DWI trace affords sharp delineation of pathologic processes, through both the removal of anisotropy of myelin fibres and the absence of contrast between grey and white matter while ADC maps allow one to get rid of the 'T_2 shine-through'.

DWI sensitivity to strokes according to their location

DWI is more accurate than CT in localizing ischemic lesions shortly after stroke onset. Admission CT does localize lesions correctly in only 53% of patients. On the other hand, conventional MRI correctly identifies acute cerebral ischemia in 71% to 80% of cases. With the addition of DWI, this

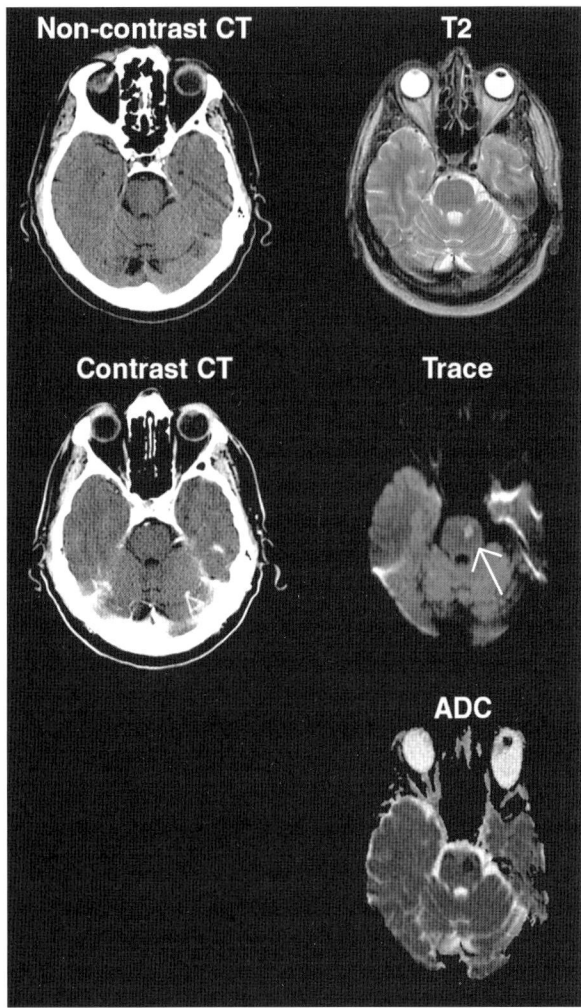

Fig. 10.1. 65-year-old male patient showing a right arm–leg hemisyndrome with a left face palsy, allowing for the suspicion of a left pontine ischemic lesion. The MR examination obtained 6 hours after onset relates the symptomatology to an acute left paramedian pontine ischemic stroke *(arrow)*, featuring hyperintensity on T_2-weighted image and DWI-trace, and hypointensity on the ADC map. Even retrospectively, this stroke could not be recognized on the admission non-contrast cerebral CT obtained 4 hours after stroke onset.

percentage increases to 94%. Interobserver agreement is better in DWI than in conventional MRI.[17–19]

DWI can show small lesions adjacent to the cerebrospinal fluid. The diagnosis of a small cortical or brainstem infarct may be difficult on T_2–WI images while DWI (Figs. 10.1–10.3) easily depicts such lesions. Fluid attenuated inversion recovery (FLAIR)

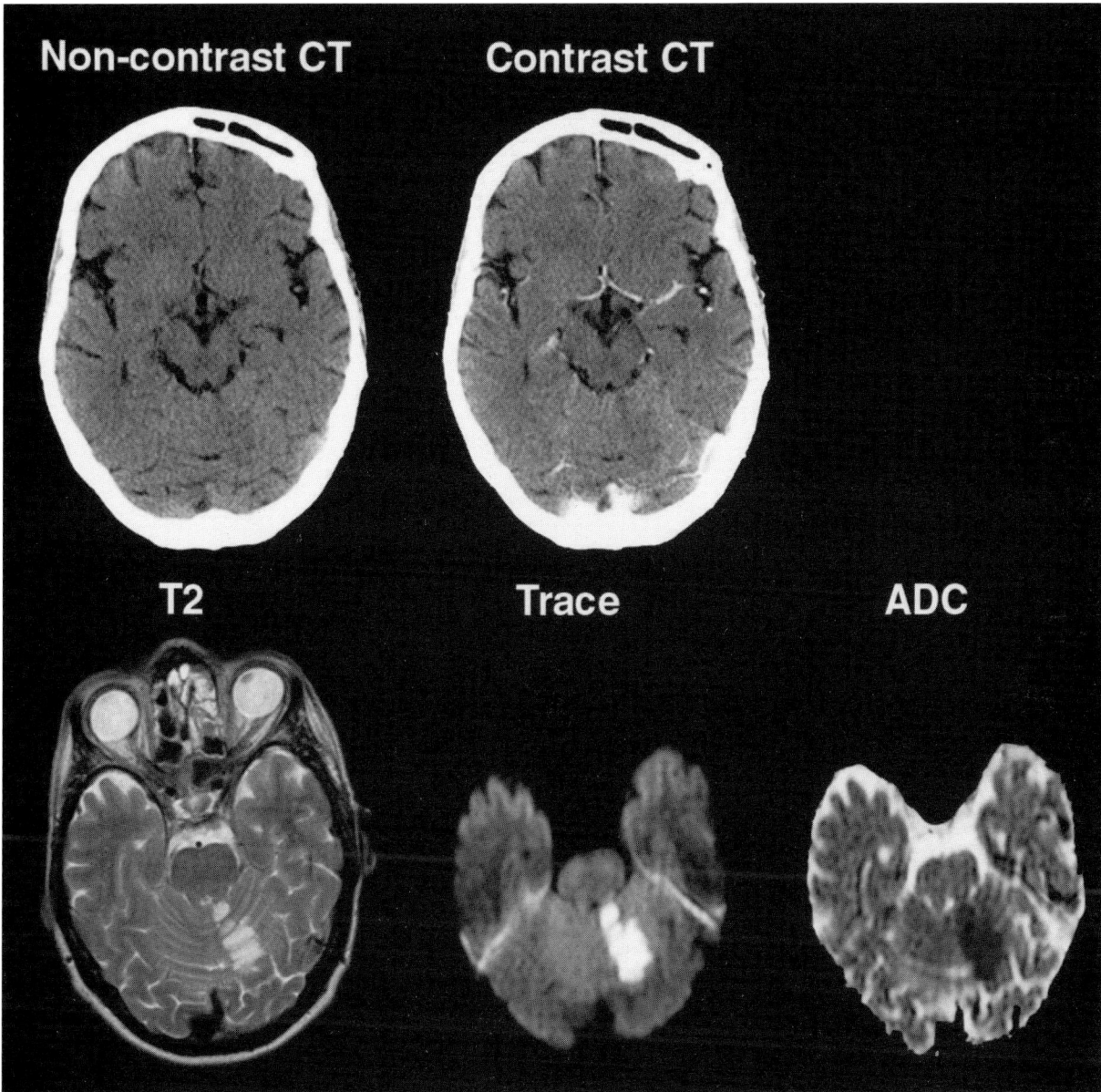

Fig. 10.2. 58-year-old female patient admitted for headaches, nausea, vomiting, vertigo and dysarthria. Physical examination let a left cerebellar stroke be suspected. The latter was demonstrated in the territory of the left superior cerebellar artery by T_2-weighted, DWI-trace and ADC obtained 24 hours after admission. On the other hand, only a slight hypodensity could be retrospectively identified in the corresponding area on the admission cerebral CT, obtained 6 hours after onset.

demonstrates similar sensitivity to ischemic lesions than DWI, but does not allow demonstration of early lesions and differentiation between new and old lesions.[20]

In the vertebro-basilar territory, there has been some concern about false-negative DWI studies, which have been reported in 19% to 31% of patients with stroke in the posterior circulation. The occurrence of false-negative DWI findings was significantly higher for small lesions and during the first 24 hours after stroke onset. In the anterior circulation, false-negative initial DWI studies are much rarer (2%).[21]

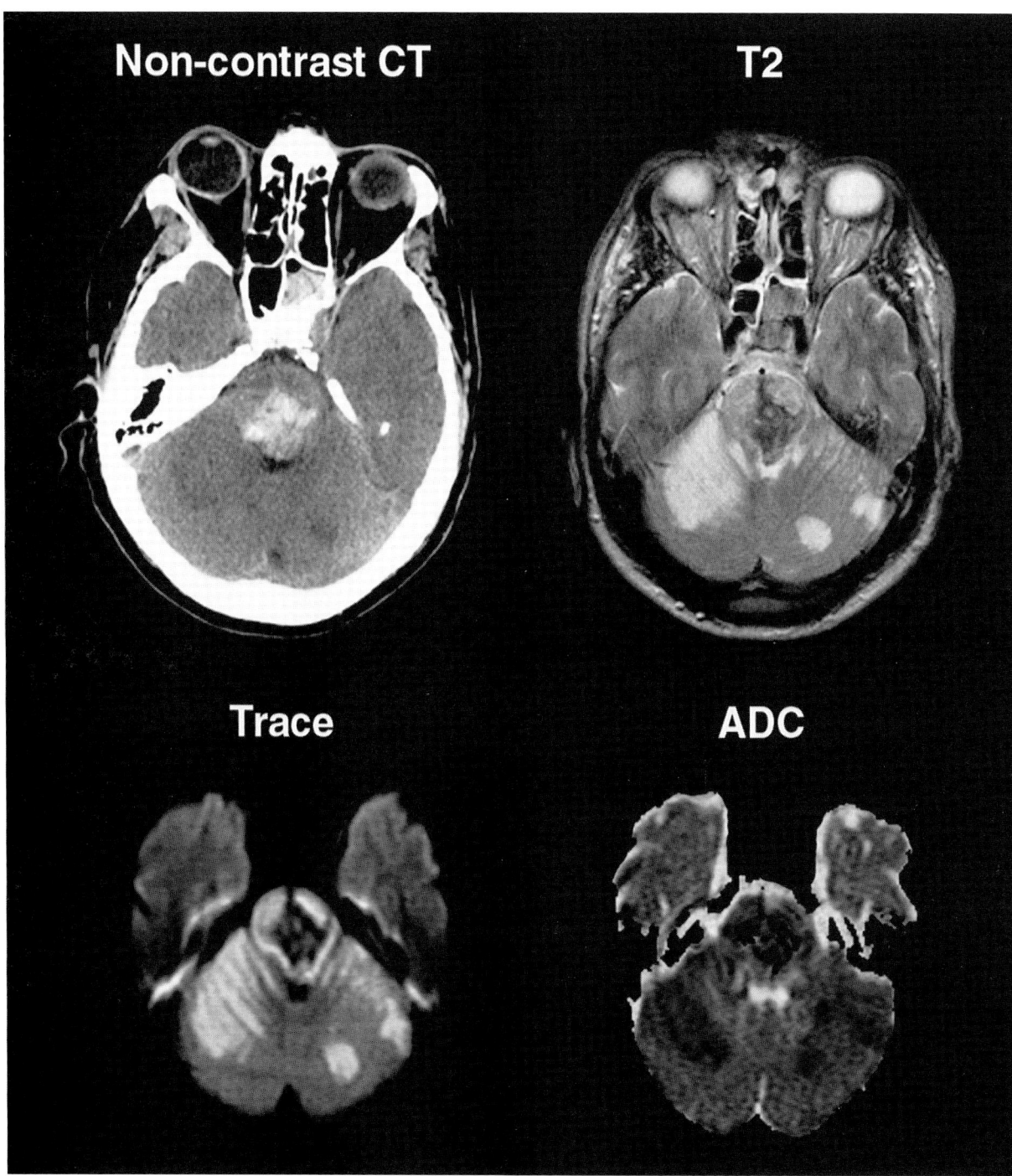

Fig. 10.3. 48-year-old male patient admitted for thrombosis of the vertebro-basilar artery responsible for a locked-in syndrome. Intra-arterial thrombolysis was attempted without success. Post-thrombolysis CT and MR examinations demonstrate hemorrhagic transformation of a complete vertebro-basilar stroke. DWI affords precise delineation of ischemic areas in both cerebellar hemispheres as well as in the brainstem. Hemorrhagic transformation is responsible for susceptibility effects, resulting in pontine hyposignal on T_2-weighted images and DWI-trace due to the T_2-shine through.

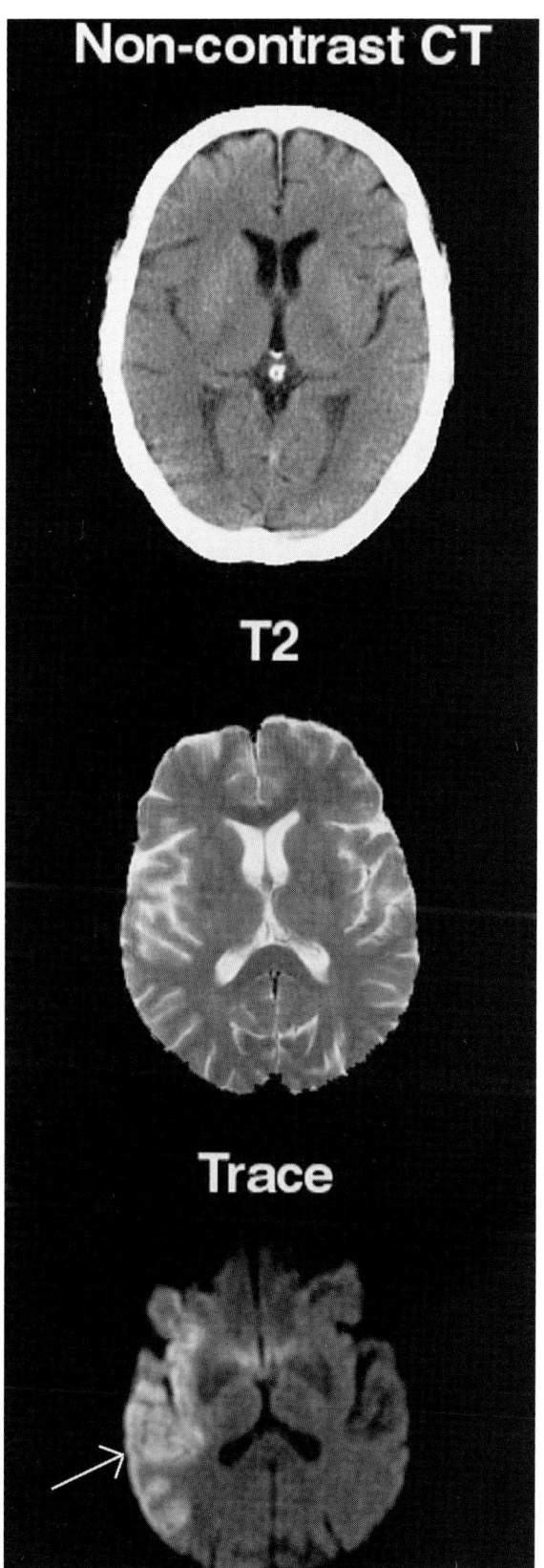

Fig. 10.4. 75-year-old male patient admitted at our institution after sudden onset of a left face–arm–leg sensitivomotor hemisyndrome. Physical examination revealed a left hemianopsia, a rightward gaze deviation, a dysarthria and a left hemineglect. The patient underwent cerebral CT and MR examinations, respectively, 2 and 3 hours after admission. The DWI-trace clearly depicts an acute stroke extending to the superficial right middle cerebral artery territory *(arrow)*, whereas the latter is much more subtle on the T_2-weighted image and especially on the non-contrast cerebral CT, where it features a 'cortical ribbon loss' sign.

DWI and stroke extent

The NINDS and ECASS studies have demonstrated an increased risk of hemorrhagic transformation in stroke patients with a large area of hypodensity on admission CT when treated with thrombolytic therapy.[22,23] The risk of hemorrhagic transformation was significantly increased for stroke involving more than one-third of the middle cerebral artery (MCA) territory.[24] However, even if hypoattenuation of more than one-third of the MCA territory was an exclusion criterion in ECASS, it often remained unidentified at the time of enrolment and 11% of the total study population with large stroke were inappropriately included in this study.[25] This observation correlated with a moderate interobserver agreement in the identification of early infarct signs involving more than one-third of the MCA territory on the admission CT.[25] During ECASS II, a special effort was made to train participating physicians to identify early infarct signs. This resulted in a reduction in the number of inappropriately randomized patients to 5%.[26]

DWI has proved to be more sensitive than CT in the assessment of the involved extent of the MCA territory (Fig. 10.4). DWI and CT sensitivity ranges between 57% and 86% and 14% and 43%, respectively. Specificity has been reported excellent for both imaging techniques and interobserver agreement has shown only moderately good in both imaging techniques (kappa: 0.6 for DWI and 0.5 for CT).[25,27] Furthermore, DWI has shown a more efficient early predictor of the volume of tissue ultimately infarcted than CT.[27]

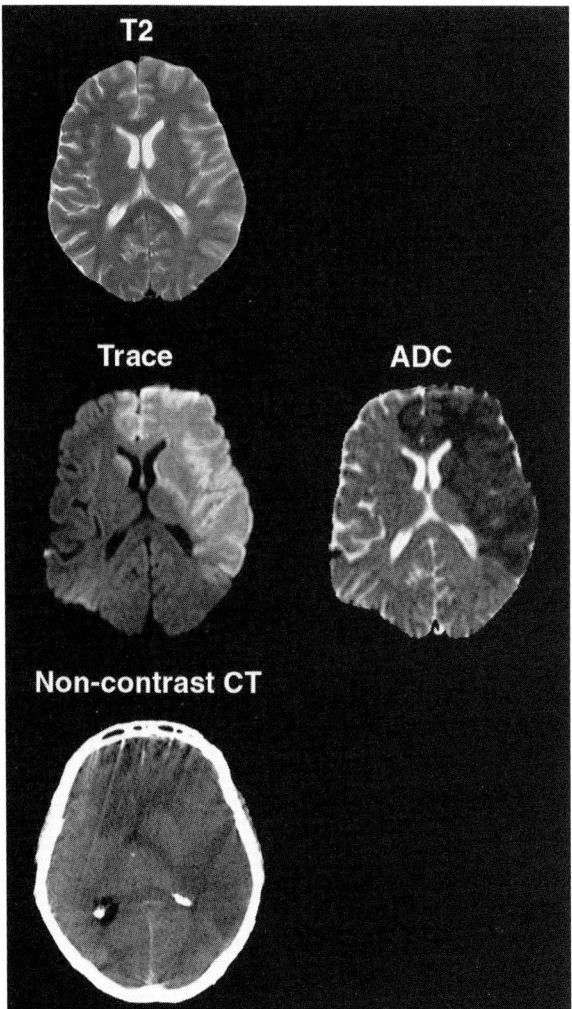

Fig. 10.5. 52-year-old male patient found unconscious at home. Admission cerebral CT was unremarkable. The patient was transferred to our institution and a cerebral MR was performed. The latter demonstrated an extensive stroke involving both anterior cerebral artey and left sylvian artery territories. The precise stroke extent was better delineated on DWI-trace and ADC than on T_2-weighted image. Follow-up cerebral CT, obtained 24 hours after cerebral MR displayed development of a malignant cerebral edema. The patient died from intracranial hypertension.

Multiple cerebral infarcts: DWI demonstrates the one responsible for the acute symptomatology

Patients with cerebrovascular diseases often have multiple ischemic lesions seen on conventional MR examination at the time of their first symptomatic event. In our registry, among 1000 consecutive patients with first-ever stroke, 3% show infarcts in multiple territories supplied by carotid arteries (Fig. 10.5), 2% display multiple infarcts in the vertebrobasilar territory (Fig. 10.6) whereas 2% show multiple infarcts in both territories. Embolism arising from aortic branch vessel atheromatosis and cardiac origin is the main cause of multiple cerebral infarcts. Whether the latter is the result of the fragmentation of a single embolism, or whether it causes multiple territory infarction by proximal occlusion of major vessels with distal hemodynamic infarction still remains unclear.[28]

Among patients with multiple cerebral ischemic lesions, 30% show multiple acute infarcts, 56% single acute infarct and multiple old infarcts, and 14% multiple acute and multiple old infarcts.[29]

One limitation of conventional MR imaging is that acute and old infarcts appear very similar. T_2-weighted images do not allow for differentiation of acute vs. chronic infarcts, whereas T_1-weighted images with gadolinium enhancement are helpful in only 12% of patients.[29] This can cause diagnostic confusion regarding which lesion is acute and symptomatic, even with the help of neurological findings, especially in elderly patients whose conventional MR examination demonstrates a large number of high-signal foci in the corona radiata, basal ganglia and brainstem on T_2-weighted images. Moreover, in such patients, it may be difficult to determine whether new neurological symptoms represent a new ischemic event, or just the unmasking of a prior deficit due to an intercurrent illness (Fig. 10.7).

DWI overcomes conventional MR imaging limitations. Indeed, DWI can easily distinguish between new and old ischemic brain injuries, as they respectively show hypo- and hypersignal on ADC maps (Fig. 10.8). On the other hand, both are hyperintense on the DWI trace, which, however, affords sharp delineation of pathologic processes through the removal of anisotropy of myelin fibres and the absence of contrast between grey and white matter. In 77% to 100% of patients with multiple cerebral infarcts, DWI not only delineates early ischemic brain injury better than conventional MR, but also

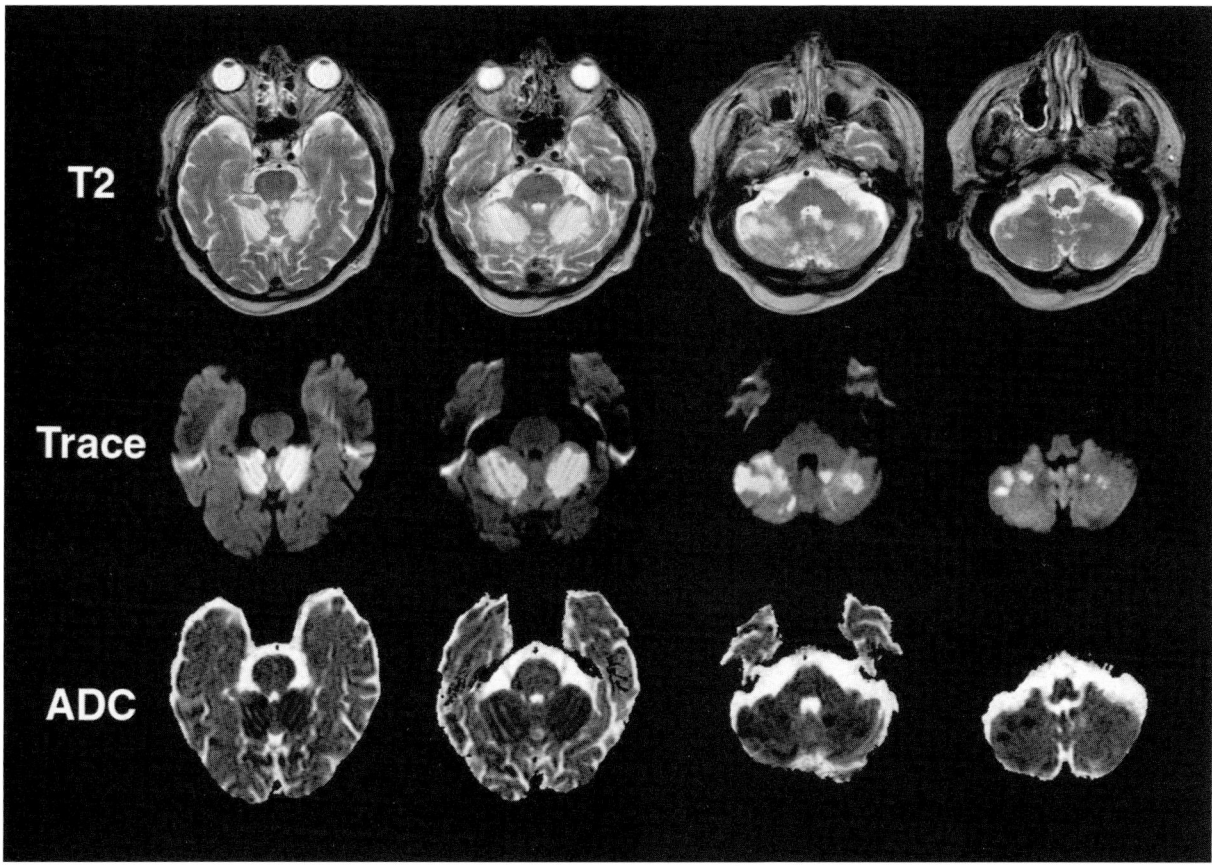

Fig. 10.6. 72-year-old male patient admitted for violent headaches. Physical examination demonstrated severely altered cerebellous tests, as well as dysarthria and bilateral corticospinal signs. MR examination obtained 10 hours after symptomatology onset related these clinical symptoms and signs with bilateral acute strokes in the territory of superior cerebellar arteries.

successfully identifies the acute lesion responsible for the clinical deficit.[20,29] Moreover, in 18% of acute stroke patients, DWI has been reported to localize the symptomatic lesion in a different vascular territory from the one suspected, which relied upon the combination of the initial clinical evaluation and the conventional MR examination. Finally, in 20% of acute stroke patients, DWI allowed to make clear that lesions thought to be acute on the conventional MR sequences were actually old (Fig. 10.9).[30]

Therapeutic impact of DWI

DWI affords accurate localization of strokes. As it successfully discriminates acute from old infarcts, it represents a remarkable tool in the study of the pathophysiology of multiple cerebral ischemic lesions and thus often provides relevant information allowing precise clinical–topographic correlations.

Identifying the origin of stroke, for instance a proximal source of embolism in the case of multiple acute lesions or a hemodynamic cause for watershed infractions, has considerable repercussions on stroke patient management, on investigations as well as on therapy.

In patients with multiple ischemic events in the anterior circulation (Fig. 10.10), imaging of the carotid bifurcation should definitely be performed because of the well-established benefits of carotid endarterectomy in surgically suitable candidates with symptomatic or significant carotid stenosis. Moreover, the benefit of carotid endarterectomy has shown considerably higher in patients with more recent ischemic symptoms.[31] For patients

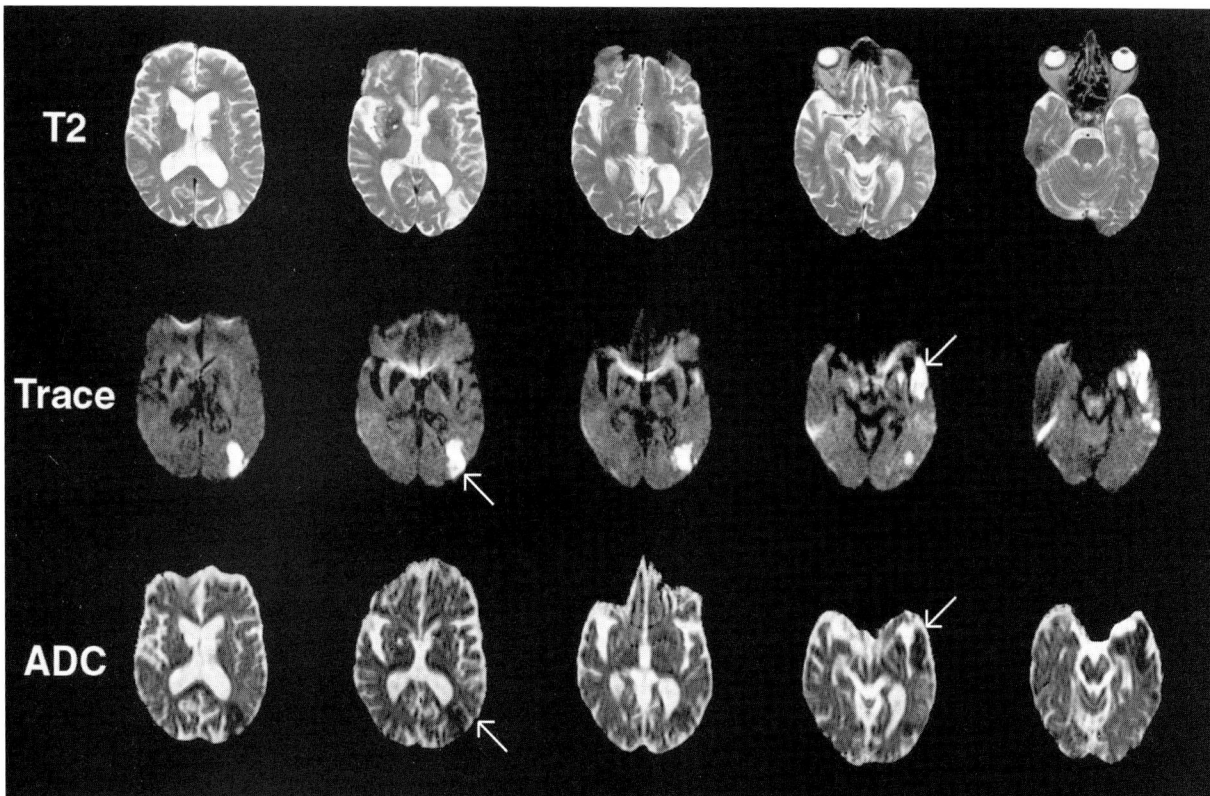

Fig. 10.7. 76-year-old male patient admitted for aphasia and visual field defect. Cerebral MR examination was obtained 4 hours after symptomatology onset. T_2-weighted images show multiple focal hyperintensities *(arrowheads)* in both basal nuclei, as well as in external capsulae. These multiple punctual lesions have high-diffusion properties, featuring hyposignal on DWI-trace and hypersignal on the ADC maps. They relate to lacunas and dilated Virchow–Robin spaces. On the other hand, more extensive acute ischemic lesions *(arrows)* can be identified in the left temporal pole and in the left parieto-occipital region. They are also hyperintense on T_2-weighted images, but demonstrate low diffusion properties, with hyper- and hyposignal on DWI-trace and ADC map, respectively.

with anterior circulation strokes who do not have marked carotid stenoses, some propose MR angiography imaging of the distal carotid or of the proximal anterior or middle cerebral arteries, conventional angiography or transcranial Doppler. If substantial intracranial lesions are identified, recent evidence suggests that anticoagulation therapy may be more beneficial than antiplatelet agents, and ongoing trials are attempting to determine the optimal therapeutic approach for these patients.[32]

If the acute symptomatic lesion is found in the posterior circulation (Fig. 10.11), diagnostic studies may focus on the vertebro-basilar system. For a symptomatic vertebro-basilar stenosis, anticoagulation may be more effective than antiplatelet agents.[32] New therapies, such as vertebral angioplasty in patients with marked posterior circulation occlusive disease, are being evaluated.[33]

Finally, DWI can more frequently differentiate a small deep subcortical infarct from a cortical (Fig. 10.12) or a combined cortical/subcortical lesion than conventional MR imaging can. In patients with small deep infarcts, many clinicians limit the diagnostic evaluation because of the relatively low yield of detailed vascular and cardiac imaging in these patients, particularly if they have predisposing risk factors.[34]

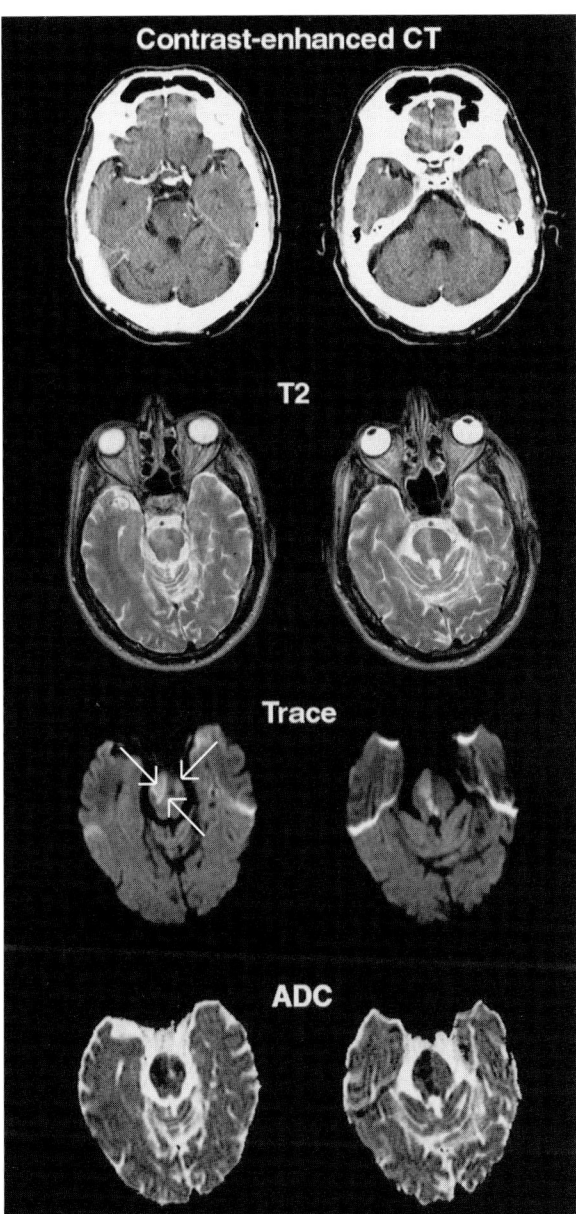

Fig. 10.8. 70-year-old male patient showing a left face–arm–leg hemisyndrome with complex oculomotricity alteration and internuclear ophthalmoplegia. Cerebral CT and MR examinations were obtained 7 and 9 hours after symptomatology onset, respectively. Cerebral MR demonstrates three ischemic lesions in the brainstem, one of them being retrospectively identified on the cerebral CT. Two of these ischemic lesions are acute. They feature hypersignal on T_2- and DWI-trace, and hyposignal on the ADC maps. They are located in the right paramedian pons and mesencephalon, and in the antero-lateral portion of the left pons *(arrows)*. On the other hand, an old lesion, also hyperintense on T_2-weighted images and ADC maps, is identified in the left central paramedian pons *(arrowhead)*. This combination explained the patient's intricate clinical picture.

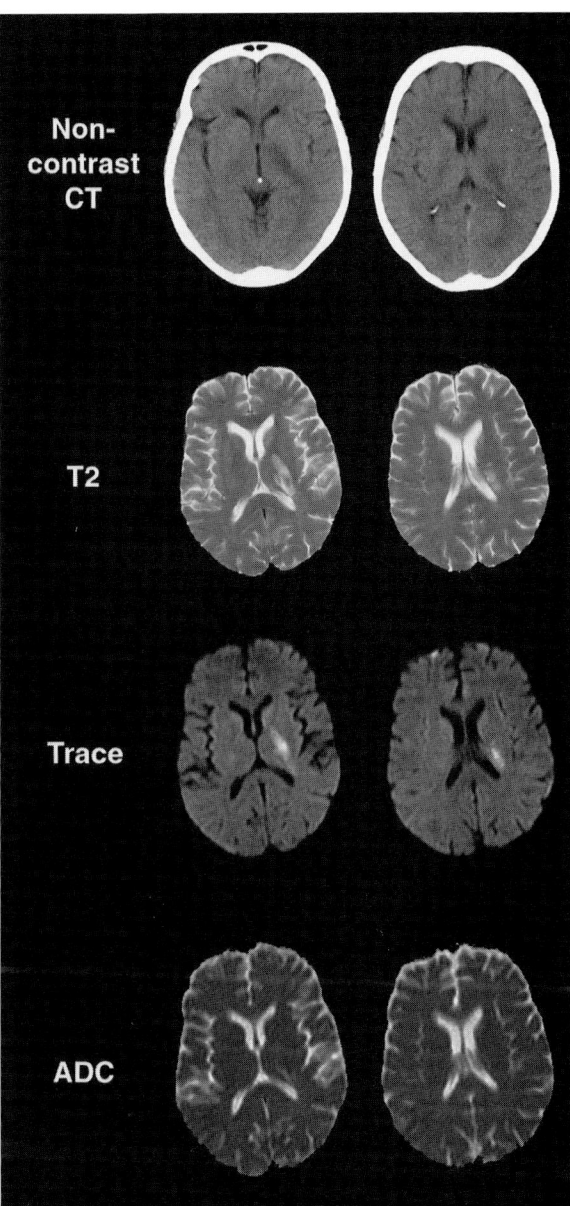

Fig. 10.9. 70-year-old female patient admitted for a right sensitivomotor face–arm–leg hemisyndrome associated with a motor aphasia. These findings were related to a left anterior choroidial stroke both by CT and MR examinations. Non-contrast cerebral CT and T_2-weighted images, as well as DWI-trace, demonstrated a signal abnormality involving the posterior arm of the left internal capsule, as well as portions of the left thalamus and lentiform nucleus, adjacent to the left lateral ventricle. ADC, displaying increased diffusion coefficients in this area, revealed this stroke to be actually evolving from at least 1 or 2 weeks.

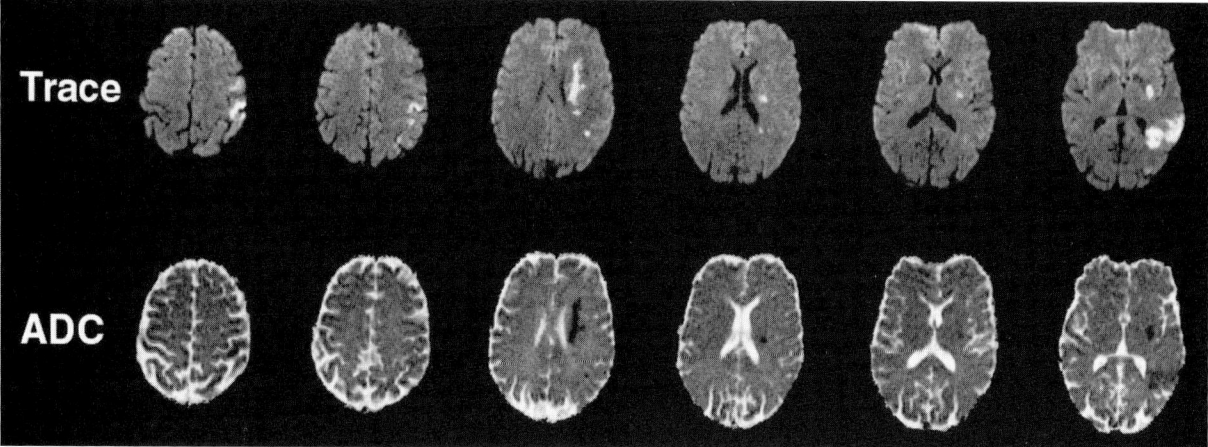

Fig. 10.10. 50-year-old male patient showing a complete right hemisyndrome. Cerebral MR examination performed 9 hours after onset attributed the symptomatology to multiple acute ischemic lesions, featuring hypersignals on DWI-trace and hyposignals on ADC maps. These lesions are distributed in the left anterior and middle cerebral artery territories. This distribution allowed for pathology of the left internal carotid artery to be suspected. Cervical angio-MR and Doppler sonography demonstrated severe atherosclerotic changes.

Conclusion

In conclusion, DWI can easily be added to conventional MR imaging. In acute stroke patients, it provides potentially relevant findings that do not show on conventional MR sequences. It improves the diagnosis of multiple brain infarcts, distinguishing between acute and old lesions. It also affords a better correlation between clinical symptoms and the site of ischemic lesions. Thus, it considerably improves stroke patient care, leading to investigations focused on the etiology of the cerebral infarct. It may sometimes result in a change of the therapeutic strategy, hopefully preventing further stroke recurrence.

REFERENCES

1. Carr HY, Purcell EM. Effects of diffusion on free precession in nuclear magnetic resonance experiments. *Phys Rev* 1954; 94: 630–638.
2. Woessner DE. Effects of diffusion in nuclear magnetic resonance spin-echo experiments. *J Chem Phys* 1961; 34: 2057–2061.
3. Stejskal EO. Use of spin echoes in a pulsed magnetic-field gradient to study anisotropic restricted diffusion and flow. *J Chem Phys* 1965; 43: 3597–3603.
4. Stejskal EO, Tanner JE. Spin diffusion measurements: spin echoes in the presence of a time-dependent field gradient. *J Chem Phys* 1965; 42: 288–292.
5. Basser PJ, Mattiello J, Le Bihan D. Estimation of the effective self-diffusion tensor from the NMR spin echo. *J Magn Reson* 1994; 103: 247–254.
6. Moseley M, Kucharczyk J, Mintorovirch J et al. Diffusion-weighted MR imaging of acute stroke: correlation with T_2-weighted and magnetic susceptibility enhanced MR imaging in cats. *Am J Neuroradiol* 1990; 11: 423–429.
7. Moseley M, Cohen Y, Mintorovitch J et al. Early detection of regional cerebral ischemia in cats: comparison of diffusion- and T_2-weighted MRI and spectroscopy. *Magn Reson Med* 1990; 14: 330–346.
8. Jones SC, Perez-Trepichio AD, Xue M, Furlan AJ, Awad IA. Magnetic resonance diffusion-weighted imaging: sensitivity and apparent diffusion constant in stroke. *Acta Neurochir* 1994; 60: 207–210.
9. Warach S, Chien D, Li W, Ronthal M, Edelman RR. Fast magnetic resonance diffusion-weighted imaging of acute human stroke. *Neurology* 1992; 42: 1717–1723.
10. Baird A, Warach S. Magnetic resonance imaging of acute stroke. *J Cereb Blood Flow Metab* 1998; 18: 583–609.
11. Beaulieu C, de Crespigny A, Tong DC, Moseley DC, Albers GW, Marks MP. Longitudinal magnetic resonance imaging study of perfusion and diffusion in stroke: evolution of lesion volume and correlation with clinical outcome. *Ann Neurol* 1999; 46: 568–578.

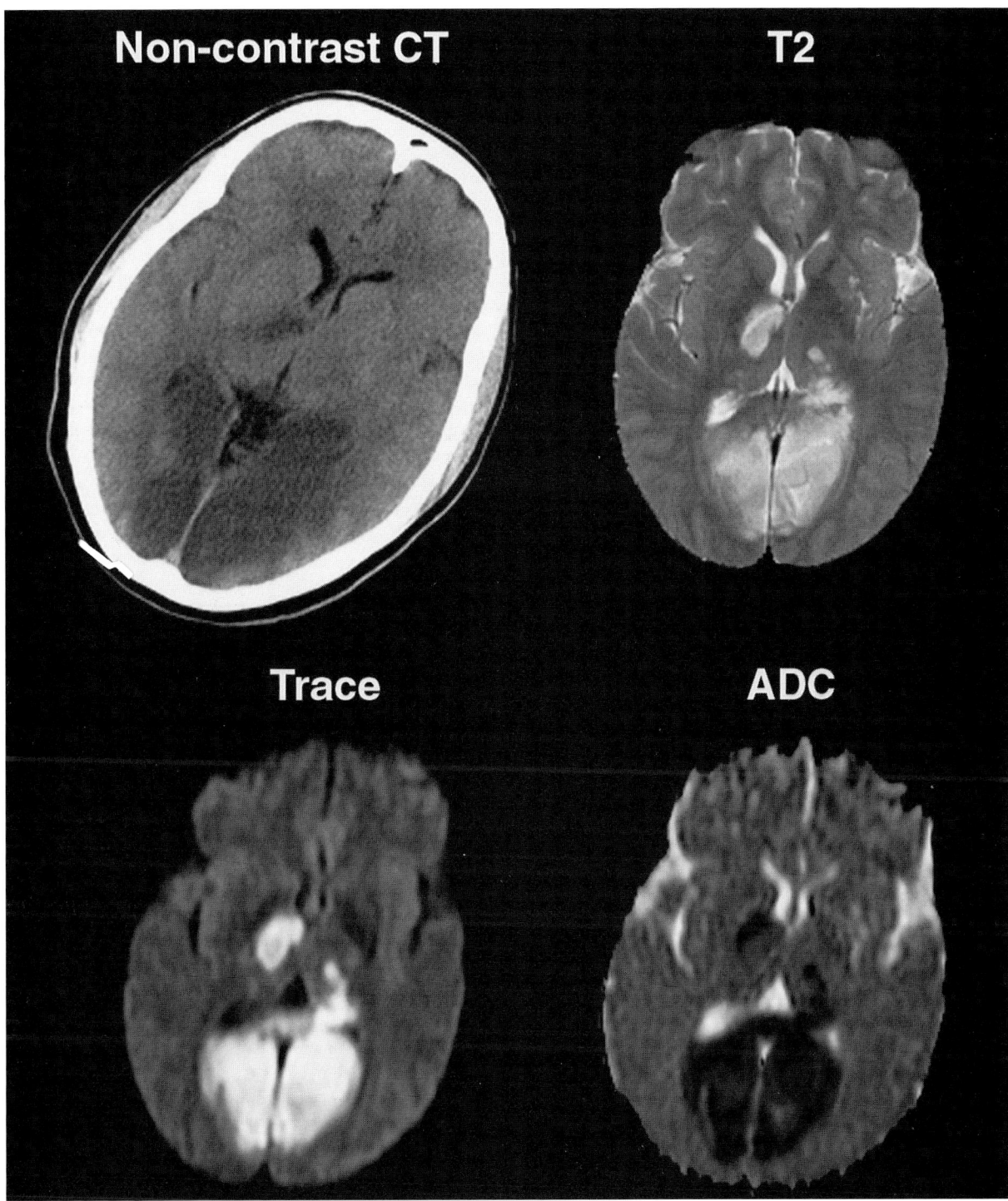

Fig. 10.11. 77-year-old male patient with sudden onset of cortical blindess and decreased level of consciousness. Cerebral CT and MR examinations were obtained 6 and 7 hours after admission. They display acute strokes in both occipital lobes, as well as in the posterior arm of the right internal capsule. MR affords better demonstration of bilateral involvement of thalami, which explained the decreased level of consciousness. Stroke occurrence in both posterior cerebral artery territories raised suspicion about a vetebro-basilar pathology in this patient. Both angio-MR and doppler-sonography demonstrated a stenosis of the distal portion of the vertebro-basilar artery.

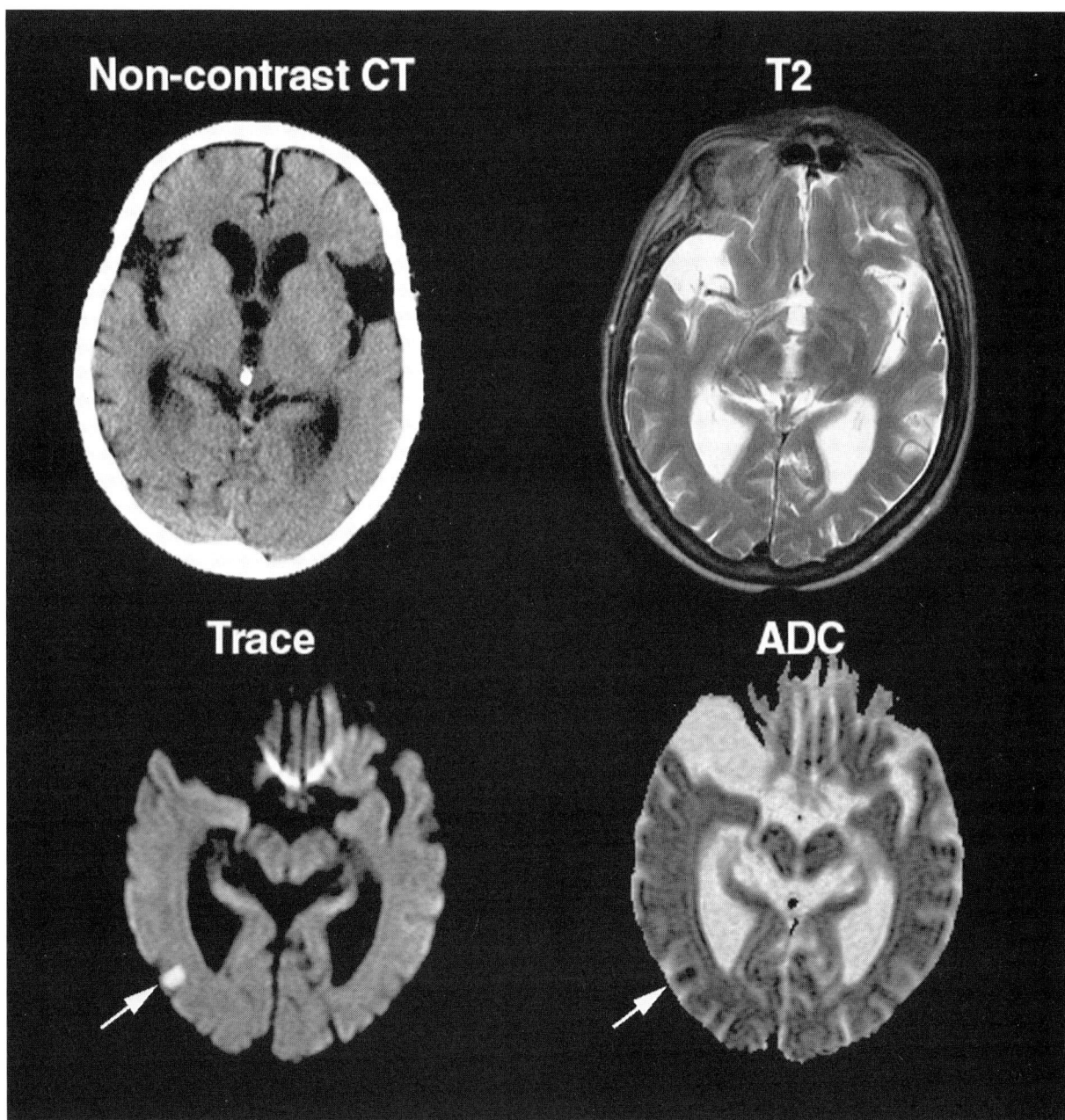

Fig. 10.12. 75-year-old male patient admitted for a left sensitivomotor hemisyndrome with aphasia. Rapid resolution of symptoms was observed, already in the emergency room. This clinical pattern was explained by a right parieto-occipital cortical infarct (arrows). The latter was demonstrated only by DWI-trace and ADC, whereas it could not be seen on cerebral CT and T_2-weighted MR examination.

12 Gonzalez RG, Schaefer PW, Buonanno F et al. Diffusion-weighted MR imaging: diagnostic accuracy in patients imaged within 6 hours of stroke symptom onset. *Radiology* 1999; 210: 155–162.

13 van Gelderen P, de Vleeschouwer MHM, DesPres D, Pekar J, van Zijl PCM, Moonen CTW. Water diffusion and acute stroke. *Magn Reson Med* 1994; 31: 154–163.

14 Ulug AM, Beauchamp N, Bryan RN, van Zijl PCM. Absolute quantitation of diffusion constants in human stroke. *Stroke* 1997; 28: 483–490.

15 Neil JJ, Shiran SI. McKinstry RC et al. Normal brain in human newborns: apparent diffusion coefficient and diffusion anisotropy measured by using diffusion tensor MR imaging. *Radiology* 1998; 209: 57–68.

16 Provenzale JR, Engelter ST, Petrella JR, Smith JS, MacFall JR. Use of MR exponential diffusion-weighted images to eradicate T2 shine-through effect. *Am J Neuroradiol* 1999; 172: 537–539.

17 Mohr JP, Biller J, Hilal SK et al. Magnetic resonance versus computed tomographic imaging in acute stroke. *Stroke* 1995; 26: 807–812.

18 Lutsep HL, Albers GW, DeCrespigny A, Kamat GN, Marks MP, Moseley ME. Clinical utility of diffusion-weighted magnetic resonance imaging in the assessment of ischemic stroke. *Ann Neurol* 1997; 41: 574–580.

19 Lansberg MG, Norbash AM, Marks MP et al. Advantages of adding diffusion-weighted magnetic resonance imaging to conventional magnetic resonance imaging for evaluation of acute stroke. *Arch Neurol* 2000; 57: 1311–1316.

20 Kumon Y, Zenke K, Kusunoki K et al. Diagnostic use of isotropic diffusion-weighted MRI in patients with ischaemic stroke: detection of the lesion responsible for the clinical deficit. *Neuroradiology* 1999; 41: 777–784.

21 Oppenheim C, Stanescu R, Dormont D et al. False-negative diffusion-weighted MR findings in acute ischemic stroke. *Am J Neuroradiol* 2000; 21: 1434–1440.

22 The NINDS t-PA Stroke Study Group. Intracerebral hemorrhage after intravenous t-PA therapy for ischemic stroke. *Stroke* 1997; 28: 2109–2118.

23 Hacke W, Kaste M, Fieschi C et al. Intravenous thrombolysis with recombinant tissue plasminogen activator for acute hemispheric stroke. The European Cooperative Acute Stroke Study (ECASS). *J Am Med Assoc* 1995; 274: 1017–1025.

24 von Kummer R, Allen KL, Holle R et al. Acute stroke: usefulness of early CT findings before thrombolytic therapy. *Radiology* 1997; 205: 327–333.

25 von Kummer R, Holle R, Gizyska U et al. Interobserver agreement in assessing early CT signs of middle cerebral artery infarction. *Am J Neuroradiol* 1996; 17: 1743–1748.

26 Hacke W, Kaste M, Fieschi C et al. Randomised double-blind trial placebo-controlled trial of thrombolytic therapy with intravenous alteplase in acute ischaemic stroke (ECASS II). Second European–Australasian Acute Stroke Study investigators. *Lancet* 1998; 352: 1245–1251.

27 Lansberg MG, Albers GW, Beaulieu C, Marks MP. Comparison of diffusion-weighted MRI and CT in acute stroke. *Neurology* 2000; 54: 1557–1561.

28 Bogousslavsky J, Van Melle G, Regli F. The Lausanne Stroke Registry: analysis of 1,000 consecutive patients with first ever stroke. *Stroke* 1988; 19: 1083–1092.

29 Altieri M, Metz RJ, Müller C, Maeder P, Meuli R, Bogousslavsky J. Multiple brain infarcts: clinical and neuroimaging patterns using diffusion-weighted magnetic resonance. *Eur Neurol* 1999; 42: 76–82.

30 Albers GW, Lansberg MG, Norbash AM et al. Yield of diffusion-weighted MRI for detection of potentially relevant findings in stroke patients. *Neurology* 2000; 54: 1562–1567.

31 The European Carotid Surgery Trial Group. Randomised trial of endarterectomy for recently symptomatic carotid stenosis: final results of the MRC European Carotid Surgery Trial (ECST). *Lancet* 1998; 351: 1379–1387.

32 The Warfarin–Aspirin Symptomatic Intracranial Disease Study Group. The warfarin–aspirin symptomatic intracranial disease study. *Neurology* 1995; 45: 1488–1493.

33 Marks MP, Marcellus M, Norbash AM et al. Outcome of angioplasty for atherosclerotic intracranial stenosis. *Stroke* 1999; 30: 1065–1069.

34 Mead GE, Wardlaw JM, Lewis SC, McDowall M, Dennis MS. Can simple clinical features be used to identify patients with severe carotid stenosis on Doppler ultrasound? *J Neurol Neurosurg Psychiatry* 1999; 66: 16–19.

MRI in transient ischemic attacks: clinical utility and insights into pathophysiology

Jeffrey L. Saver and Chelsea Kidwell

UCLA Stroke Center, Los Angeles, CA, USA

The brain responds dynamically to transient episodes of ischemic insult. Standard brain imaging techniques, computed tomography (CT) and conventional magnetic resonance imaging (MRI), are insensitive to dynamic and regionally varying neural parenchymal responses to tissue ischemia. In contrast, the novel MRI techniques of perfusion and diffusion imaging permit visualization of these critical tissue processes, and have afforded new insights into the physiopathology of human cerebral ischemia. In addition, clinical studies have demonstrated that magnetic resonance imaging is of substantial clinical utility in patients with transient ischemic attacks (TIAs).

Overview

The current conventional definition of transient ischemic attack is neurologic symptoms due to focal cerebral ischemia that resolve completely within 24 hours (Special Report from the National Institute of Neurological Disorders and Stroke, 1990). Defects of this definition, already apparent in the CT era, have been demonstrated even more pointedly by MRI investigations. We will consequently propose a new definition of TIA, informed by MRI findings, at the conclusion of this chapter. Nonetheless, all MRI studies to be reviewed in this chapter have employed this conventional definition.

Recent studies in animal models and in human patients with conventionally defined TIAs have identified three distinct tissue patterns on MRI, reflecting three somewhat dissimilar ischemic episodes that can underlie clinically similar TIAs. A very brief or low-intensity period of focal ischemia may disrupt synaptic transmission and produce transient neurologic deficits without causing early cytotoxic edema or permanent tissue injury. In these cases, perfusion MRI may show focally reduced cerebral blood flow, but both acute diffusion MRI, sensitive to early cytotoxic edema, and late T_2 imaging, sensitive to increased water content, a marker of permanent parenchymal injury, will be unrevealing. A somewhat more severe transient ischemic insult may sufficiently disrupt cellular energetic state to impair maintenance of ionic gradients across cell membranes, producing cytotoxic edema, but not cause advanced bioenergetic failure. Early restoration of blood flow may permit cellular re-energization and restoration of ionic gradients, with edema resolution. In this setting, acute perfusion MRI during the episode and diffusion MRI close to the time of the episode will be abnormal, but late T_2 imaging will be unrevealing. A more profound ischemic insult may produce loss of cell membrane integrity, in addition to failure of synaptic transmission and cytotoxic edema, with resulting permanent parencyhmal injury. However, early recruitment of alternative neural circuitry and synaptic outgrowth, neuroplasticity and neurorepair, may allow rapid resolution of clinical deficits. In this setting, patients with rapidly transient neurologic signs may exhibit early perfusion, early diffusion, and late T_2 abnormalities on MRI imaging.

Standard MR imaging studies in patients with transient ischemic attacks

Patients with clinical TIAs frequently have had prior cerebral ischemic events, both clinically manifest and silent. Conventional MRI is more sensitive than standard CT in identifying these pre-existing lesions, with MR in different studies showing evidence of at least one infarct somewhere in the cerebrum in 81% of TIA patients,[1] vs. 0–68% in CT series. Some of these infarcts are in locations that could have accounted for the deficits observed during the TIA. Among patients meeting clinical criteria for TIA, 31–39% demonstrate neuroanatomically relevant infarcts on conventional magnetic resonance imaging[1,2] and 2–48% on standard computed tomography.[3–8] It is difficult with conventional MRI and CT to determine what proportion of these appropriately localized infarcts occurred at the time of the index TIA, and what proportion existed prior to the presenting event.

The earliest report of MRI findings in TIA patients came from Awad and colleagues.[7] This group studied 22 patients with both MRI and CT. They found 77% of patients had focal ischemic changes on MRI compared to 32% on CT. However, the majority of lesions did not correlate with symptomatology.

Fazekas and colleagues reported the results of routine MR imaging in 62 patients with hemispheric TIAs.[1] Forty-five of these patients also had contrast-enhanced studies. They found that 81% of their cohort had MRI evidence of focal ischemic injury, and reported that 31% demonstrated evidence of an acute TIA-associated infarct. The definition Fazekas and colleagues employed for acute TIA-associated infarcts was: lesions (i) located in a vascular territory potentially corresponding to the patient's TIA symptoms, (ii) having signal characteristics of appearing hyperintense on T_2-weighted scans and isointense or only minimally hypointense on T_1-weighted scans, and (iii) showing regional swelling or contrast enhancement. This definition is problematic, as many lesions remote in time may demonstrate this T_2/T_1 pattern and the accuracy of rater discrimination of swelling for small lesions is uncertain. The majority of infarcts identified as acute (68%) were < 1.5 cm in diameter and 58% were purely cortical. Thirty-seven per cent of the acute infarcts were multiple in nature. Contrast enhancement occurred in 5 of the 45 patients studied, but in only 2 patients contributed to the delineation of the acute lesion. Evidence of infarction in these patients was associated with higher frequency of significant vascular or cardiac disorders.

Bhadelia and colleagues studied 100 TIA patients from the Cardiovascular Health Study imaged with standard MRI sequences.[9] Brain infarcts were demonstrated in 46% of the TIA patients compared to 28% of patients without a history of TIA. In stepwise logistic regression analysis, diastolic blood pressure and internal carotid intima-media thickness were predictive of infarction on MRI. These authors also found an increased frequency of cortical infarcts and multiple infarcts in the TIA patients.

In their study of 64 patients with carotid territory TIAs studied with MRI, Kimura and colleagues found 16 of 41 patients demonstrated contrast enhancement.[2] The majority of contrast-enhancing lesions were cortical (81%). Aphasia or confusional state, hypertension and presence of an emboligenic cardiac or arterial source were more frequently observed in patients with enhancement. The increased rate of contrast enhancement in this study compared to the Fazekas report may be related to differences in patient characteristics and timing of the MRI studies.

Walters and colleagues performed serial MRI studies over a 2-year period in 125 TIA patients and compared the results to 75 controls. They found that 47% of the TIA patients demonstrated evidence of new asymptomatic lesions on follow-up imaging compared to 12% of controls. Thirteen TIA patients had new cerebral transient symptoms, of which two had new relevant MRI lesions. In addition, four TIA patients had experienced a stroke during the follow-up period (three ischemic events, one intracerebral hemorrhage). Factors that correlated with an increased risk of a new ischemic lesion included diastolic blood pressure, male sex, age, and initial severity of MRI ischemic lesions. Also of note, these authors found that TIA patients had an accelerated rate of brain atrophy compared to controls.

MR spectroscopy in transient ischemic attacks

MR spectroscopy is an interesting new application of MRI for the study of patients with TIA. A preliminary report by Giroud and colleagues of 5 TIA patients found no differences in NAA/creatine ratio, but did find an increase in lactate/creatine ratio. Further studies are needed to confirm and clarify the significance of these findings.

Diffusion MRI in transient ischemic attacks

Studies from several groups have demonstrated that diffusion MR imaging provides a more sensitive and specific evaluation of ischemic insult in TIA patients as compared to standard CT and MRI studies.[10–13]

UCLA study

We studied consecutive TIA patients using diffusion MR imaging and compared them to a group of contemporaneous completed stroke patients to determine: (i) the incidence of diffusion-weighted imaging (DWI) and apparent diffusion coefficient (ADC) abnormalities in TIA patients compared to standard T_2-weighted MRI sequences; (ii) whether the presence of a diffusion MR imaging abnormality correlates with the duration, location or mechanism of symptoms; (iii) whether the diffusion MR imaging signature in TIA differs from that in completed stroke; and (iv) the impact of diffusion imaging data on clinical diagnosis of TIA localization and mechanism.[10]

Clinical, conventional MRI, and diffusion MRI data were collected on consecutive patients presenting to the UCLA Medical Center over a 6-month period with symptoms of a transient ischemic attack. TIAs were defined as symptoms of presumed ischemic cerebrovascular etiology lasting less than 24 hours. Patients with brainstem and/or hemispheric symptoms were included while patients with isolated amaurosis fugax were excluded. All MRI scans were obtained within 3 days of symptom onset. During the enrolment period, 61 patients were admitted to our university hospital with symptoms suggestive of a cerebral TIA. Forty-two underwent MRI scanning and 19 did not, due to metal implant (5), refused/claustrophobia (6), MRI technical difficulty (3), and non-stroke attending preference (5).

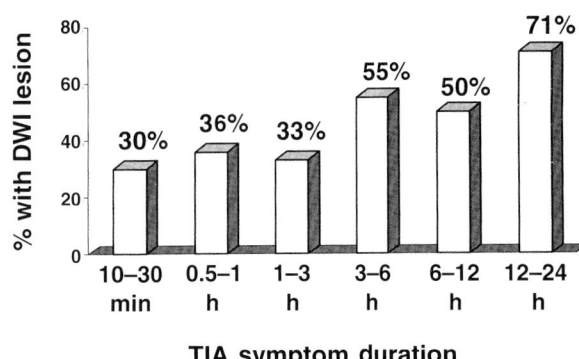

Fig. 11.1. Relation of TIA symptom duration to presence or absence of DWI abnormality among 42 consecutive patients in UCLA series. (From UCLA Stroke Center.)

Among the 42 clinical TIA patients, 20 (48%) demonstrated a focal abnormality on diffusion-weighted imaging, consistent with acute neural bioenergetic compromise. In five (25%) of these 20 patients, there was no lesion correlate on initial T_2-weighted (T_2W) sequences (example of a more recent similar patient is shown in Fig. 11.1). The remaining 15 patients did exhibit T_2-weighted lesion abnormalities in the same regions as DWI alterations (example of a more recent similar patient is shown in Fig. 11.2). Two patients with visible but very small DWI abnormalities did not have a measurable ADC volume. There was a strong correlation between ADC and DWI volumes ($r = 0.77$). There were no significant differences between patients who demonstrated DWI abnormalities and those who did not, in age, sex, and presence of hypertension, diabetes, tobacco use, hypercholesterolemia, or history of prior stroke or TIA.

A precise estimation of TIA duration (all were unequivocally less than 24 hours) was available for 15 of the 20 patients with DWI abnormalities and 17 of the 22 without DWI abnormalities. Duration of TIA symptoms for patients without a DWI

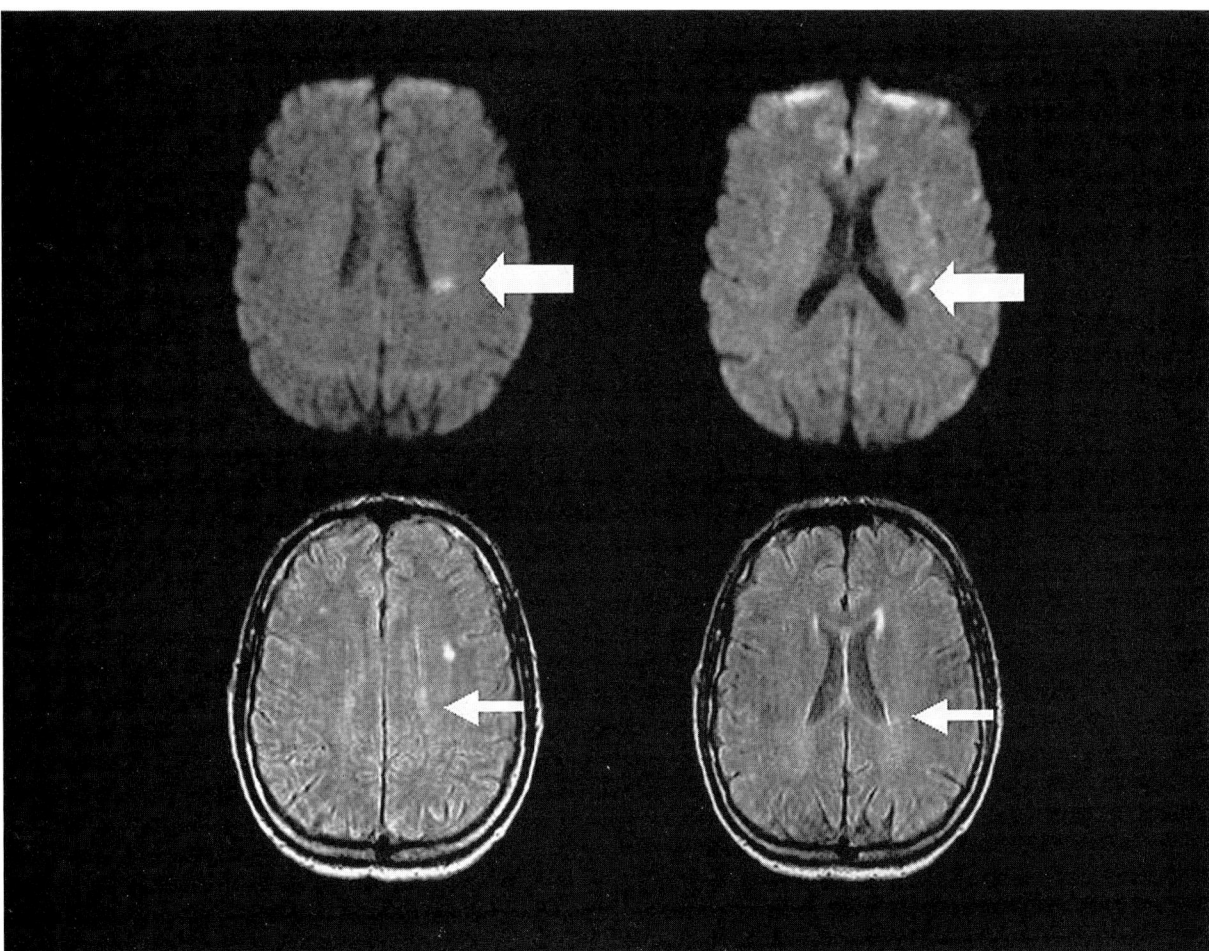

Fig. 11.2. A 63-year-old male presented with right arm weakness lasting 30 minutes. Top row shows consecutive axial DWI sequences demonstrating left corona radiata lesion (thick arrows) not obviously apparent on FLAIR sequences (bottom row, thin arrows). (From UCLA Stroke Center.)

abnormality was mean 3.2 hours (± 4.7 hours standard deviation), median 0.5 hours vs. mean 7.3 hours (± 6 hours standard deviation), median 4.0 hours for patients with a DWI abnormality (t test for difference in means, $P = 0.03$). The percentage of patients with a DWI abnormality within various symptom duration intervals increased as the total duration of symptoms increased (Fig. 11.3).

The mean time from symptom onset to MRI study for all TIA patients was 17 hours (range 1.25–73 hours), and did not significantly differ between the two groups (mean 15.8 hours for DWI-negative patients, mean 19.5 hours for DWI-positive patients). One patient in the group without DWI lesions was still symptomatic at the time of the MR imaging, while two in the DWI positive category were still symptomatic at the time of MR imaging. Interval from time of resolution of TIA symptoms to time of MRI for patients with a DWI abnormality was mean 12.7 hours, median 8.8 hours vs. mean 12.9 hours, median 5.1 hours in patients without a DWI abnormality (rank sums test for difference in medians, $P = 0.7$).

In the 20 patients with diffusion MRI abnormalities, DWI signal changes were localized to the brainstem in four patients, the cerebellum in two patients, subcortical hemispheric structures in seven patients, and cortical regions in seven patients. Vascular territories affected were superficial middle cerebral artery in six patients, deep

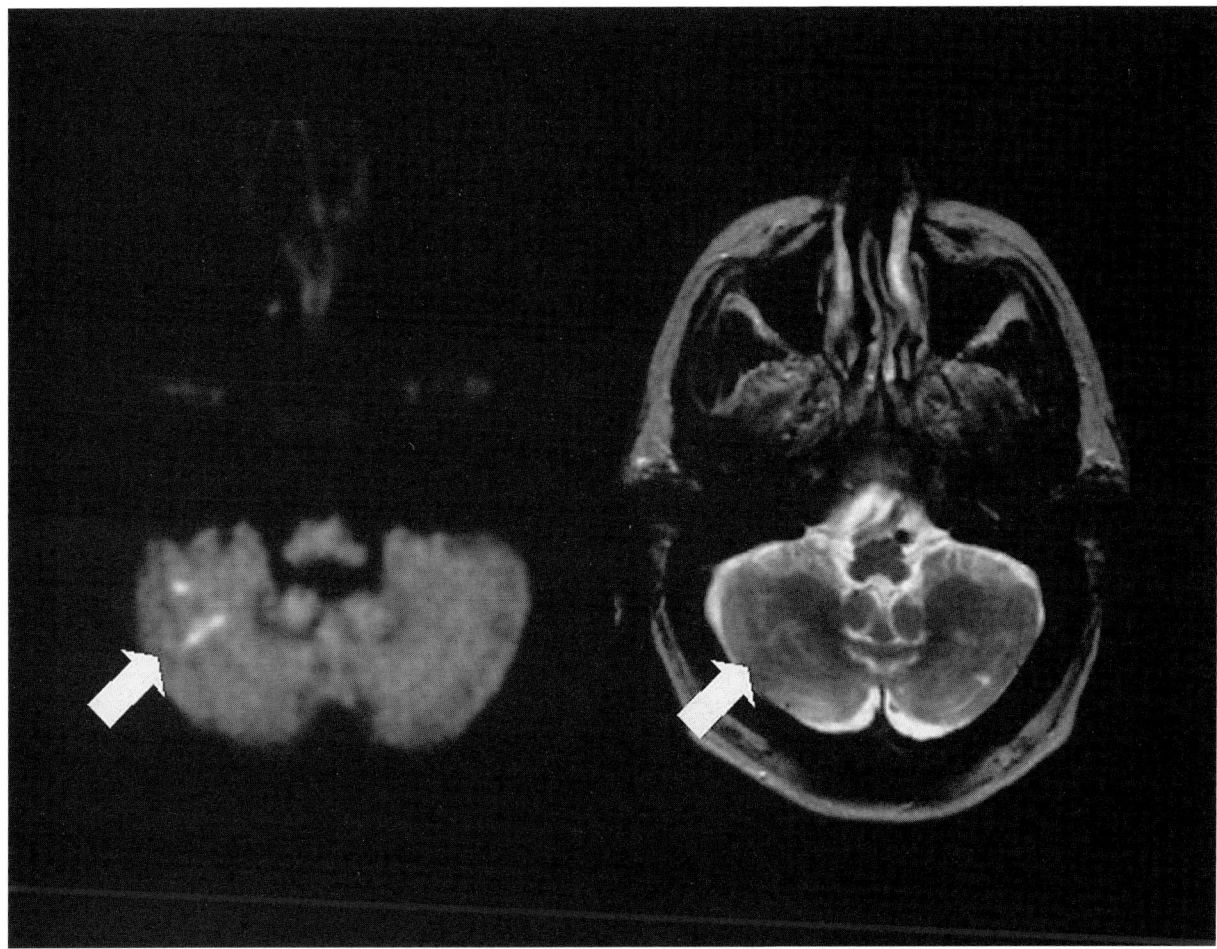

Fig. 11.3. A 79-year-old patient presented with dysarthria and bilateral arm incoordination lasting one hour. DWI (left image) sequence showing right cerebellar lesions, also subtly evident on T_2-weighted sequence (right image). (From UCLA Stroke Center.)

middle cerebral artery in six patients, brainstem perforators in four patients, and posterior cerebral arteries in two patients. In these 20 patients, final etiologic mechanism was felt to be small vessel lacunar in nine patients, large vessel atherothrombotic in four patients, and cardioembolic in seven patients.

DWI results altered the attending physician's opinion regarding vascular localization in 7/20 patients, anatomical localization in 8/20 patients and probable TIA mechanism in 6/20 patients. The types of alterations in diagnosis were quite varied and no single pattern predominated. For example, among etiological diagnoses, of four patients initially suspected to have large artery atherothrombotic mechanisms, one changed post-DWI to likely cardioembolic and one changed to likely small vessel; of seven initial cardioembolic diagnoses, one changed to likely large vessel atherothrombotic and one changed to likely small vessel; and of nine initial small vessel diagnoses, one changed to likely large vessel atherothrombotic and one changed to likely cardioembolic.

There were significant differences in the DWI and ADC MR signatures between the TIA patients with DWI abnormalities and the patients with completed stroke (Table 11.1). Completed stroke patients had larger volumes and greater intensities of ADC and DWI alteration than TIA patients.

Table 11.1. Comparison of DWI signature between TIA patients with diffusion MR abnormality and patients with completed stroke

	TIA patients ($n=20$) mean (SEM)	Completed stroke patients ($n=23$) mean (SEM)	P value
DWI lesion volume (cm^3)	2.9 (8.4)	22.2 (7.8)	0.0002[a]
ADC volume (cm^3)	0.7 (3.4)	10.5 (3.2)	0.0001[a]
DWI intensity	35% (5%)	62% (5%)	0.001[b]
Mean ADC value (μm^2/s)	442 (6.7)	409 (6.1)	0.009[b]

Notes:
[a] Rank Sums Test
[b] T test. Modified, with permission, from reference 10.

Table 11.2. Time intervals and yield of diffusion MRI in transient ischemia attack patients: three series

Series	TIA duration (mean) (h)	Time from TIA onset to MRI (mean) (h)	Frequency of positive DWI findings on MRI (%)
UCLA ($n=42$)	3.2[a]	17	48
Duke ($n=40$)	4.8	37	35
MGH ($n=57$)	1.9	39	46

Note:
[a] Median duration was 2.0 hours.

All 20 TIA patients demonstrating DWI abnormalities were contacted for a follow-up MRI, and nine of these patients agreed to return for repeat neuroimaging. Three patients were studied with head CT and six with brain MRI 2–7 months post event. Of these nine patients, five (three MRI, two CT) demonstrated a subsequent infarct in the region corresponding to the original DWI abnormality while four (three MRI, 1 CT) did not. Five of the 22 patients without a DWI abnormality underwent follow-up imaging (three MRI, two CT), 2 weeks to 15 months post event. None demonstrated a subsequent relevant infarct.

Duke, Massachusetts General Hospital and additional studies

Studies of diffusion MRI in TIA patients performed by investigators at Duke University, Massachusetts General Hospital (MGH), and by Takayama and colleagues have confirmed and extended our findings.[12,13] Though differing somewhat in cohort characteristics and timing of MRIs, the four series show convergent results regarding the frequency of DWI positivity among TIA patients, ranging from 35% in the Duke cohort, 37% in the Takayama cohort, 46% in the MGH cohort, and 48% in the UCLA cohort (Table 11.2). Aggregating the four series, among 158 TIA patients studied, 42% exhibited diffusion MRI abnormalities. The Duke investigators found that in their cohort, as in ours, TIAs of longer clinical duration were more likely to be DWI positive. Among DWI positive patients, mean TIA duration was 7.1 hours in the Duke cohort and 7.3 hours in the UCLA cohort; in DWI negative patients mean TIA duration was 3.2 hours in both cohorts. In contrast, TIA duration was not a predictor of DWI positivity in the MGH series. In part, this discrepancy may be due to the briefer average duration of TIAs and the longer interval from TIA offset to MR imaging in the MGH study. The MGH investigators did find that prior, non-stereotyped

TIAs, identified stroke etiology, and cortical symptoms were independent clinical predictors of DWI positivity. These clinical factors seem to index larger, more severe ischemic episodes, as does longer duration of clinical deficits, and this underlying physiologic factor is likely to be the most critical for the appearance of DWI abnormality.

Takayma and colleagues studied 19 TIA patients with diffusion imaging and found that seven (37%) demonstrated DWI positivity. On follow-up imaging, all of the DWI lesions had evolved to persistent T_2 lesions.

In addition to the above series, there are two case reports in the literature of DWI lesions associated with TIAs, both reporting reversibility of the DWI abnormalities on follow-up imaging.[14,15] In one of these patients, reversal of an initial perfusion abnormality was also demonstrated.[15]

Discussion of diffusion MR findings

These studies of diffusion MRI in transient ischemic attack provide important new insights into the pathophysiology of TIAs and the clinical utility of new MRI sequences in TIA patients. Across all series, more than two of every five cerebral TIA patients demonstrated diffusion MRI evidence of acute bioenergetic compromise. In the UCLA study, among TIA patients with early DWI abnormalities who had follow-up imaging, approximately one-half exhibited late CT or MRI evidence of established infarction. Together, these data suggest that approximately one quarter of cerebral TIA patients actually have cerebral infarction with transient signs. We, and others, also identified a distinct subset of TIA patients, representing about one fifth of TIA cases, who had early DWI abnormalities but no late evidence of established infarction. This finding in TIA patients suggests that DWI abnormalities may be reversible in humans if early restoration of blood flow is obtained. This observation has been confirmed, with important additional complexities, by MRI studies in patients undergoing reperfusion after thrombolytic stroke therapy.[16]

In TIA patients, the ADC volume, mean ADC value, DWI volume and DWI signal intensity were all significantly less abnormal than in acute stroke patients. These differences support the concept that the cerebral ischemia experienced by patients with TIAs is lesser in volume and severity than that experienced by patients with clinically completed stroke syndromes.

Both the UCLA and Duke series found a strong statistical correlation between duration of TIA symptoms and presence of a lesion on DWI. This correlation, however, was not absolute. DWI lesions appeared in patients with clinical episodes as brief as 10 minutes, while some patients in the DWI negative group had symptoms lasting more than 12 hours. DWI abnormalities do appear to be uncommon, if present at all, in patients with clinical symptoms lasting less than 5 minutes.

In addition to improving our understanding of the underlying pathophysiological processes that occur with TIAs, these data add to a growing body of evidence demonstrating the clinical utility of DWI.[17,18] A variety of studies have demonstrated that the diagnosis of TIA is often difficult, especially for the non-neurologist.[19,20] Kraaijeveld and colleagues found kappa measures of inter-rater agreement of only 0.65 among eight experienced neurologists diagnosing 56 TIA patients and of only 0.31 for determination of the vascular territory involved.[21] The size, appearance and location of DWI lesion(s) in TIA may help guide physicians in determining the underlying etiologic mechanism and in choosing the optimal therapeutic regimen to reduce the probability of recurrent TIAs or completed stroke in the future.

In the UCLA study, information obtained from the DWI study led to a change in the suspected anatomical localization, vascular localization and TIA mechanism in over one third of patients. In addition to clarifying the site and source of ischemia in patients with clinically definite TIAs, diffusion imaging also can be quite helpful in patients with atypical transient neurologic symptoms, when it is unclear whether the event was a TIA vs. migraine, hyperventilation, brief seizure, or other TIA mimic. Although DWI abnormalities have rarely been reported in TIA mimics, a visualized diffusion abnormality in these cases generally provides supportive evidence of the diagnosis of TIA.

The observation that DWI alone was positive in

25% of patients, while 75% had correlative lesions identified retrospectively on T_2-weighted imaging underestimates the diagnostic impact of DWI. Even in the patients with T_2 visible lesions, the diffusion imaging provided added clinical utility. Many of the T_2 positive patients had multiple foci of increased T_2 signal, and determining which, if any, T_2 foci were new and related to the recent TIA may not have been possible without the DWI sequences. Standard T_2-weighted sequences alone are generally incapable of reliably differentiating acute from chronic events.

Identifying which patients have a new infarct on imaging may have important prognostic value.[22] In the Dutch TIA trial, evidence of any cerebral infarct on CT was an independent risk factor for subsequent stroke, myocardial infarction, or vascular death.[23,24] Evans and colleagues reported that in TIA patients, CT verified infarction increased the risk of death by 109% over a 10-year period following the TIA.[5] However, this study did not correlate the risk with evidence of a new, appropriately located TIA related infarct. Eliasziw and colleagues did not find an increased risk of ipsilateral stroke in a group of TIA patients with severe carotid stenosis treated medically as part of the North American Symptomatic Carotid Endarterectomy Trial; however, these results cannot be generalized to all TIA patients.[25] Only larger series with long-term follow-up will be able to distinguish if there is a difference in prognosis in TIA patients without diffusion abnormalities, TIA patients with transient diffusion abnormalities but no eventual T_2 lesion, and patients with diffusion abnormalities and a subsequent T_2 lesion.

Several issues require further study. The clinical prognostic significance of finding an associated DWI abnormality in a patient with a TIA remains uncertain. We concur with the general view advanced by Caplan that all TIA patients are at significant risk of subsequent vascular events and it is the underlying mechanism rather than the duration of symptoms that is most critical to determine.[26] However, it may be that within each mechanism category, longer duration of a TIA or presence of a DWI abnormality identifies a subgroup at increased risk. How often patients with DWI abnormalities are experiencing ongoing ischemia will need to be clarified by large series of concurrent perfusion studies. The severity and size of the perfusion deficit might also be an indicator of the reversibility of the diffusion abnormality. Finally, the pathologic correlates of DWI changes in TIA require investigation, including how often signal abnormalities reflect, at the histopathologic level, absence of infarction, incomplete infarction, or complete infarction.[27]

A new, tissue-based definition of transient ischemic attacks

Time-based definitions for TIA first arose in the 1950s as an imprecise means to distinguish between those cerebral ischemic episodes that caused brain injury and those that did not, in the absence of imaging or other laboratory measures that could directly determine tissue parenchymal status. Proposed time cutoffs varied widely. A 1958 NIH committee on classification of cerebrovascular disease suggested that TIAs could last as long as 1 hour.[28] Acheson and Hutchinson, in 1964, also employed a 1-hour threshold to distinguish TIA from stroke.[29] However, also in 1964, Marshall employed a 24-hour limit in defining TIA, although his data showed that symptoms lasted less than 1-hour in three-fourths of his patients.[30] In the 1975 revision of the NIH classification document, a 24-hour limit for TIAs was adopted.[31]

Accumulating evidence suggests that any time cutoff for TIA is inaccurate in reflecting end organ injury. The current 24-hour operational definition is especially misleading. Large-scale studies have clarified our understanding of the typical duration of TIAs, showing that most TIAs resolve within 10–60 minutes rather than lasting several hours.[32,33] Moreover, diffusion MR findings of diffusion change in patients with spells as brief as 10 minutes challenge the simplistic assumption that, because clinical TIA symptoms rapidly resolve, significant ischemic tissue injury must not occur.

MR imaging studies have demonstrated the untenability of any definition of TIA based solely on clinical manifestations and an arbitrarily assigned time window, rather than tissue changes and physiologic processes. While the likelihood of DWI alterations is directly related to the duration of symptoms, some patients with spells as brief as 10 minutes will show parenchymal changes on diffusion imaging and some with spells exceeding 12 hours will show no diffusion alteration. There is not likely to be a fundamental biologic difference between a patient whose symptoms last 59 minutes and a patient whose symptoms last 61 minutes, or between 23 hour 59 minute spells and 24 hour 1 minute spells.

Accordingly, we propose the following new definition of transient ischemic attacks, based on fundamental physiologic processes indexed by imaging or other laboratory measures, rather than a strict time limit: *A TIA is a brief episode of neurologic dysfunction due to focal cerebral ischemia, that is not associated with permanent brain injury.* Although most TIAs last 1 minute to 2 hours, a minority last up to 24 or more hours.

Under this definition, the diagnosis of TIAs may be rendered on clinical grounds alone. However, for research purposes, it is useful to have a more detailed, strictly operationalized definition, again based on the presence or absence of tissue injury rather than time interval. We propose the following:

- A TIA is a brief episode of neurological dysfunction, presumed to be due to focal cerebral ischemia, that is not associated with permanent brain injury. Although most TIAs last 1 minute to 2 hours, a minority last up to 24 or more hours.
- Highly probable TIA: transient neurological dysfunction presumed to be due to focal cerebral ischemia, imaging evidence of focal hypoperfusion during episode, no laboratory/imaging evidence of tissue injury.
- Probable TIA: transient neurological dysfunction presumed to be due to focal cerebral ischemia, perfusion imaging not performed during episode, no laboratory/imaging evidence of tissue injury.
- Possible TIA: transient neurological dysfunction presumed to be due to focal cerebral ischemia, perfusion imaging not performed during episode, no sensitive laboratory/imaging test of tissue injury performed.

This research definition recognizes three levels of strength of evidence for a spell being a TIA. The lowest level is clinical criteria alone. The next level higher is clinical criteria plus a supportive test showing that no parenchymal tissue injury occurred during the spell. The supportive test should be highly sensitive to subtle brain parenchymal injury, such as diffusion MR. Conventional CT and MR are insufficient. Serum biomarkers of brain parenchymal injury, such as the S-100 protein and neuron specific enolase,[34,35] may be useful alternative laboratory measures for this definition. The highest level of evidence additionally includes imaging evidence of focal hypoperfusion during the spell. This finding helps to exclude seizures, compressive neuropathies, and other TIA mimics and rules in focal hypoperfusion as the etiology of the episode. Any of the wide variety of perfusion imaging modalities available could provide the data required for this level of evidence, including CT perfusion imaging, xenon CT, perfusion MR, single positron emission tomography (SPECT), positron emission tomography (PET), transcranial Doppler ultrasound, and cerebral angiography.

Conclusion

Magnetic resonance imaging has fundamentally altered our understanding of the pathophysiology of transient ischemic attack. The spectrum of ischemic tissue alterations underlying transient clinical symptoms is now understood to variably include synaptic transmission failure, cytotoxic edema and permanent tissue injury, and these processes are easily delineated in individual patients on MR imaging. In routine clinical practice, MR permits confirmation of focal ischemia rather than another process as the cause of a patient's deficit, improves accuracy of diagnosis of the vascular localization and etiology of TIA, and assesses the extent of pre-existing cerebrovascular injury. Accordingly, MRI, including diffusion sequences, should now be considered a preferred diagnostic test in the investigation of the patient with potential transient ischemic attacks.

ACKNOWLEDGEMENTS

We are grateful to our collaborators in the UCLA Magnetic Resonance Imaging in Human Cerebral Reperfusion Study Group: Jeffrey R. Alger, PhD, Gary Duckwiler, MD, Y. Pierre Gobin, MD, Reza Jahan, MD, James Mattiello, PhD, Sidney Starkman, MD, Pablo Villablanca, and Fernando Vinuela, MD.

REFERENCES

1. Fazekas F, Fazekas G, Schmidt R, Kapeller P, Offenbacher H. Magnetic resonance imaging correlates of transient cerebral ischemic attacks. *Stroke* 1996; 27: 607–611.
2. Kimura K, Minematsu K, Wada K, Yonemura K, Yasaka M, Yamaguchi T. Lesions visualized by contrast-enhanced magnetic resonance imaging in transient ischemic attacks. *J Neurol Sci* 2000; 173: 103–108.
3. Dennis M, Bamford J, Sandercock P, Warlow C. Prognosis of transient ischemic attacks in the Oxfordshire Community Stroke Project. *Stroke* 1990; 21: 848–853.
4. Koudstaal PJ, van Gijn J, Frenken CW et al. TIA, RIND, minor stroke: a continuum, or different subgroups? Dutch TIA Study Group. *J Neurol Neurosurg Psychiatry* 1992; 55: 95–97.
5. Evans GW, Howard G, Murros KE, Rose LA, Toole JF. Cerebral infarction verified by cranial computed tomography and prognosis for survival following transient ischemic attack. *Stroke* 1991; 22: 431–436.
6. Bogousslavsky J, Regli F. Cerebral infarct in apparent transient ischemic attack. *Neurology* 1985; 35: 1501–1503.
7. Awad I, Modic M, Little JR, Furlan AJ, Weinstein M. Focal parenchymal lesions in transient ischemic attacks: correlation of computed tomography and magnetic resonance imaging. *Stroke* 1986; 17: 399–403.
8. Davalos A, Matias-Guiu J, Torrent O, Vilaseca J, Codina A. Computed tomography in reversible ischaemic attacks: clinical and prognostic correlations in a prospective study. *J Neurol* 1988; 235: 155–158.
9. Bhadelia RA, Anderson M, Polak JF et al. Prevalence and associations of MRI-demonstrated brain infarcts in elderly subjects with a history of transient ischemic attack. The Cardiovascular Health Study. *Stroke* 1999; 30: 383–388.
10. Kidwell CS, Alger JR, Di Salle F et al. Diffusion MRI in patients with transient ischemic attacks. *Stroke* 1999; 30: 1174–1180.
11. Engelter ST, Provenzale JM, Petrella JR, Alberts MJ. Diffusion MR imaging and transient ischemic attacks [letter; comment]. *Stroke* 1999; 30: 2762–2763.
12. Ay H, Buonanno FS, Schaefer PW et al. Clinical and diffusion-weighted imaging characteristics of an identifiable subset of TIA patients with acute infarction (Abstract). *Stroke* 1999; 30: 235A.
13. Takayama H, Mihara B, Kobayashi M, Hozumi A, Sadanaga H, Gomi S. [Usefulness of diffusion-weighted MRI in the diagnosis of transient ischemic attacks]. *No To Shinkei* 2000; 52: 919–923.
14. Lecouvet FE, Duprez TP, Raymackers JM, Peeters A, Cosnard G. Resolution of early diffusion-weighted and FLAIR MRI abnormalities in a patient with TIA. *Neurology* 1999; 52: 1085–1087.
15. Neumann-Haefelin T, Wittsack HJ, Wenserski F et al. Diffusion- and perfusion-weighted MRI in a patient with a prolonged reversible ischaemic neurological deficit. *Neuroradiology* 2000; 42: 444–447.
16. Kidwell CS, Saver JL, Mattiello J et al. Thrombolytic reversal of acute human cerebral ischemic injury shown by diffusion/perfusion magnetic resonance imaging. *Ann Neurol* 2000; 47: 462–469.
17. Lee LJ, Kidwell CS, Alger J, Starkman S, Saver JL. Impact on stroke subtype diagnosis of early diffusion-weighted magnetic resonance imaging and magnetic resonance angiography. *Stroke* 2000; 31: 1081–1089.
18. Lutsep HL, Albers GW, DeCrespigny A, Kamat GN, Marks MP, Moseley ME. Clinical utility of diffusion-weighted magnetic resonance imaging in the assessment of ischemic stroke. *Ann Neurol* 1997; 41: 574–580.
19. Ferro JM, Falcao I, Rodrigues G et al. Diagnosis of transient ischemic attack by the nonneurologist. A validation study. *Stroke* 1996; 27: 2225–2229.
20. Calanchini PR, Swanson PD, Gotshall RA et al. Cooperative study of hospital frequency and character of transient ischemic attacks. IV. The reliability of diagnosis. *J Am Med Assoc* 1977; 238: 2029–2033.
21. Kraaijeveld CL, van Gijn J, Schouten HJ, Staal A. Interobserver agreement for the diagnosis of transient ischemic attacks. *Stroke* 1984; 15: 723–725.
22. Toole JF. The Willis lecture: transient ischemic attacks, scientific method, and new realities. *Stroke* 1991; 22: 99–104.

23 The Dutch TIA Trial Study Group. Predictors of major vascular events in patients with a transient ischemic attack or nondisabling stroke. The Dutch TIA Trial Study Group. *Stroke* 1993; 24: 527–531.

24 van Swieten JC, Kappelle LJ, Algra A, van Latum JC, Koudstaal PJ, van Gijn J. Hypodensity of the cerebral white matter in patients with transient ischemic attack or minor stroke: influence on the rate of subsequent stroke. Dutch TIA Trial Study Group. *Ann Neurol* 1992; 32: 177–183.

25 Eliasziw M, Streifler JY, Spence JD, Fox AJ, Hachinski VC, Barnett HJ. Prognosis for patients following a transient ischemic attack with and without a cerebral infarction on brain CT. North American Symptomatic Carotid Endarterectomy Trial (NASCET) Group. *Neurology* 1995; 45: 428–431.

26 Caplan LR. Are terms such as completed stroke or RIND of continued usefulness? *Stroke* 1983; 14: 431–433.

27 Li F, Liu KF, Silva MD et al. Transient and permanent resolution of ischemic lesions on diffusion-weighted imaging after brief periods of focal ischemia in rats : correlation with histopathology. *Stroke* 2000; 31: 946–954.

28 Ad Hoc Committee on Cerebrovascular Disease of the Advisory Council of the National Institute of Neurological Disease and Blindness. A classification of and outline of cerebrovascular diseases. *Neurology* 1958; 8: 395–434.

29 Acheson J, Hutchinson EC. Observations on the natural history of transient cerebral ischaemia. *Lancet* 1964; 2: 871–874.

30 Marshall J. The natural history of transient ischaemic cerebrovascular attacks. *Q J Med* 1964; 33: 309–324.

31 NIH. A classification and outline of cerebrovascular diseases. II. *Stroke* 1975; 6: 564–616.

32 Levy DE. How transient are transient ischemic attacks? *Neurology* 1988; 38: 674–677.

33 Dyken ML, Conneally M, Haerer AF et al. Cooperative study of hospital frequency and character of transient ischemic attacks. I. Background, organization, and clinical survey. *J Am Med Assoc* 1977; 237: 882–886.

34 Elting JW, de Jager AE, Teelken AW et al. Comparison of serum S-100 protein levels following stroke and traumatic brain injury. *J Neurol Sci* 2000; 181: 104–110.

35 Persson L, Hardemark HG, Gustafsson J et al. S-100 protein and neuron-specific enolase in cerebrospinal fluid and serum: markers of cell damage in human central nervous system. *Stroke* 1987; 18: 911–918.

Perfusion-weighted MRI in stroke

William A. Copen[1] and A. Gregory Sorensen[2]

[1]Massachusetts General Hospital Department of Radiology, Boston, USA
[2]Massachusetts General Hospital NMR Center, Charlestown, USA

Introduction

Perfusion is the circulation of blood through living tissue via a capillary bed that permits transport of oxygen, nutrients and other substances to and from the bloodstream. Correspondingly, perfusion-weighted magnetic resonance imaging (PWI) encompasses a set of techniques that create images depicting hemodynamics at the microvascular level. This is in contrast to vascular imaging studies such as magnetic resonance angiography that show changes occurring in larger arteries and veins. The pathological event initiating ischemic stroke often originates in such larger vessels. However, infarction is directly caused by an impairment of perfusion, that is, an inadequacy of circulation through the capillary bed of affected brain tissue. Therefore, PWI offers the opportunity to study the pathophysiological events that lead most directly to ischemic damage. In some cases, these events are largely or completely undetected by techniques that study only larger vessels. Furthermore, when brain tissue is threatened but not irreversibly damaged by impaired perfusion, the cerebral vasculature exhibits characteristic and identifiable responses that can be identified by PWI. For this reason, PWI may play an important role in guiding therapeutic rescue of tissue that is threatened by ischemia.

This chapter first reviews the techniques employed in PWI, beginning with the role of contrast agents, and the MR pulse sequences that are usually chosen. The postprocessing algorithms that are used to convert raw data into clinically interpretable perfusion-weighted images are then presented. Finally, the clinical interpretation of perfusion-weighted images is discussed.

Contrast agents in PWI

Any cross-sectional imaging technique that studies brain perfusion must detect the presence of blood in vessels much smaller than the tissue voxels that correspond to individual image pixels. In PWI, as with non-MR-based techniques relying on X-ray computed tomography or nuclear imaging, this is accomplished by measuring local concentrations of a contrast agent, or tracer, that is dissolved in the blood. Performing PWI with MRI rather than some other imaging modality offers the theoretical advantage that the contrast agent can be either an endogenous contrast agent that is naturally present in the blood, or an exogenous one that is injected for the purpose of obtaining images.

Two approaches to using endogenous contrast agents have been successful experimentally, though they are not yet optimized for clinical imaging in the setting of stroke. In the first, the contrast agent is hemoglobin. Deoxyhemoglobin is a paramagnetic compound, and therefore has effects on MR images similar to those of other paramagnetic contrast agents such as gadolinium. This observation is the basis of techniques such as BOLD (blood oxygen level dependent) imaging,[1-3] which has been used successfully in numerous experimental studies of brain activation. These changes do reflect brain perfusion to some degree. Unfortunately, the signal changes produced by deoxyhemoglobin are small, in the order of 1% at usual field strengths, and they are difficult to produce uniformly in the brain, and may depend not just on brain perfusion but brain utilization of oxygen; this is an area of active investigation. Consequently, techniques using hemoglobin as an intrinsic contrast agent are not usually used clinically.

A second approach utilizes the protons within flowing blood as an endogenous contrast agent. In this method, called arterial spin labelling (ASL), an additional magnetic pulse, sometimes from a second radiofrequency coil, is performed in the region of an artery supplying the brain, such as an internal carotid artery. This additional pulse is used to excite or tag in some way the protons ('spins') in the blood as they flow by. These excited, or 'labelled' spins then serve as a contrast agent as they enter the brain's capillaries, enabling generation of perfusion-weighted images.[4–6] ASL shows great promise as a PWI technique of the future, and offers several potential advantages. These include lesser expense, lack of side effects from exposure to exogenous contrast agents, the potential for absolute measurement of cerebral blood flow, and the ability to label easily only those spins passing through a particular artery, so that the perfusion territory of a particular artery can be demarcated. Unfortunately, with currently available technology, the signal-to-noise resolution of ASL techniques is much lower than that of methods using exogenous contrast agents. This means that ASL requires image acquisition times that are unacceptably long in the clinical setting in order to produce perfusion-weighted images of comparable quality. Furthermore, these techniques may have artefacts and shortcomings particularly in patients with disturbed cerebral perfusion that have not yet been fully characterized.

Because of the above limitations, PWI techniques now used for imaging stroke patients generally rely on exogenously administered contrast agents. All currently approved MRI contrast agents contain the gadolinium ion, which has a particularly high magnetic moment because of its seven unpaired 4f suborbital electrons. It is this property that makes gadolinium a useful MRI contrast agent.

The free gadolinium ion is toxic, and is therefore always administered in one of several available chelated forms. After intravenous injection, any of the gadolinium chelates rapidly equilibrate throughout the extracellular space in most organs of the body. However, the chelate is too large a complex to pass through the intact blood–brain barrier. Therefore, the contrast agent normally enters the brain parenchyma via small arteries several seconds after injection, passes through the capillary bed, and then exits through small veins within a matter of seconds. Very little gadolinium remains within parenchymal regions with an intact blood–brain barrier.

Conventional contrast-enhanced brain MRI exploits this fact in order to highlight regions in which the blood–brain barrier is absent or damaged. This is accomplished by acquiring T_1-weighted images several minutes after intravenous injection of a gadolinium-based contrast agent, at a time when the agent has been washed out of normal brain tissue. The gadolinium persists in the interstitial spaces of regions without an intact blood–brain barrier. When water molecules whose protons have been excited during an MRI pulse sequence pass very close to the gadolinium ion, they are able to transfer some of their excess energy to the gadolinium ion, in a process alternatively known as spin-lattice relaxation, longitudinal relaxation, or T_1 relaxation. The relaxation process occurs spontaneously in any substance whose protons have been excited, whether or not an exogenous contrast agent is present. The process is accelerated, however, in the presence of gadolinium, because transfer of energy from excited spins is more efficient when the energy acceptor is one with a large magnetic moment such as gadolinium. This 'relaxivity effect' of gadolinium results in shortened T_1, and increased signal intensity on T_1-weighted images.

Though PWI uses the same contrast agents as conventional contrast-enhanced MRI techniques, PWI relies on two fundamentally different principles. First, in PWI, the contrast agent is injected as a rapid bolus, and sequential images are acquired *during* the intravascular transit of that bolus, rather than some time later. In this way, local concentrations of the agent can be measured as they rise and fall rapidly within regions of brain tissue whose blood–brain barrier is intact. Second, PWI techniques generally rely upon gadolinium's 'susceptibility effect' on MR images, rather than the relaxivity effect discussed above.

The susceptibility effect occurs because gadolinium ions and other paramagnetic substances are more magnetically susceptible than diamagnetic substances, meaning that the former behave as small magnets in the presence of an externally applied magnetic field, causing non-uniform microscopic variations in that field. These variations alter the precession frequencies of nearby excited magnetic spins, so that they lose their phase coherence more quickly. This is manifested as loss of signal intensity in T_2- or T_2^*-weighted images. The same susceptibility effect is responsible for loss of signal intensity in the vicinity of hemorrhagic blood breakdown products, metallic hardware such as aneurysm clips, and other highly susceptible substances within the brain. In PWI, loss of signal in T_2- or T_2^*-weighted images due to magnetic susceptibility is exploited in order to measure the local concentration of gadolinium dynamically during intravascular transit.

PWI techniques are usually designed to rely on gadolinium's susceptibility effect rather than its relaxivity effect, chiefly because these effects are exhibited over different ranges. The relaxivity effect requires that an excited hydrogen nucleus approach a gadolinium ion very closely, within several angstroms, in order for transfer of energy to occur. The magnitude of the relaxivity effect falls off with the sixth power of the distance between the two species. Although signal in MR images comes mostly from hydrogen nuclei within water molecules, which are distributed among all tissue compartments, the intact blood–brain barrier limits gadolinium to the intravascular compartment, which occupies only about 4% of tissue volume in grey matter, and 2% in white matter. Therefore, if PWI were to use T_1-weighted images, and measure gadolinium concentration based on relaxivity-related increases in signal intensity, at most about 4% of excited spins would be affected, and the contrast agent would produce only small changes in signal intensity.

Gadolinium's magnetic susceptibility effect, however, operates over much longer ranges. If present in large concentration, such as during its first pass through the cerebral vasculature, gadolinium within a small blood vessel accelerates spin dephasing within a radius approximately equal to the diameter of the vessel. This means that, when PWI is accomplished using T_2- or T_2^*-weighted pulse sequences that are sensitive to gadolinium's susceptibility effect, all of the spins in each tissue voxel are potentially affected by the presence of the contrast agent. Consequently, larger changes in signal intensity are produced, more precise measurements of gadolinium concentration are possible, and more accurate perfusion-weighted images can be generated.

Pulse sequences

For the reasons discussed above, PWI is accomplished most effectively using T_2- or T_2^*-weighted pulse sequences, which are sensitive to the spin dephasing caused by gadolinium's magnetic susceptibility. Elsewhere in clinical practice, T_2^*-weighted gradient echo pulse sequences are often employed when susceptibility effects are of paramount interest, such as when evaluating for the presence of blood breakdown products remaining from previous hemorrhage. Gradient echo pulse sequences can be used in PWI, and demonstrate excellent sensitivity to gadolinium's susceptibility effect. However, clinical experience has shown that spin echo sequences may be more useful, despite such sequences' smaller sensitivity to magnetic susceptibility. This is because signal changes in spin echo images are more dependent on gadolinium concentrations within the capillary bed and other microscopic vessels, whereas gradient echo images assign relatively more weighting to larger vessels. Tissue metabolism is most directly dependent on capillary-level hemodynamics, so spin echo images are more suited to depicting the conditions that determine tissue viability. Furthermore, perfusion-weighted images based on gradient echo pulse sequences are so dominated by large vessels that subtle but important differences in parenchymal perfusion can be difficult to appreciate.

Table 12.1. Sample imaging parameters for perfusion-weighted imaging.

TR: 1500 ms.
TE: 70 ms
Field of view: 20 cm × 20 cm
Matrix size: 128 × 128
Slice thickness: 5 or 6 mm
Interslice gap: 1 mm or interleaved
Number of sequential images for each slice: 45
Number of slices: 11
Total imaging time: 68 seconds (45 images × 1.5 seconds)
Timing of bolus injection: 10 seconds after beginning of imaging
Gadolinium dose: 0.2 mmol/kg
Rate of injection: 5 ml/s
Saline flush: 25 ml
Rate of injection of saline flush: 5 ml/s
Size of intravenous catheter: ideally 18 gauge or larger.

Notes:
These parameters have been used extensively with a 1.5 tesla General Electric scanner, with an echo planar imaging modification by Advanced NMR Systems.

Table 12.1 lists sample image acquisition parameters that have been used successfully in spin echo pulse sequences used for PWI. Note that, because spin echo sequences are less sensitive than gradient echo sequences in detecting the magnetic field inhomogeneities that result from magnetic susceptibility, the usual dose of gadolinium required is 0.2 mmol per kg of body weight, double that used in conventional contrast-enhanced imaging.

Successful implementation of PWI requires that sequential images be acquired rapidly, with a temporal interval of less than 2 seconds, in order to sample adequately the effects of the contrast agent as it passes through the vasculature. This can be accomplished by almost any medium-field scanner in clinical use today. However, multislice PWI requires the use of fast imaging techniques such as echo planar imaging, which can be implemented only on scanners with high performance gradient systems.

Figure 12.1 shows a sequence of images acquired during the intravascular transit of a gadolinium-based contrast agent. Note that the image darkens as the contrast agent enters the cerebral circulation, then lightens again as the agent is washed out of the brain. Qualitatively speaking, the degree to which each part of the brain darkens reflects the regional perfusion of that part of the brain. The next section describes the computational methods that are used to transform raw images such as those in Fig. 12.1 into perfusion-weighted images that convey quantitative information about brain perfusion.

Image postprocessing

In conventional MR images, each pixel's brightness reflects the magnitude of the radiofrequency signal that was emitted by a corresponding voxel of tissue. In PWI, these signal-intensity-based images must undergo an additional processing step, in which one of several computational methods is employed in order to produce images that depict one of a variety of perfusion-related parameters.

The simplest of these parameters to measure is regional cerebral blood volume, or rCBV. Consider, for example, the images marked '0 s' and '9 s' in Fig. 12.1. The 0 s image was acquired just as the bolus of contrast agent reached the brain. Because of the pulse sequence used, it is a predominantly T_2^*-weighted image. The 9 s image, however, was acquired while the contrast agent was present in the cerebral vasculature. It is, therefore, both a T_2-weighted and rCBV-weighted image. This is because, relative to the original 0 s image, each voxel's signal intensity in the 9 s image has fallen by an amount related to the quantity of gadolinium within that voxel, due to accelerated T_2 relaxation. The change in the rate of relaxation, $\Delta R2$, is linearly proportional to the quantity of gadolinium within the voxel, and therefore to the volume of blood in that voxel. So, for each voxel,

$rCBV = k\Delta R2$

where k is a constant, and $\Delta R2$ is the change in the rate of T_2 relaxation. The change in signal intensity that results from T_2 relaxation is an exponential

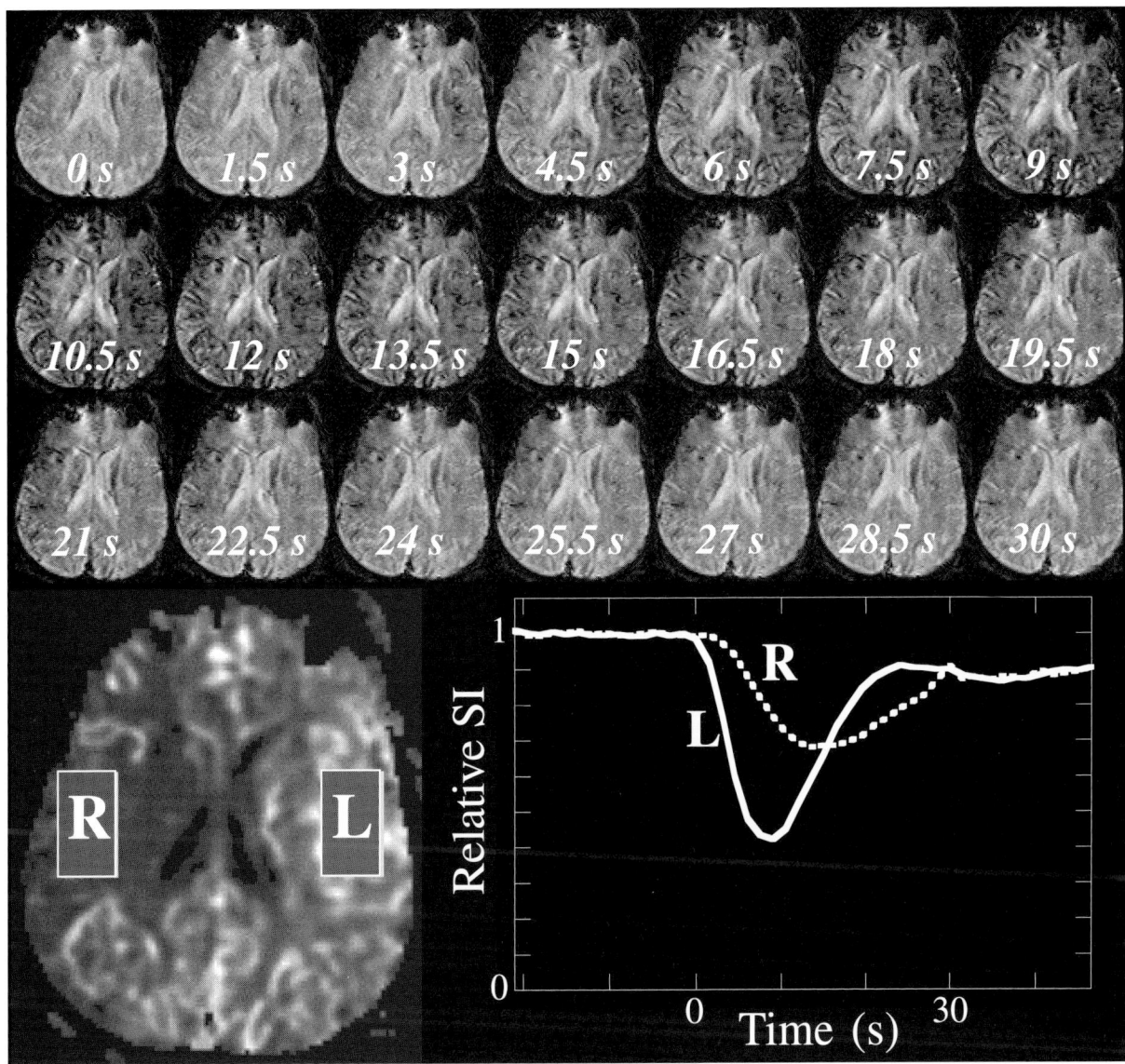

Fig. 12.1. Sequential axial T_2^*-weighted images acquired during intravascular transit of a bolus of gadolinium. The smaller images were acquired every 1.5 seconds, and were used to generate the larger map of rCBF at lower left. The graph at lower right shows how mean pixel signal intensity (relative to baseline pre-gadolinium signal intensity) varied with time in regions of interest placed in the left (L) and right (R) hemispheres. The locations of these regions of interest are shown on the rCBF map at lower left.

process, so the above equation can be converted into one incorporating signal intensities as follows:

$$rCBV_t = -k' \ln\left(\frac{S_t}{S_0}\right)$$

where $rCBV_t$ is the volume of blood within a given voxel at time t, k is a new constant, S_t is the signal intensity at time t and S_0 is the signal intensity that was present at time zero, before the arrival of the contrast agent. Note that only relative rCBV can be calculated, because the value of the constant k depends on numerous factors that are difficult to monitor, including, for example, the delivery of gadolinium to the brain and its subsequent clearance.

The above equation allows calculation of rCBV in each voxel, provided that at least two images are acquired: a baseline image acquired before the arrival of the contrast agent, and a second image acquired while the contrast agent is in the cerebral vasculature. Nevertheless, rCBV is usually calculated using far more than two images. One reason for this is that acquiring multiple images allows more precise estimation of rCBV, simply because more precise estimations of any quantity can be obtained by averaging repeated measurements. Another reason is that the contrast agent is usually injected as a rapid bolus, rather than a steady-state infusion (see below). This means that the agent is not homogeneously dissolved in the blood pool. Depending on differences in regional hemodynamics, the bolus may arrive in different parts of the brain at slightly different times. If only one postcontrast image were acquired, erroneously higher rCBV would be assigned to regions through which the contrast bolus happened to be arriving at the time of image acquisition. Using multiple images helps to minimize this effect by averaging values obtained during the entire passage of the bolus through every voxel.

Customarily, approximately ten to twenty pre-contrast images are acquired before the arrival of the contrast agent in the brain, and averaged to obtain each pixel's baseline S_0 value. Subsequently, approximately 20 to 40 more images are acquired while the contrast agent passes through the brain. For each pixel, rCBV is calculated in each image, and the average rCBV value over time is assigned to each pixel to create a calculated 'map' of rCBV in each part of the brain (see Figs. 12.3, 12.4, and 12.5).

As mentioned above, the contrast agent in PWI is usually injected as a single rapid bolus, rather than as a constant infusion. While it may seem that either injection method would be acceptable, there are two reasons why rapid bolus injection is preferable. First, in order for gadolinium's T_2 relaxivity effects to extend outside of the blood vessels in which it is contained, it must be present in fairly high concentration. At low concentrations, gadolinium's T_1 effects predominate instead. Sufficiently high serum concentrations are difficult to achieve for a prolonged length of time, because gadolinium-based contrast agents are rapidly cleared from the blood in organs other than the brain, where they quickly exit into the interstitial space. About 20% of an injected dose of contrast agent can be lost in its first pass through the lungs alone. Slow infusion would preclude attainment of adequate gadolinium concentrations within the cerebral vasculature.

Rapid bolus injection of gadolinium is also preferable because this allows computation of perfusion parameters other than rCBV. Two such parameters can be intuitively appreciated by visual inspection of the two signal-intensity-vs.-time curves in the lower right portion of Fig. 12.1. It is clear that signal intensity falls more gradually (meaning that gadolinium concentration rises more gradually) in the right hemisphere, which is undergoing infarction, than in the left hemisphere, which is normal. Physiologically, this is because blood flow to the right hemisphere is abnormally low. It is also clear that gadolinium remains in the right hemisphere for a longer time than in the left hemisphere. Physiologically, this is because the mean transit time of any particular small volume of blood through the brain's vasculature is longer in the right hemisphere. Regional cerebral blood flow (rCBF) and mean transit time (rMTT) are perfusion parameters that, along with rCBV, may be useful in guiding stroke therapy. Like rCBV, they can be computed from concentration-vs.-time curves like those in Fig. 12.1. Unlike rCBV, however, their computation is mathematically dependent upon bolus rather than steady-state injection of a contrast agent. Computation of rCBF and rMTT also is more mathematically complex than computation of rCBV.

Before proceeding to the calculations necessary to compute rCBF and rMTT, it will be worthwhile to consider the qualitative examples in Fig. 12.2, which illustrates conceptually some of the difficulties of determining rCBF using PWI. The top row of Fig. 12.2 (part (*a*)) of Fig. 12.2 depicts an idealized PWI examination, in which the entire quantity of gadolinium that enters a voxel of brain tissue

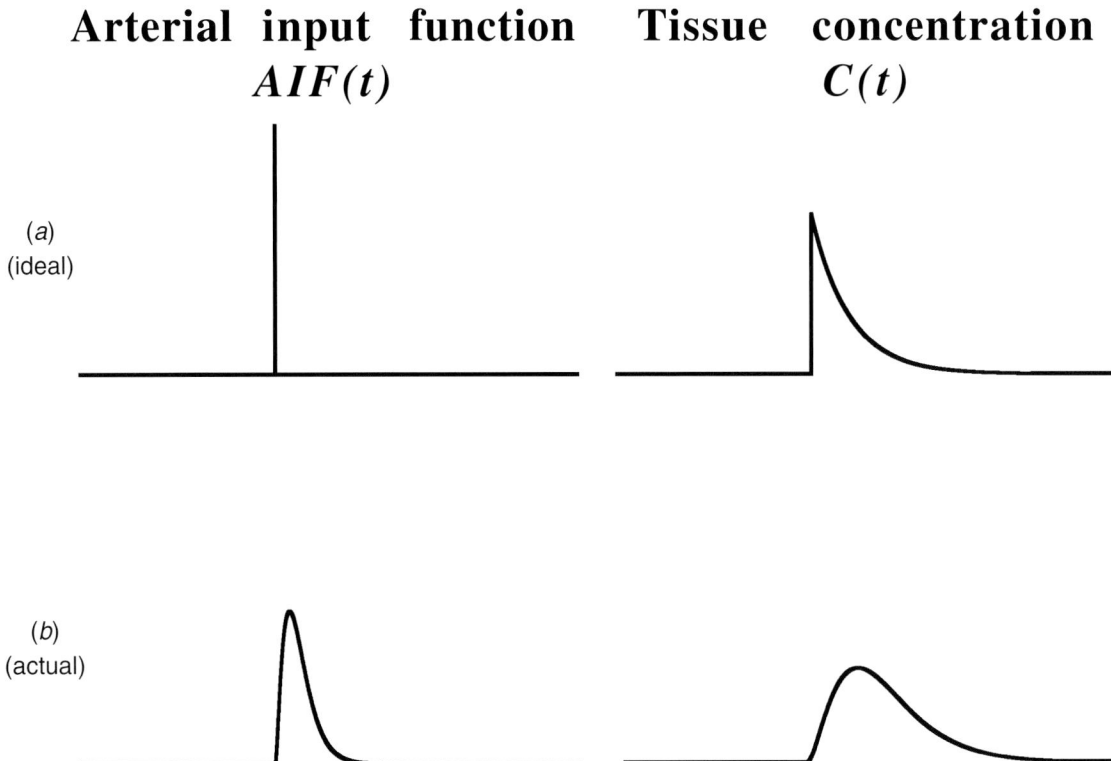

Fig. 12.2. Ideal and actual arterial input function and tissue concentration curves. In these four curves, time is measured on the *x*-axis, and gadolinium concentration on the *y*-axis. The two curves on the left are arterial input functions, depicting the delivery of a bolus of gadolinium to a hypothetical tissue voxel as a function of time. The two curves on the right depict the concentration of gadolinium in that voxel as a function of time. Ideally, as in (*a*) the entire gadolinium bolus is delivered during a single instant in time. In this case, tissue concentration immediately reaches its maximum, and rCBF in each voxel is proportional to the initial maximum value attained in that voxel. (*b*) depicts a more realistic situation, in which the bolus of gadolinium is delivered over a brief but not instantaneous period of time. In this case, tissue concentration rises and falls more gradually, and rCBF must be calculated by deconvolution (see text).

arrives at the same instant in time, as shown by the arterial input function, AIF(t), on the left. In this idealized case, the concentration function, C(t), which describes the concentration of gadolinium in the voxel as a function of time, reaches its maximum immediately, and then falls gradually as the gadolinium bolus leaves the voxel via the venous system. In this case, computation of rCBF is straightforward and maximally accurate; it is proportional to the gadolinium concentration at the instant when the bolus arrives.

In reality, it is impossible to achieve instantaneous arrival of the entire gadolinium bolus. Even mechanical power injectors are limited in the rate at which they can deliver contrast agents into the bloodstream. Furthermore, for practical reasons, the gadolinium must be injected into a vein, rather than directly into an artery supplying the brain. As the bolus travels through the venous system, the right heart, the pulmonary vasculature, and finally the arteries supplying the brain, it is dispersed in the blood, so that the arrival of gadolinium in a brain voxel is dispersed in time. This dispersion is amplified by slower injection of the contrast agent bolus, or in patients whose cardiac output is low.

The bottom row of Fig. 12.2 (part (*b*)) depicts this noninstantaneous arrival of the tracer bolus that occurs in reality, and the effect that it has on C(t). In this case, computation of rCBF in this voxel is no longer straightforward. This is because C(t) is now mathematically dependent not only on rCBF, but also on two other functions: AIF(t), and R(t), a 'residue function' that describes the proportion of tracer remaining in the voxel as a function of time. The residue function is not shown explicitly in Fig. 12.2, but has exactly the same shape as the concentration function in part A. Mathematically, it can be said that C(t) is the product of rCBF and the convolution of AIF(t) and R(t). In order to calculate rCBF, R(t) must be determined, using a somewhat complex process called deconvolution. A number of algorithms for deconvolution exist. We have used singular value decomposition, which is relatively robust, in that it works well in a variety of situations in which perfusion is altered.[7,8]

All deconvolution methods are similar in that they require that AIF(t) be supplied along with C(t). Generally, one AIF to be used for all image pixels is obtained by selecting manually several pixels that lie adjacent to a major cerebral artery, and therefore can be used to sample the concentration of tracer within the artery. A middle cerebral artery is typically used, because much of its course is usually visualized within a single axial image section, and this makes selection of adjacent pixels easier. Note that pixels that lie within the artery cannot be used, because, for technical reasons, the relationship between signal intensity and gadolinium concentration is more complex for those pixels than for pixels just outside the artery. Pixel selection can be performed by a physician, technologist, or other trained personnel in a few minutes, or can be done by an automated or semiautomated computer program.

Selection of pixels to sample arterial flow is based both on location and on signal characteristics. The ideal pixels to choose are those that demonstrate the characteristics of flow in a major artery rather than microvascular flow, i.e. early arrival of the tracer, large signal drop during tracer passage, and rapid return to baseline signal intensity. After several such pixels have been chosen, their signal intensities at each time point are averaged, and the resulting signal-intensity-vs.-time curve is converted to a concentration-vs.-time curve, which is used as AIF(t). The automated deconvolution process then takes several more minutes, depending on available computing resources, to generate maps of rCBF. After rCBF has been calculated for each image pixel, calculation of rMTT is straightforward, because rCBV, rCBF, and rMTT are related by the central volume theorem:

$$rMTT = \frac{rCBV}{rCBF}$$

Because deconvolution is computationally intensive and requires calculation of an arterial input function, some centres have used more mathematically simple approximations of rCBF and rMTT. For example, the slope of the increase in gadolinium concentration after bolus arrival can be used as an approximation of rCBF. The width of the concentration curve when it reaches half of its maximum value can be used as an approximation of rMTT. While such approximations lack the mathematical rigor of quantities determined by deconvolution, their calculation is more straightforward.

Interpretation of perfusion-weighted images

When rCBV, rCBF, and rMTT are evaluated together, considerable information regarding regional cerebral perfusion is available. This is because these quantities illuminate not only the degree and physical location of ischemic insult, but also the nature of the cerebrovascular response.

The fundamental determinant of cerebral perfusion is cerebral perfusion pressure, or CPP. The blood vessels of the brain adapt to changes in CPP by adjusting vascular resistance so that, within a wide range of local CPP values, rCBF is maintained close to its normal value of about 50 cm^3 of blood per 100 g of brain tissue per minute in grey matter, and somewhat less in white matter. When decreases in CPP are so great that this autoregulatory process begins to fail, rCBF falls. However, the vasculature is still able to compensate with further reductions in vascular recruitment and vasodilation. This tends to preserve or even increase rCBV. Importantly, because the effective cross-sectional area of the microvasculature is increased, the velocity of blood flow is reduced. Consequently, MTT of blood within each capillary is increased. When red blood cells spend a greater amount of time in each capillary, brain tissue is able to extract a larger amount of oxygen, possibly enough to survive for some period of time despite impaired rCBF. In light of these effects, elevations in rMTT can be seen as indications of the brain's attempts to compensate for ischemic insult. Accordingly, a drop in rCBV could signify exhaustion of the vasculature's autoregulatory reserve.

Understanding of cerebrovascular hemodynamics suggests several potential roles for PWI in caring for stroke patients. PWI is of greatest clinical interest in acute stroke, when timely therapeutic reperfusion may result in the preservation of ischemically threatened tissue that otherwise would undergo infarction. In this setting, PWI is most often performed along with diffusion-weighted magnetic resonance imaging, or DWI. DWI is much more accurate than other imaging modalities in identifying damaged tissue very early after stroke onset.[9–11] However, infarcts often enlarge over time to encompass more tissue than initially appears abnormal on DWI.[12–18]

Now that thrombolytic therapy is commonly employed in acute stroke management, predicting the extent to which acute infarcts will grow in the days following presentation is increasingly important. Intravenous or intra-arterial thrombolysis is capable of saving substantial quantities of brain tissue that otherwise would have undergone infarction, resulting in marked reduction of permanent neurologic deficits. However, thrombolysis also carries considerable risk of catastrophic intracranial hemorrhage. The decision of whether or not to accept this risk and proceed with thrombolysis is a highly individualized one. In making that decision, clinicians, patients and their families would benefit from an informed estimation of how much brain tissue will be affected, and how severe neurological deficits are likely to be, if thrombolytic therapy is not initiated.

PWI can help to identify tissue that is at risk of inclusion into growing infarcts. This tissue may be represented by regions of 'diffusion-perfusion mismatch', i.e. that portion of the brain in which abnormalities are seen on acute-stage PWI, but not on DWI. Infarcts are more likely to grow substantially when the area of diffusion–perfusion mismatch is large.[13,18–20]

This observation raises the question of how information from the various kinds of perfusion-weighted images should be integrated in order to identify tissue at risk and predict lesion enlargement. One study found that volumes of abnormalities on initial rCBV images provide the best estimate of final lesion volumes, though slightly underestimating those volumes. That study found that abnormalities on initial rCBF or rMTT images are often much larger, and may overestimate the amount of tissue that will be involved.[18] Another study also found that rCBF abnormalities tended to be larger than final infarct volumes, but found that, among patients with a large region of diffusion–perfusion mismatch, abnormalities on rCBF maps provided the best single estimate of final infarct progression.[20]

These studies are consistent with the view that reduced rCBF represents ischemic threat to brain tissue, increased rMTT represents the brain's active response to that threat, and reduced rCBV may represent failure of that response to meet metabolic needs. In this view, regions of reduced rCBV represent tissue that is very likely destined for infarction, but regions of abnormal rCBF or rMTT may or may not proceed to infarction (see Fig. 12.3 and Fig. 12.4). There have been efforts to develop models that combine all three of these parameters, along with other imaging measurements, in order to predict the probability of infarction of any given tissue voxel.[21]

Besides informing the decision of whether or not to proceed to thrombolysis by identifying tissue that is at risk, PWI has also been used to determine whether reperfusion has occurred,

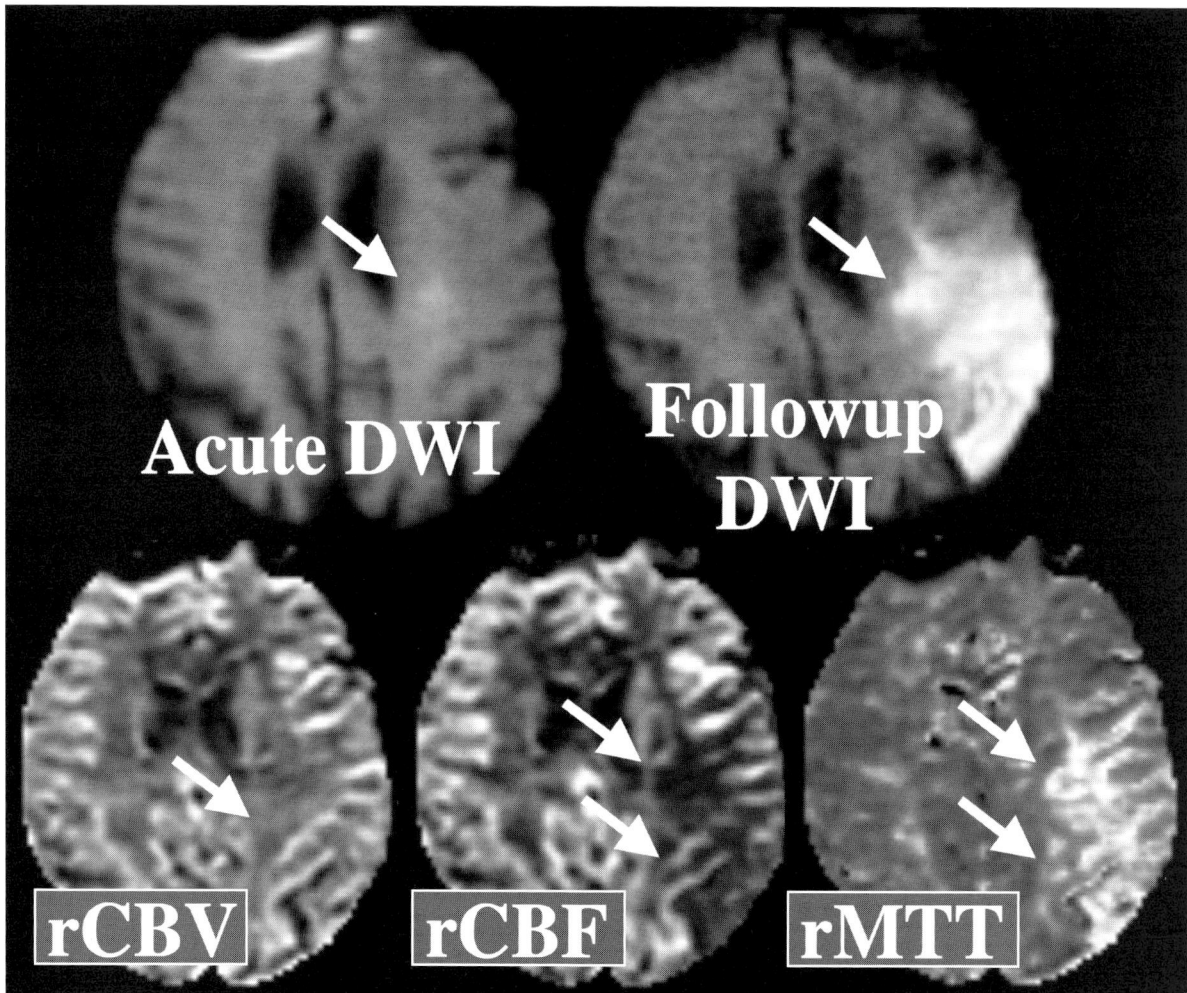

Fig. 12.3. Extension of an acute infarct into an area of abnormal perfusion. In this patient, acute-stage diffusion-weighted imaging (DWI) showed a small, subtle ischemic lesion in the left centrum semiovale. A map of rCBV, acquired during the same examination, showed a matching small, subtle region of decreased rCBV. However, the other two PWI maps showed a much larger region of decreased rCBF and increased rMTT. Abnormal regions in each image are marked by arrows. A follow-up DWI image obtained one day later shows that the infarct had grown to encompass much of the ischemically threatened tissue identified in the rCBF and rMTT maps.

either spontaneously or as a result of thrombolytic therapy.[22,23] Figure 12.5 provides an example of an acute stroke patient in whom spontaneous reperfusion occurred prior to imaging. In this patient, thrombolytic therapy would confer no potential benefit, while conferring a significant risk of hemorrhage.

As clinical experience with PWI in acute stroke accrues, it is likely that more precisely formulated guidelines will emerge for interpreting information that already is contained in currently available perfusion-weighted images.

Conclusions

PWI describes a set of techniques in which sequential magnetic resonance images of the brain are acquired during intravascular transit of a bolus of a gadolinium-based exogenous contrast agent, in order to

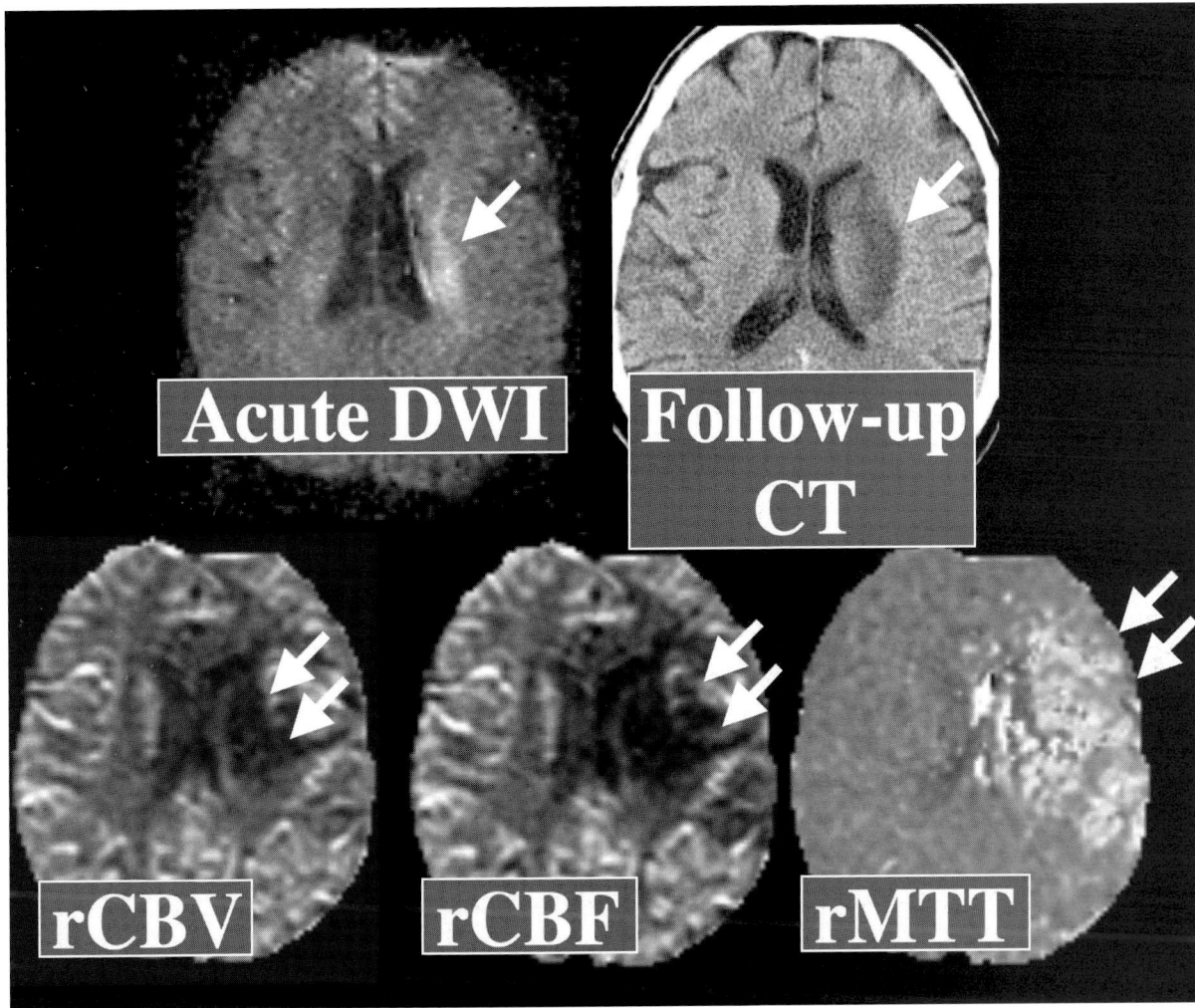

Fig. 12.4. Failure of an acute infarct to extend into an area of abnormal perfusion. In this patient, acute-stage DWI showed a small ischemic lesion involving the left corona radiata. PWI showed larger regions of abnormal rCBV, rCBF, and rMTT. Abnormal regions in each image are marked by arrows. A follow-up CT image obtained 2 days later shows that the infarct had not grown significantly into the region of acutely impaired perfusion.

produce images that depict hemodynamics at the microvascular level. Although PWI can be accomplished with most scanners in clinical use today, multislice PWI requires fast imaging pulse sequences such as echo planar imaging. The raw images obtained during intravascular transit of the contrast agent are used to generate images depicting regional variations in any of several perfusion-related parameters, which may include cerebral blood volume, cerebral blood flow and mean transit time. These are most useful in acute stroke, when information about regional perfusion may help to guide decisions regarding thrombolytic therapy. Tissue that demonstrates abnormal perfusion, without abnormal appearance on acute-stage diffusion-weighted imaging, may be tissue that is at risk of inclusion into a growing infarct, and therefore tissue that may be rescued by timely therapeutic reperfusion. PWI can also identify cases in which spontaneous or therapeutic reperfusion of ischemic areas has occurred, so that further thrombolytic therapy would be dangerous and without potential benefit. Additional clinical experience with PWI will enable more precise and detailed definition of the role of PWI in stroke management.

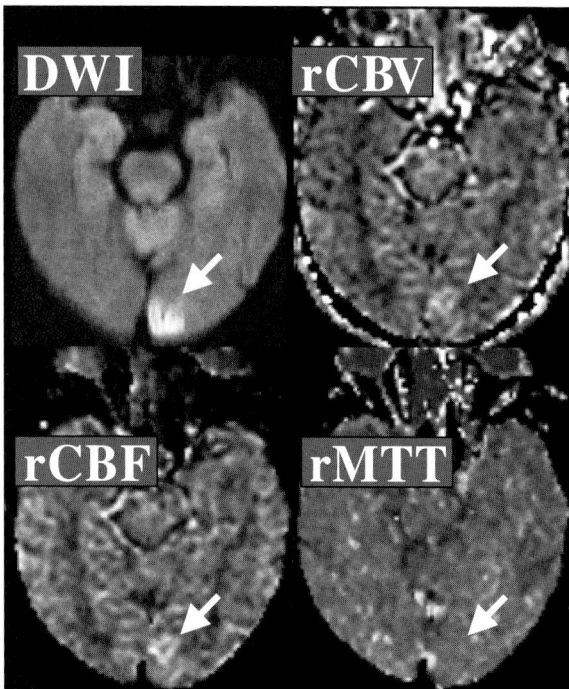

Fig. 12.5. Spontaneous reperfusion. In this patient, acute-stage DWI showed an ischemic lesion in the left occipital lobe (*arrow*). PWI showed that rCBV and rCBF were not decreased, but rather elevated (arrows) in this region, signifying the characteristic hyperemia or 'luxury perfusion' that often follows spontaneous reperfusion of ischemic brain tissue. There was no definite rMTT abnormality. In this patient, thrombolytic therapy would pose a significant risk of hemorrhage, probably without potential gain.

REFERENCES

1 Ogawa S, Lee TM. Magnetic resonance imaging of blood vessels at high fields: in vivo and in vitro measurements and image simulation. *Magn Reson Med* 1990; 16: 9–18.

2 Ogawa S, Lee TM, Kay AR, Tank DW. Brain magnetic resonance imaging with contrast dependent on blood oxygenation. *Proc Natl Acad Sci USA* 1990; 87: 9868–9872.

3 Ogawa S, Lee TM, Nayak AS, Glynn P. Oxygenation-sensitive contrast in magnetic resonance image of rodent brain at high magnetic fields. *Magn Reson Med* 1990; 14: 68–78.

4 Detre JA, Subramanian VH, Mitchell MD et al. Measurement of regional cerebral blood flow in cat brain using intracarotid $2H_2O$ and ^2H NMR imaging. *Magn Reson Med* 1990; 14: 389–395.

5 Williams DS, Detre JA, Leigh JS, Koretsky AP. Magnetic resonance imaging of perfusion using spin inversion of arterial water. [erratum appears in *Proc Natl Acad Sci USA* 1992 May 1; 89(9): 4220]. *Proc Natl Acad Sci USA* 1992; 89: 212–216.

6 Edelman RR, Siewert B, Darby DG et al. Qualitative mapping of cerebral blood flow and functional localization with echo-planar MR imaging and signal targeting with alternating radio frequency. *Radiology* 1994; 192: 513–520.

7 Østergaard L, Weisskoff RM, Chesler DA, Gyldensted C, Rosen BR. High resolution measurement of cerebral blood flow using intravascular tracer bolus passages. Part I: Mathematical approach and statistical analysis. *Magn Reson Med* 1996; 36: 715–725.

8 Østergaard L, Sorensen AG, Kwong KK, Weisskoff RM, Gyldensted C, Rosen BR. High resolution measurement of cerebral blood flow using intravascular tracer bolus passages. Part II: Experimental comparison and preliminary results. *Magn Reson Med* 1996; 36: 726–736.

9 Lövblad KO, Laubach HJ, Baird AE et al. Clinical experience with diffusion-weighted MR in patients with acute stroke. *Am J Neuroradiol* 1998; 19: 1061–1066.

10 Singer MB, Chong J, Lu D, Schonewille WJ, Tuhrim S, Atlas SW. Diffusion-weighted MRI in acute subcortical infarction. *Stroke* 1998; 29: 133–136.

11 Gonzalez RG, Schaefer PW, Buonanno FS et al. Diffusion-weighted MR imaging: diagnostic accuracy in patients imaged within 6 hours of stroke symptom onset. *Radiology* 1999; 210: 155–162.

12 Sorensen AG, Buonanno FS, Gonzalez RG et al. Hyperacute stroke: evaluation with combined multi-section diffusion-weighted and hemodynamically weighted echo-planar MR imaging. *Radiology* 1996; 199: 391–401.

13 Baird AE, Benfield A, Schlaug G et al. Enlargement of human cerebral ischemic lesion volumes measured by diffusion-weighted magnetic resonance imaging. *Ann Neurol* 1997; 41: 581–589.

14 Barber PA, Darby DG, Desmond PM et al. Prediction of stroke outcome with echoplanar perfusion- and diffusion-weighted MRI. *Neurology* 1998; 51: 418–426.

15 Schwamm LH, Koroshetz WJ, Sorensen AG et al. Time course of lesion development in patients with acute stroke: serial diffusion- and hemodynamic-weighted magnetic resonance imaging. *Stroke* 1998; 29: 2268–2276.

16 van Everdingen KJ, van der Grond J, Kappelle LJ, Ramos LM, Mali WP. Diffusion-weighted magnetic resonance imaging in acute stroke. *Stroke* 1998; 29: 1783–1790.

17 Rordorf G, Koroshetz WJ, Copen WA et al. Regional ischemia and ischemic injury in patients with acute middle cerebral artery stroke as defined by early diffusion-weighted and perfusion-weighted MRI. *Stroke* 1998; 29: 939–943.

18 Sorensen AG, Copen WA, Østergaard L et al. Hyperacute stroke: simultaneous measurement of relative cerebral blood volume, relative cerebral blood flow, and mean tissue transit time. *Radiology.* 1999; 210: 519–527.

19 Neumann-Haefelin T, Wittsack HJ, Wenserski F et al. Diffusion- and perfusion-weighted MRI. The DWI/PWI mismatch region in acute stroke. *Stroke* 1999; 30: 1591–1597.

20 Parsons MW, Yang Q, Barber PA et al. Perfusion magnetic resonance imaging maps in hyperacute stroke: relative cerebral blood flow most accurately identifies tissue destined to infarct. *Stroke* 2001; 32: 1581–1587.

21 Wu O, Koroshetz WJ, Ostergaard L et al. Predicting tissue outcome in acute human cerebral ischemia using combined diffusion- and perfusion-weighted MR imaging. *Stroke* 2001; 32: 933–942.

22 Marks MP, Tong DC, Beaulieu C, Albers GW, de Crespigny A, Moseley ME. Evaluation of early reperfusion and i.v. tPA therapy using diffusion- and perfusion-weighted MRI [see comments]. *Neurology* 1999; 52: 1792–1798.

23 Kidwell CS, Saver JL, Mattiello J et al. Thrombolytic reversal of acute human cerebral ischemic injury shown by diffusion/perfusion magnetic resonance imaging. *Ann Neurol* 2000; 47: 462–469.

Perfusion imaging with arterial spin labelling

David C. Alsop[1] and John A. Detre[2]

[1]Department of Radiology,
Beth Israel Deaconess Medical Center and Harvard Medical School, USA
[2]Departments of Neurology and Radiology
University of Pennsylvania Medical Center, USA

Introduction

Unlike diffusion imaging, which is unique to MRI, imaging of cerebral blood flow is possible with a number of tomographic techniques including PET,[1] SPECT,[2] and X-ray CT.[3,4] Relative to these other approaches, blood flow imaging with MRI can be advantageous because of its speed, spatial resolution, lack of ionizing radiation, and MRI's ability to obtain other, spatially registered images such as diffusion, MR angiography, or even MR spectroscopy within the same study.

Imaging of hemodynamic parameters such as time to peak, mean transit time, relative blood flow, and relative blood volume is possible with the bolus injection of a contrast agent.[5,6] This dynamic susceptibility contrast (DSC) approach yields a large signal change, which permits the sensitive characterization of the passage of the bolus through the vasculature. It is particularly good at delineating very delayed or extended transit of the bolus through a region of tissue and has thus been widely applied to the study of stroke in animals and humans.

While clearly a powerful technique, hemodynamic MRI with contrast injection is not without weaknesses. First, it requires a well-timed i.v. injection of a contrast agent. The injection increases the cost of the study significantly, requires good venous access, preferably a power injector, and limits the short term repeatability of the study. Second, because it is an intravascular tracer, quantification of perfusion can be confused by pathologic conditions such as delayed flow or collateral flow through multiple paths.[7] Third, measurements of absolute blood flow and volume are not readily possible. Finally, motion during the bolus is a frequent problem because of poor patient cooperation and discomfort from the injection. Motion is an inherent problem with most imaging techniques, but those that depend upon changes in a larger background signal intensity are most prone to error.

An alternative technique for the measurement of perfusion MRI known as arterial spin labelling (ASL) shows promise for addressing many of the limitations of bolus contrast for perfusion assessment.[8,9] This approach employs electromagnetic fields to non-invasively label the nuclear spins of water in the inflowing arterial blood. These labelled spins then enter the tissue where the labelling causes an attenuation of signal proportional to perfusion. While the signal change resulting from labelling is much smaller than with bolus contrast injection, ASL offers a flexibility of acquisition and quantification strategies that can be advantageous in numerous applications.

Arterial spin labelling methods

The spatially selective radiofrequency (RF) excitation and inversion capabilities of magnetic resonance make possible a totally non-invasive method for perfusion imaging, which is known as arterial spin labelling. The basic principle of ASL perfusion imaging is simple, (see Fig. 13.1). If blood flows

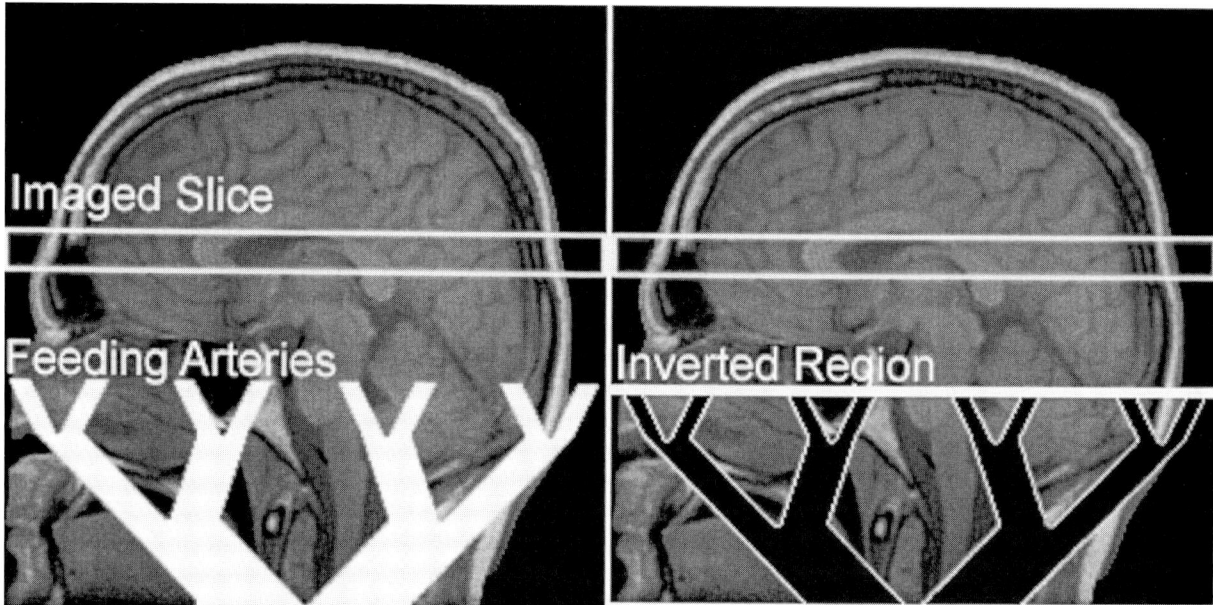

Fig. 13.1. The arterial spin labelling technique. Normally positive nuclear spins flow from feeding arteries into the slice of tissue being imaged, left. Spatially selective inversion can be applied inferior to the slice to be imaged such that the sign of the spins in the feeding arteries is changed. This negative signal flows into the imaged slice and decreases the signal intensity.

through a region of tissue, then it must be supplied by an artery which comes from outside of the region. Any spatially selective alteration of signal outside of the region will change the spins in the feeding artery. If time is allowed for these changed spins to enter the tissue, then there will be a change in the spins within the tissue.

ASL is a competition between T_1 decay and inflow of new spins. With f (the flow or perfusion) being the rate of inflow and $1/T_1$ being the rate of decay, the fractional change in the image intensity due to ASL tends to be approximately $f \times T_1$. For a T_1 of 1 second and a flow of 60 ml/100 g/min, equal to 1 ml/100 g per s ($= 0.01/s$), the ratio is 1%. Typically, ASL signal changes in human grey matter are of this order and white matter flow is considerably smaller. Compared to DSC imaging, the signal change in ASL is quite small and one might initially consider the signal unmeasurable. However, with modern scanners equipped with fast imaging hardware to minimize motion related noise, images of the perfusion-related signal can readily be measured, albeit at lower spatial resolution than typically used for clinical MRI.

The small size of the ASL effect means that it is virtually impossible to obtain an ASL measurement without first subtracting out the unwanted, perfusion unrelated background signal. This is typically achieved by acquiring one image with some perturbation of the inflowing arterial spins, the labelled image, and a second image with no perturbation of the arterial spins, the control image. Subtraction of the two images yields a perfusion sensitive image (Fig. 13.2) As with DSC imaging, there would be no signal in this subtraction image without perfusion but quantification of perfusion requires further analysis

Labelling strategies for ASL

The simplicity of the ASL approach has been somewhat muddled by the introduction of a number of different approaches to labelling, each with its own acronym. The clearest distinction between labelling approaches is between continuous ASL and pulsed ASL. In continuous ASL,[9] spins are continuously inverted at a specific location before they enter the tissue. Thus spins which enter the tissue first are

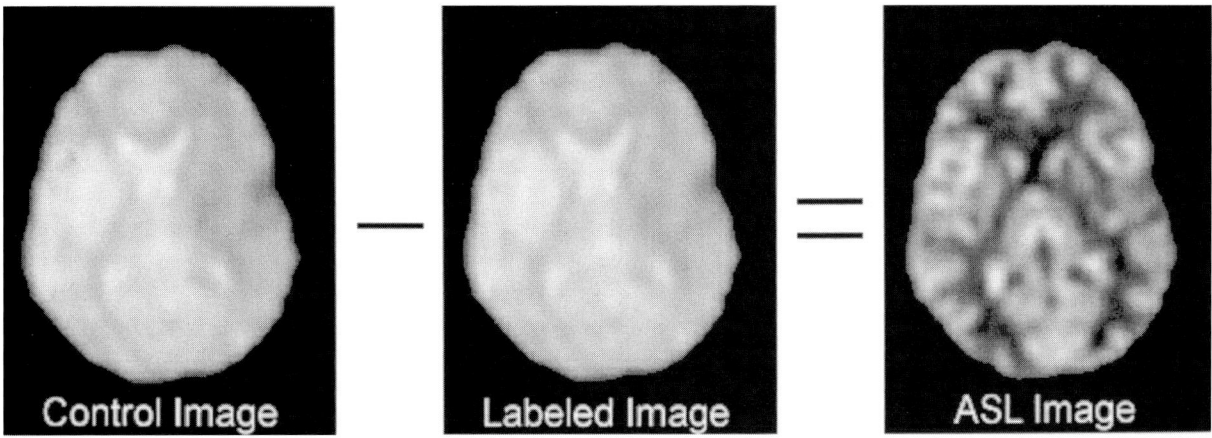

Fig. 13.2. The subtraction method used for most ASL imaging. An image acquired with labelling is subtracted from an image without labelling, the control. The resulting very small difference, typically less than 1% of the image intensity, reflects perfusion.

labelled first and spins which enter later are labelled later. In contrast, the pulsed labelling techniques[10,11] apply a single perturbing pulse to the spins outside the slice and then wait as the spins enter the tissue. Because spins which enter the tissue later are perturbed earlier than in the continuous technique, there is additional T_1 decay of the label and generally the signal change with pulsed techniques is smaller than with continuous techniques.[12,13] Nevertheless, pulsed techniques employ more traditional RF and gradient strategies and can produce excellent images. For simplicity, the pulsed techniques will be discussed first.

In pulsed techniques, an RF pulse is applied at a time approximately 1 second before imaging. Almost always an inversion RF pulse is used because it creates the largest change in the arterial magnetization and, by analogy to inversion recovery, the time before imaging is referred to as TI. Two images are obtained, one with the region containing the inflowing artery inverted and one where it is not inverted. The only differences between all of the pulsed labelling strategies is what inversions are applied to other tissue, including the imaged region, and what is done to insure that the differences between the two RF preparations do not cause direct effects on the image which are independent of perfusion. Such direct effects can result from imperfect inversion slice profiles[14] and differences in the magnetization transfer effects of the two preparation sequences.[15,16]

Edelman et al.[10] were the first to apply pulsed techniques in humans. They employed a slab selective inversion pulse inferior to the imaged brain region to label arterial spins and a superior inversion slab during the control image preparation. The most distinct alternative strategy employs a non-selective inversion pulse for the labelling and a slab selective inversion containing the entire imaged region for a control. This inversion technique was first proposed by Kwong et al.[11] Because any slight difference in the flip angle of the two pulses will have a big effect upon the measured signal, special RF pulses with low sensitivity to variations in RF amplitude and very sharp slice profiles must be employed.[17]

Continuous ASL usually employs a special RF labelling scheme known as flow driven adiabatic inversion.[18] One can approximate continuous saturation[8] of spins as they flow past a certain plane by applying a series of thin saturation pulses repeatedly, but trying the same strategy with inversion pulses is problematic; some spins may remain within the saturation slab for two or more inversions and get doubly inverted. Because inversion provides a stronger signal change in ASL, it is considered highly desirable to use a continuous inversion technique. Flow-driven adiabatic inversion is a simple technique because it requires only turning on a constant gradient and R; however, the concept of flow driven adiabatic inversion is foreign to most MRI practitioners who typically use only pulsed RF.

For the purposes of perfusion imaging, however, it is only necessary to understand that the technique defines a plane such that all spins flowing through the plane get inverted at the time they flow through.

The greatest attraction of continuous ASL is that it can achieve a signal approximately two to three times larger than with pulsed ASL.[12] To achieve this large a signal change, however, the labelling must be left on for many seconds. The decreased number of averages achievable per unit time with this large signal change partially offsets the signal advantage.[19] Still, continuous ASL is generally more sensitive than pulsed techniques and has some advantages in the details of implementation. The greatest disadvantages of the continuous labelling approach are the unusual RF requirements of the labelling. First, many scanners are designed specifically for brief, widely spaced pulses of RF at high power. Flow-driven adiabatic inversion requires weaker RF for an extended period of time, so implementation on some scanners may be difficult. The long duration of the labelling can also lead to high RF power deposition in the subject that can approach the FDA limits. Nevertheless, continuous labelling can be performed on many mainstream clinical scanners at power levels well within the FDA limits.[13]

Quantification of perfusion with ASL

ASL perfusion measurement differs from DSC imaging in several important ways. First, the tracer, water spins, can readily diffuse into tissue.[20] This makes it impossible to measure venous blood volume with ASL but it also makes ASL insensitive to the vessel permeability issues that affect DSC perfusion imaging when the blood–brain barrier is damaged. Another important difference is that the tracer is rapidly decaying. Finally, the tracer is 'injected' into the arteries right near the tissue, so deconvolution of an intravenous bolus is unnecessary. Typically, the arterial input function is assumed based upon the labelling applied whether pulsed or continuous.

Because the tracer is rapidly decaying, it is important to know the decay rate, T_1. T_1 of blood can be taken from literature values[21] or an attempt can be made to measure it in vivo. Likewise, the tissue T_1 can be measured, since it may be different than the T_1 of blood. Including the effects of the different T_1's complicates the discussion,[13] so for now, assume T_1 of blood and tissue are the same.

For pulsed experiments, the effect of the inversion is to create a bolus of labelled spins that is of duration t_b. If we wait long enough for the bolus to enter the tissue, a time TI, before imaging, then the labelled signal will be just the perfusion times the duration of the bolus times a decay factor for T_1 decay over TI.

If we had not waited long enough, then some of the labelled blood destined for the tissue would still be in the feeding vessels and the perfusion would be underestimated. One of the challenges of pulsed ASL quantification is that t_b is not known because the inversion pulse inverts a thickness of tissue containing arteries, not a duration. Wong and collaborators[22] applied a saturation pulse at a certain time after the inversion to eliminate any labelled blood still remaining in the inverted slab. This makes the t_b always be equal to TI–Tsat.

For continuous ASL experiments the perfusion quantification is slightly different. Since the spins are not all labelled at the same time we have to average the T_1 decay of the duration of the bolus. Often the term TI is not used for continuous experiments. Instead w, a postlabelling delay is defined such that $TI = t_b + w$.[13] As with the pulsed experiment, flow will be underestimated unless one waits long enough for all of the bolus to enter the tissue.

If the T_1 of tissue and blood are significantly different, then there will be added uncertainty in the quantification of perfusion. Generally, if one uses the T_1 of blood in the above equations and T_1 of tissue is shorter, the perfusion will be underestimated, and if the T_1 of tissue is longer, then perfusion will be overestimated.[13]

Motion artefacts and ASL

While the small signal level of ASL reduces the signal-to-noise ratio of ASL perfusion images, surprisingly good images can be obtained if motion artefacts can be reduced and eliminated. Though

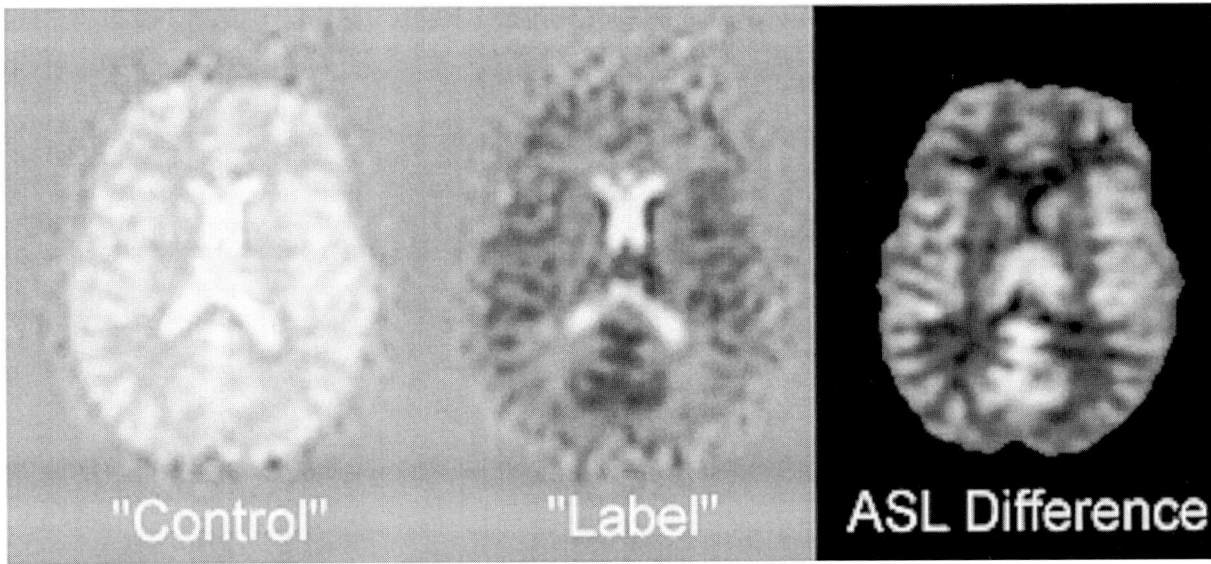

Fig. 13.3. Background suppressed ASL. The background signal has been attenuated to less than the grey matter perfusion signal such that the negative ASL contribution changes the sign of the labelled image. The difference image, right, is much less sensitive to motion artefact than in traditional ASL.

snapshot imaging is typically used for ASL studies, the subtraction of images acquired at different times still can be sensitive to motion. Experience with patient studies has shown, however, that good image quality can be obtained with simple strategies to reduce motion and recent developments suggest even greater robustness to motion is possible.

Typically imaging of perfusion with ASL requires multiple averages to achieve an acceptable signal-to-noise ratio. If the label and control images are interleaved, i.e. first a control, then a label, then a control, then a label, etc., the time difference between the two sets of images will be only one TR, even if the averaging continues for many minutes. This rapid alternation between label and control tends to give improved robustness to motion and other sources of noise in the scanner, such as drifts in sensitivity. In normal subjects and reasonably cooperative volunteers, this subtraction strategy is sufficient to achieve good quality images.[23] Robustness to motion can be further improved by using postprocessing methods to reduce motion. Using one particular strategy[24] we have been able to drastically reduce residual motion in ASL perfusion images of acute stroke patients and demented patients, even when subjects were speaking during the scan.

Further reduction of motion artefacts is possible by suppression of the background signal, which is normally much larger than the perfusion related signal change. A very successful strategy for suppression was first proposed by Dixon et al.[25] First apply a highly selective 90 degree pulse to the tissue to be imaged. Next perform the labelling pulse. Later, apply one or more non-selective inversion pulses timed to null the tissue signal at the imaging time. In the absence of inflow, there will be zero signal from the tissue but the inflowing blood signal will be the same magnitude.

Such a strategy was employed by Ye et al.[26] to reduce noise from the motion of the background signal in an ASL experiment by a factor of 10. We have found that optimization of inversion timing for suppression over a broad range of T_1's can produce suppression of the background signal by a factor of greater than 100. This makes the signal from ASL larger than the background signal and greatly reduces concerns of motion artefact (Fig. 13.3). Background suppression changes the relative motion sensitivity of the two MR perfusion imaging techniques. Background suppressed ASL is much less sensitive to motion than DSC imaging.

Background suppression can be adapted to most

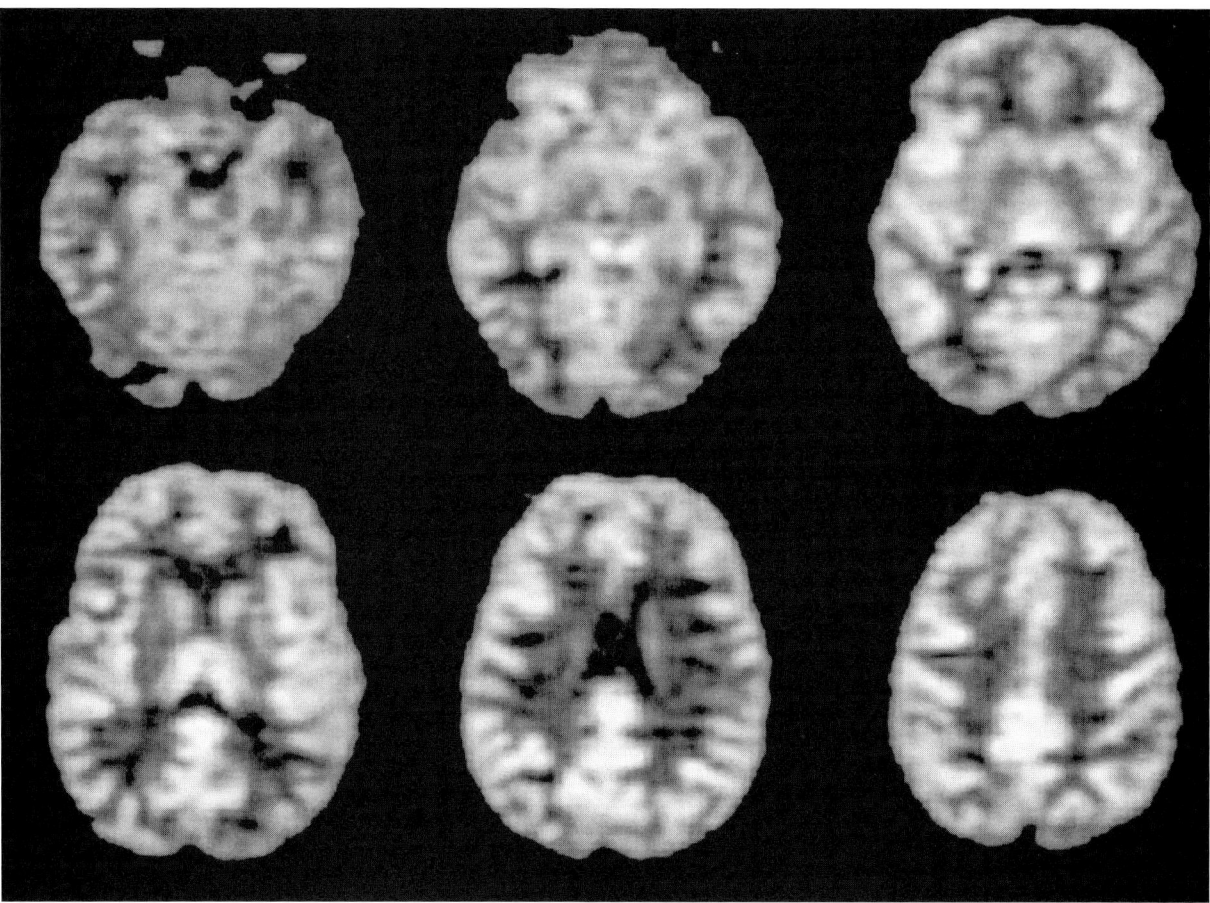

Fig. 13.4. ASL difference images acquired with background suppression, continuous labelling, and a 3D fast spin echo imaging sequence.

ASL imaging sequences. For continuous labelling sequences, some of the inversion pulses must be spatially selective with their boundary located exactly at the labelling plane. Inversion of the spins past the labelling plane will change the sign of the accumulating label so the continuous labelling must be switched between label and control after each inversion.[27] Example continuous ASL images obtained with background suppression are shown in Fig. 13.4.

Multislice ASL imaging

In principle, acquiring more than one slice with ASL is straightforward, but in practice there are a number of complications. Since ASL benefits from averaging, acquiring one slice at a time would make the imaging of the whole brain an unacceptably long process. Just as with traditional imaging, interleaving of slice acquisition is the obvious solution. This approach is challenging for several reasons. First, the ASL label decays with T_1. Acquiring images over a period of time comparable to T_1 will cause loss of signal, and signal-to-noise ratio, in the later images, relative to single slice acquisition. Second, it may take longer for blood to enter a thick slab than to enter a thin one. This longer transit time will necessitate longer waits before imaging and consequently some signal decay due to T_1. Finally, it is harder to control for systematic differences in the direct effects of the labelling RF on the tissue signal across a thick slab.

The first problem requires that the different slices be acquired as rapidly as possible so that T_1 decay of the label is not a concern. A reasonable number of slices can be acquired with very fast imaging systems, but the 20 or more slices required for whole brain coverage probably cannot be satisfactorily achieved this way. Imaging time per preparation sequence can be reduced by using multishot versions of the single-shot sequences currently being used for ASL. Alternatively, three-dimensional acquisition can be used so that all of the slices are acquired at exactly the same time after labelling. Multishot and three-dimensional scans could increase the noise in a perfusion study because motion-related phase errors can cause ghosts and other artefacts. The use of background suppression can help a great deal with this approach.[26]

The longer transit into a thick slab of tissue is an unavoidable result of imaging a thicker region of tissue. If the flow into the thick slab is so slow that a very long wait has to be used, then the signal-to-noise ratio may suffer dramatically. In such a case, a series of sequential single slice scans may give comparable or superior results. Usually, however, a large volume of tissue is perfused by a relatively large and fast feeding artery, so flow is not markedly delayed in transit. If there is a stenotic vessel, then delay in the large vessel could be more of a serious issue.

Finally direct labelling effects on the measured signal must be eliminated for accurate results. A number of strategies to control for direct effects of RF only work perfectly when there is one, thin slice.[9] Generally, RF can affect tissue directly in two ways, either through imperfect slice profiles[14] or magnetization transfer.[15]

All of the discussion above has assumed that one could perfectly invert or saturate a square slab of tissue with a very fast boundary. In practice, there is a transition region between the inversion and no inversion area. Depending on the RF pulse used, the transition may be very broad. For a slice near the end of an imaged slab, the transition region will pass directly through the slice and systematic errors can occur. To overcome these errors, very carefully engineered inversion pulses have been used. Two adiabatic pulses, the hyperbolic secant pulse and, more recently, the FOCI pulse[17] have become popular for multislice pulsed ASL experiments because of their sharp slice profiles as well as insensitivity to B1 variations. The FOCI pulse in particular can be made to have very sharp boundaries and has helped a great deal with pulsed labelling studies.

Magnetization transfer is a physical process that can cause attenuation of tissue magnetization by RF at a considerable offset in frequency from the slice. Even if the slice profile is perfect, the magnetization transfer effects of two different inversion pulses need not be perfectly matched. Magnetization transfer is an especially important issue for adiabatic labelling since the RF is on for a long time. RF must be applied during the preparation period of the control image in order to avoid a large systematic error. Single-slice studies simply moved the labelling plane above the slice instead of below the slice.[9] This serves only as a good control for one slice. A second, small RF coil can be used for the labelling that produces only a weak RF field in the imaged region and thus minimizes magnetization transfer effects[28,29] but this does require a favourable labelling geometry and special hardware. We have shown[30] that sinusoidal modulation of the amplitude of the RF pulse during the control period can mimic the magnetization transfer effects of the labelling while allowing most of the blood spins to pass uninverted. Sinusoidal modulation can be thought of as splitting the inversion plane into two separate inversion planes that doubly invert the inflowing blood. The efficiency of the scheme is not perfect, however, and an improved control for multislice continuous ASL would be desirable. Talagala et al.[31] have proposed a strategy that controls for magnetization transfer near the centre slice better than the original superior slice strategy,[9] making possible the imaging of a thin slab near the centre slice. We are currently evaluating a promising alternative strategy, which involves modulation of both the gradient and RF amplitudes.[32]

MT can also be a significant but smaller problem for pulsed labelling, especially when adiabatic RF pulses are used. Several groups have suggested strategies involving double pulses with altered properties that can help to eliminate MT systematic errors.[15,16]

Validation of ASL perfusion MRI

ASL methods have been validated against existing methods for quantifying cerebral perfusion. CBF values obtained using continuous ASL have been validated against microspheres in a rat model of middle cerebral artery occlusion[33] and against 15O-PET scanning in humans.[34]

Applications to cerebrovascular disease

Perfusion mapping in animal models

One important role for ASL is in the study of animal models of acute stroke.[35–37] A large body of investigation has defined ischemic thresholds in animal models using diffusible tracers,[38] and these results are directly comparable to values obtained using ASL methods. In addition, because no injection is required, ASL can be repeatedly performed to map blood flow over the course of infarction and reperfusion treatments. Perfusion maps can easily be acquired every few minutes for many hours of lesion evolution. Alternatively, ASL perfusion can be interleaved with other measures of stroke physiology including diffusion and spectroscopic MRI so that comparisons of perfusion deficits and energetics can be made. These methods can be used to evaluate the mechanisms of MRI measures in humans and to further the understanding of stroke physiology. Animal MRI scanners, such as for rats and mice, are relatively inexpensive and already widely available in the imaging research community.

Clinical applications in stroke

Patients presenting with neurological symptoms on an ischemic basis should manifest regional hypoperfusion, and the distribution of observed hypoperfusion with respect to known vascular distributions should be diagnostically informative. In principle, perfusion imaging should provide the greatest sensitivity for stroke detection because hypoperfusion occurs in advance of metabolic and subsequently structural changes. The measurement of cerebral perfusion using MRI, in combination with diffusion MRI, is becoming an important part of the evaluation of acute stroke. These data are used to confirm the diagnosis of stroke, to establish a baseline against which stroke therapies can be assessed, and to contribute to prognosis. Perfusion imaging may be particularly valuable in the triage of patients for thrombolytic therapy, where patients with normal perfusion might be spared the risks of thrombolysis, while patients with perfusion deficits in the absence of significant structural change might be afforded the benefits of thrombolysis even outside the accepted temporal window.

ASL perfusion MRI provides a means of non-invasively quantifying cerebral perfusion in the acute setting without contrast administration and is ideal in instances where intravenous access is difficult to obtain or where serial perfusion measurements are required. The use of contrast-enhancement in magnetic resonance angiography can greatly improve the visualization of luminal profiles, but requires no prior contrast administration during the scanning session. This represents another setting in which an ability to obtain perfusion images without contrast administration is advantageous.

We have reliably obtained interpretable data from patients with acute stroke using continuous ASL perfusion MRI[39] (Fig. 13.5). Perfusion deficits corresponding to the vascular distribution of the patients' symptoms were observable, and ranged from small focal deficits of a similar size to diffusion lesions, to large deficits extending well beyond the diffusion lesion. In some instances, bright linear features were present in ASL perfusion MRI scans, suggesting effects of delayed arterial transit. While ASL arterial transit effects are probably most problematic in the acute setting, it remains possible to identify areas of hemodynamic compromise and transit effects themselves may provide diagnostically relevant information. We have begun to compare the characteristics of DSC and ASL perfusion images to assess the strengths and limitations of both techniques (Fig. 13.6).

While embolism rather than primary hypoperfusion has been considered to be the cause of most cerebrovascular symptoms, patients presenting

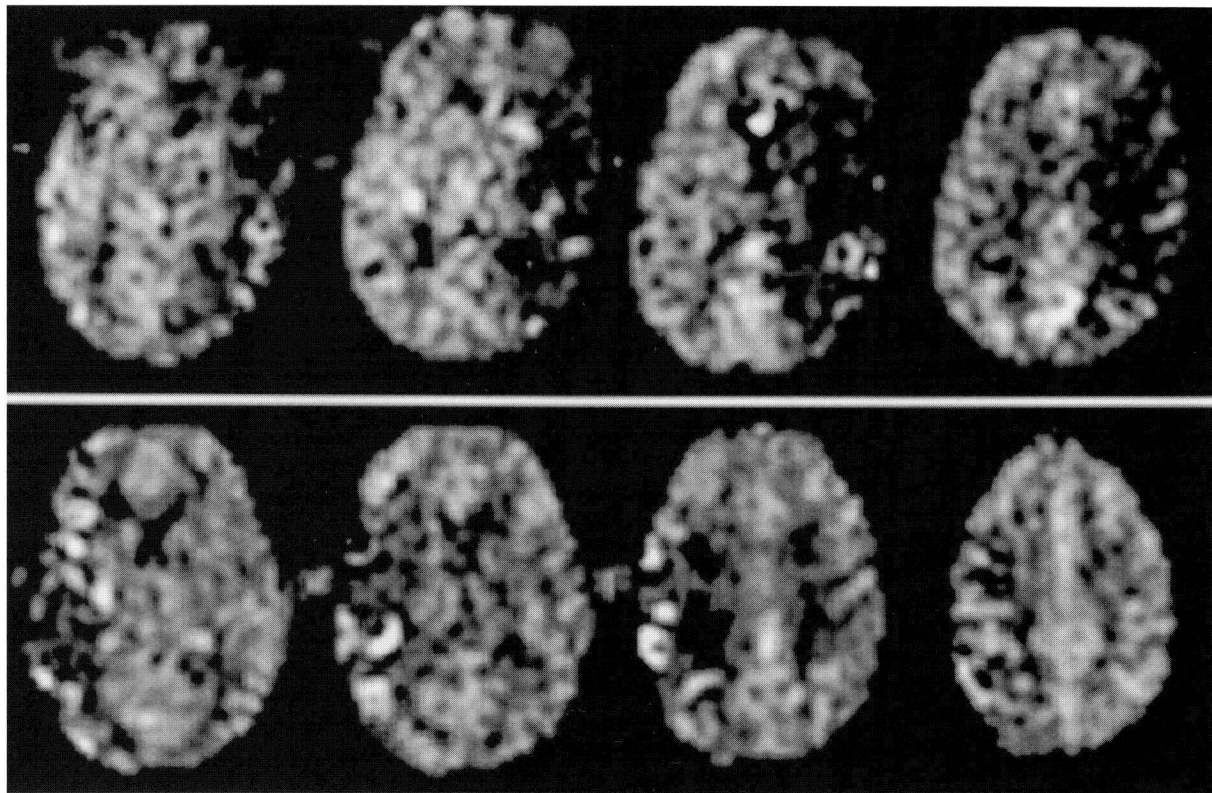

Fig. 13.5. Quantitative perfusion images in two patients with acute stroke. Unilateral hypoperfusion is apparent in both cases. Residual bright signal in vessels, most apparent in the bottom case, indicates labelled blood has not reached the tissue. ASL underestimates perfusion in such cases but signal in vessels can be used as an indicator of collateral flow.

with stroke, transient ischemic attack (TIA), or severe carotid stenosis may have clinical features suggesting hypoperfusion. Our studies using continuous ASL perfusion MRI in such a cohort suggest that resting perfusion abnormalities are indeed prevalent,[40] particularly in patients with high grade stenotic lesions of the cerebral vasculature, (Fig. 13.7). These findings are consistent with other reports correlating cerebral perfusion or perfusion reserve with the presence of extracranial stenoses of the carotid arteries. Although most studies have failed to clearly implicate primary hypoperfusion as a cause of large vessel stroke, hypoperfusion has been found to be predictive of recurrent stroke. This discrepancy has begun to be reconciled through the hypothesis that hypoperfusion may influence the outcome from cerebral embolization.[41] This hypothesis, if true, suggests an increasingly important role for perfusion imaging in predicting cerebrovascular ischemia, particularly in situations of increased embolization such as cardiovascular surgery.

CBF is maintained over a broad range of perfusion pressures by a property of the cerebrovascular system termed 'autoregulation'. Because autoregulatory mechanisms in the cerebral vasculature can maintain CBF through vasodilatation, it has been suggested that CBF alone is an inadequate measure of hemodynamic compromise. Thus, while resting reductions in perfusion are clearly abnormal, alterations in hemodynamic reserve are also significant because they suggest that the autoregulatory capacity of the cerebral vasculature may be exhausted. Cerebrovascular reserve is tested by measuring the increase in CBF induced by carbon dioxide inhalation or acetazolamide administration ('cerebrovascular reactivity'). A number of studies have demonstrated that cerebrovascular reserve

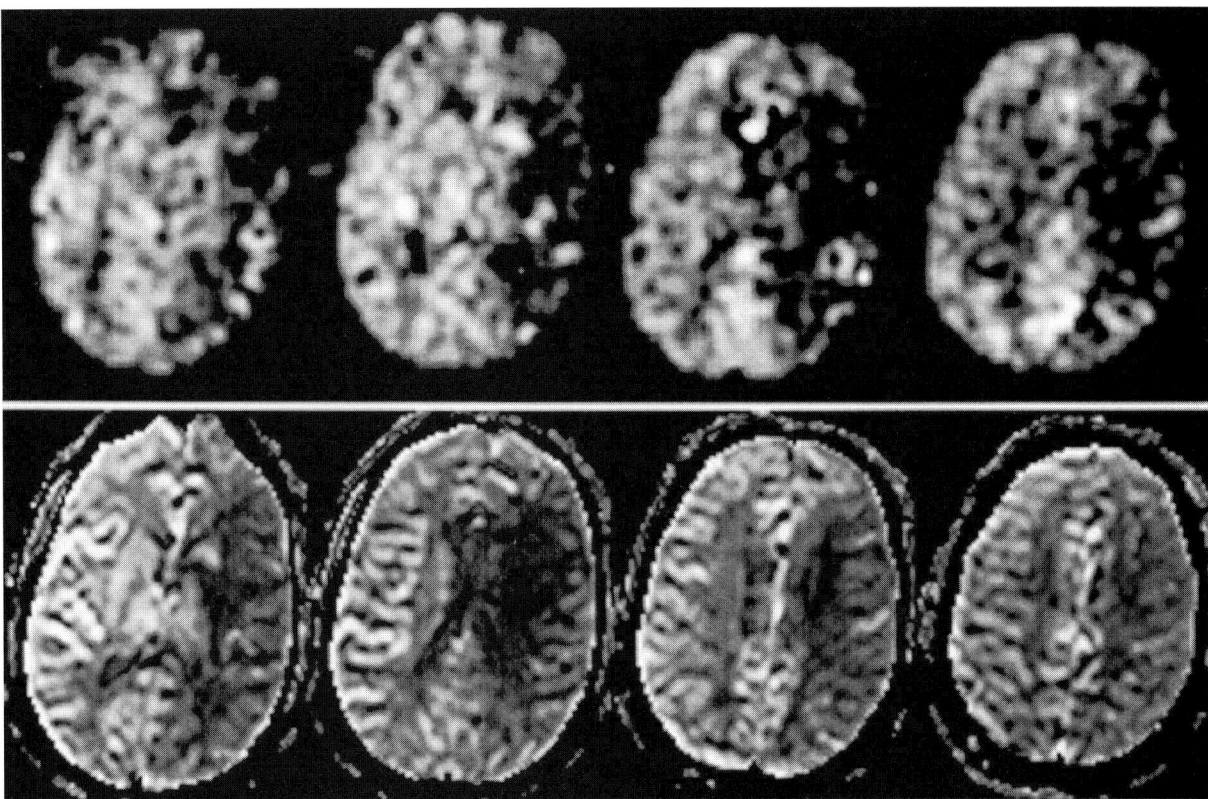

Fig. 13.6. Comparison of ASL and DSC perfusion imaging in acute stroke. The pattern of hypoperfusion is similar in both approaches.

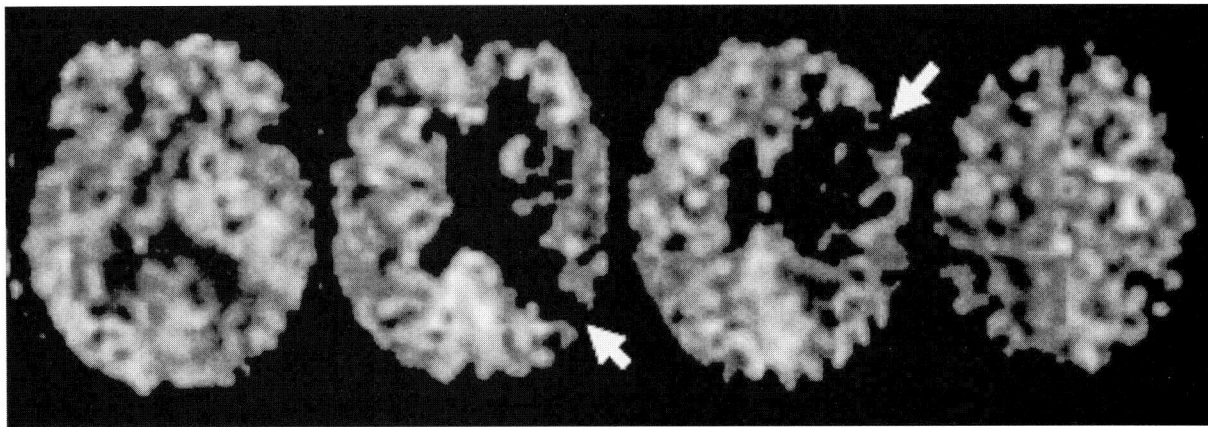

Fig. 13.7. Resting perfusion imaging in a patient with left carotid stenosis. Borderzone hypoperfusion as indicated by arrows, is apparent in a subset of patients with symptomatic cerebrovascular disease.

impairment is particularly significant in patients with borderzone ischemia, and that abnormalities in augmentation are predictive of stroke. Perfusion MRI provides a convenient method for quantitatively and non-invasively measuring the effects of pharmacological augmentation throughout the brain.[42] An example of fractional augmentation maps made with ASL perfusion is shown in Fig.

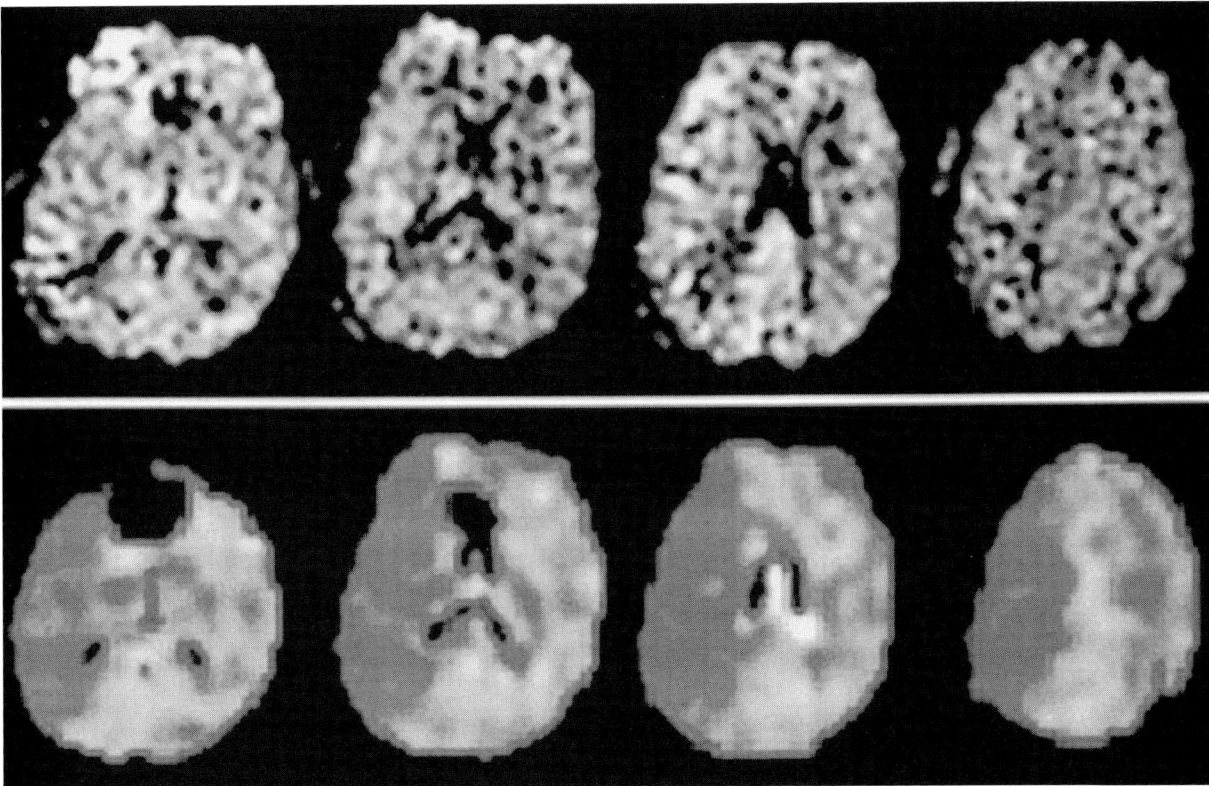

Fig. 13.8. Characterization of cerebrovascular reserve with ASL and acetazolamide challenge. Resting ASL images, top, show little abnormality but maps of fractional augmentation of flow, bottom, show impaired reserve in the right MCA distribution.

13.8, and demonstrates impaired cerebrovascular reserve in the vascular distribution of a right middle cerebral artery stenosis.

Measurement of regional CBF is likely to have several other applications in cerebrovascular disease and stroke. Management of hypertension has been widely recognized as the most important intervention in stroke prevention.[43] While clear benefits have been demonstrated for even modest reductions in systolic or diastolic blood pressure, the lower bounds for such reductions have not been established, and many patients with chronic hypertension may have alterations in CBF autoregulation. Non-invasive and repeatable perfusion imaging could allow antihypertensive therapy to be titrated based on resulting CBF values. Perfusion imaging can also help to distinguish between embolic and hemodynamic mechanisms of ischemic symptoms, since this may be difficult to determine clinically yet may suggest differing treatment strategies. A recent hypothesis posits that hypoperfusion may reduce clearance of microemboli and exacerbate their ischemic consequences,[41] in which case perfusion imaging may be used to predict ischemic complications during cardiovascular surgery.

Discussion

ASL perfusion MRI can be a useful tool for the assessment of stroke both in model systems and in the clinical setting. Relative to other perfusion measurement techniques, the greatest weakness of ASL for clinical applications is the rapid decay of the tracer. If blood takes a long time to reach the tissue, then a loss of signal is unavoidable. While the use of a postlabelling delay can be used to minimize the systematic effect of the transit time on the measured perfusion, the signal-to-noise ratio will be badly compromised. This effect was observed in both our study of acute stroke[39] and in cases with severe intracranial stenosis.[40] ASL studies at higher fields strengths should improve perfusion quantification in these situations due to longer T_1 values at higher fields. It can be argued that the ASL perfusion images provide much the same information as qualitative time-to-peak DSC images: the identification of regions with abnormal vascular supply. It is also interesting to note that the transit delays observed in some of our acute stroke studies exceeded the 1.5 second postlabelling delay we employed. These delays are comparable to the normal mean transit times of intravascular tracers. Attempts to quantify perfusion with DSC using deconvolution or fitting techniques[5,44] will also be inaccurate in the presence of such long delays.

Because of the acquisition flexibility of ASL, it is possible to alter the labelling to overcome transit time limitations. If labelling is performed within one cm or less of the imaged region, then inflow of blood to the tissue occurs through small nearby vessels. Such a labelling strategy would eliminate the effects of large vessel stenosis or tortuous collateral flow on the observed images. This labelling strategy can be approximated by single slice studies where all the blood inflowing from very nearby the slice is labelled. While single slice acquisitions are less efficient than multislice when the transit time through the brain is short, they can become competitive when the transit time is long. For example, a continuous labelling experiment with a postlabelling delay of 1.5 seconds suffers more than a factor of 3 loss of signal due to the decay of the label during that time relative to an acquisition with no delay and zero transit time. Ten slices can be acquired sequentially with the same signal-to-noise ratio and in the same time-period as the multislice acquisition if moving the label very close to the slice eliminates the long transit time into the tissue. Future developments such as selective labelling of blood based on velocity[45] rather than spatial position may also overcome these transit limitations.

While DSC MRI is certainly a powerful method for assessing hemodynamic abnormalities, ASL offers a number of advantages, which, with improved implementation and optimization, may make it preferable for perfusion measurement in some studies of stroke and cerebrovascular disease. Three great advantages of ASL are non-invasiveness, repeatability and absolute quantification. Traditional ASL implementations may be more motion sensitive than DSC, but the use of new background suppression techniques can make ASL less sensitive than DSC. Preliminary clinical studies indicate that traditional ASL is already useful in the assessment of acute stroke. Further technical developments promise to address most of the challenges of acute stroke evaluation with ASL.

REFERENCES

1 Matthew E, Andreason P, Carlson RE et al. Reproducibility of resting cerebral blood flow measurements with $H_2^{15}O$ positron emission tomography in humans. *J Cereb Blood Flow Metab* 1993; 13: 748–754.

2 Waldemar G. Functional brain imaging with SPECT in normal aging and dementia. *Cereb Brain Metab Rev* 1995; 7: 89–130.

3 Axel L. Cerebral blood flow determination by rapid-sequence computed tomography. *Radiology* 1980; 137: 676–686.

4 Yonas H, Darby JM, Marks EC, Durham SR, Maxwell C. CBF measured by Xe–Ct–approach to analysis and normal values. *J Cereb Blood Flow Metab* 1991; 11: 716–725.

5 Ostergaard L, Sorensen AG, Kwong KK, Weisskoff RM, Gyldensted C, Rosen BR. High resolution measurement of cerebral blood flow using intravascular tracer bolus passages .2. Experimental comparison and preliminary results. *Magn Reson Med* 1996; 36: 726–736.

6 Rosen BR, Belliveau JW, Buchbinder BR et al. Contrast agents and cerebral hemodynamics. *Magn Reson Med* 1991; 19: 285–292.

7 Calamante F, Gadian DG, Connely A. Delay and dispersion effects in dynamic susceptibility contrast MRI: simulations using singular value decomposition. *Magn Reson Med* 2000; 44: 466–473.

8 Detre JA, Leigh JS, Williams DS, Koretsky AP. Perfusion imaging. *Magn Reson Med* 1992; 23: 37–45.

9 Williams DS, Detre JA, Leigh JS, Koretsky AP. Magnetic resonance imaging of perfusion using spin inversion of arterial water. *Proc Natl Acad Sci USA* 1992; 89: 212–216.

10. Edelman RR, Siewert B, Darby DG et al. Qualitative mapping of cerebral blood flow and functional localization with echo-planar MR imaging and signal targeting with alternating radio frequency. *Radiology* 1994; 192: 513–520.
11. Kwong KK, Chesler DA, Weisskoff RM et al. MR Perfusion studies with T_1-weighted echo planar imaging. *Magn Reson Med* 1995; 34: 878–887.
12. Buxton RB, Frank LR, Wong EC, Siewert B, Warach S, Edelman RR. A general kinetic model for quantitative perfusion imaging with arterial spin labeling. *Magn Reson Med* 1998; 40: 383–396.
13. Alsop DC, Detre JA. Reduced transit-time sensitivity in non-invasive magnetic resonance imaging of human cerebral blood flow. *J Cereb Blood Flow Metab* 1996; 16: 1236–1249.
14. Frank LR, Wong EC, Buxton RB. Slice profile effects in adiabatic inversion: application to multislice perfusion imaging. *Magn Reson Med* 1997; 38: 558–564.
15. Golay X, Stuber M, Pruessmann KP, Meier D, Boesiger P. Transfer insensitive labeling technique (TILT): application to multislice functional perfusion imaging. *J Magn Reson Imaging* 1999; 9: 454–461.
16. Edelman RR, Chen G. EPISTAR MRI: multislice mapping of cerebral blood flow. *Magn Reson Med* 1998; 40: 800–805.
17. Yongbi MN, Branch CA, Helpern JA. Perfusion imaging using FOCI RF pulses. *Magn Reson Med* 1998; 40: 938–943.
18. Dixon WT, Du LN, Faul DD, Gado M, Rossnick S. Projection angiograms of blood labeled by adiabatic fast passage. *Magn Reson Med* 1986; 3: 454–462.
19. Wong EC, Buxton RB, Frank LR. A theoretical and experimental comparison of continuous and pulsed arterial spin labeling techniques for quantitative perfusion imaging. *Magn Reson Med* 1998; 40: 348–355.
20. Raichle ME, Eichling JO, Straatmann MG, Welch MJ, Larson KB, Ter-Pogossian MM. Blood–brain barrier permeability of ^{11}C-labeled alcohols and ^{15}O-labeled water. *Am J Physiol* 1976; 230: 543–552.
21. Bryant RG, Marill K, Blackmore C, Francis C. Magnetic relaxation in blood and blood clots. *Magn Reson Med* 1990; 13: 133–144.
22. Wong EC, Buxton RB, Frank LR. Quantitative imaging of perfusion using a single subtraction (QUIPSS and QUIPSS II). *Magn Reson Med* 1998; 39: 702–708.
23. Siewert B, Bly BM, Schlaug G et al. Comparison of the BOLD- and EPISTAR-technique for functional brain imaging by using signal detection theory. *Magn Reson Med* 1996; 36: 249–255.
24. Alsop DC, Detre JA. Reduction of excess noise in fMRI using noise image templates (abstr). *Proc Int Soc Magn Reson Med* Fifth Scientific Meeting and Exhibition. Berkeley, CA: International Society for Magnetic Resonance in Medicine, 1997: 1687.
25. Dixon WT, Sardashti M, Castillo M, Stomp GP. Multiple inversion recovery reduces static tissue signal in angiograms. *Magn Reson Med* 1991; 18: 257–268.
26. Ye FQ, Frank JA, Weinberger DR, McLaughlin AC. Noise reduction in 3D perfusion imaging by attenuating the static signal in arterial spin tagging (ASSIST). *Magn Reson Med* 2000; 44: 92–100.
27. Alsop DC, Detre JA. Background suppressed 3D RARE ASL perfusion imaging. *Proc Int Soc Magn Reson Med*. Seventh Scientific Meeting, Philadelphia, 1999.
28. Silva AC, Zhang WG, Williams DS, Koretsky AP. Multislice MRI of rat-brain perfusion during amphetamine stimulation using arterial spin-labeling. *Magn Reson Med* 1995; 33: 209–214.
29. Zaharchuk G, Ledden PJ, Kwong KK, Reese TG, Rosen BR, Wald LL. Multislice perfusion and perfusion territory imaging in humans with separate label and image coils. *Magn Reson Med* 1999; 41: 1093–1098.
30. Alsop DC, Detre JA. Multisection cerebral blood flow MR imaging with continuous arterial spin labeling. *Radiology* 1998; 208: 410–416.
31. Talagala SL. Multi-slice perfusion MRI using continuous arterial spin labeling: controlling for MT effects with simultaneous proximal and distal RF. *Proc Int Soc Magn Reson Med*. Sixth Scientific Meeting and Exhibition. Berkeley, CA: International Society for Magnetic Resonance in Medicine, 1998: 381.
32. Alsop DC. Improved efficiency for multi-slice continuous arterial spin labeling using time varying gradients. *Proc Int Soc Magn Reson Med*. Ninth Scientific Meeting and Exhibition. Berkeley, CA: International Society for Magnetic Resonance in Medicine, 2001: 1562.
33. Walsh EG, Minematsu K, Leppo J, Moore SC. Radioactive microsphere validation of a volume localized continuous saturation perfusion measurement. *Magn Reson Med* 1994; 31: 147–153.
34. Ye FQ, Berman KF, Ellmore T et al. $H_2^{15}O$ PET validation of steady-state arterial spin tagging cerebral blood flow measurements in humans. *Magn Reson Med* 2000; 44: 450–456.
35. Wang Y, Hu WX, Perez-Trepichio AD et al. Brain tissue sodium is a ticking clock telling time after arterial occlusion in rat focal cerebral ischemia. *Stroke* 2000; 31: 1386–1391.

36 Lythgoe MF, Thomas DL, Calamante F et al. Acute changes in MRI diffusion, perfusion, T-1, and T-2, in a rat model of oligemia produced by partial occlusion of the middle cerebral artery. *Magn Reson Med* 2000; 44: 706–712.

37 Jiang Q, Zhang RL, Zhang ZG, Ewing JR, Divine GW, Chopp M. Diffusion-, T-2–, and perfusion-weighted nuclear magnetic resonance imaging of middle cerebral artery embolic stroke and recombinant tissue plasminogen activator intervention in the rat. *J Cereb Blood Flow Metab* 1998; 18: 758–767.

38 Hossman KA. Viability thresholds and the penumbra of focal ischemia. *Ann Neurol* 1994; 36: 557–565.

39 Chalela JA, Alsop DC, Gonzalez-Atavales JB, Maldjian JA, Kasner SE, Detre JA. Magnetic resonance perfusion imaging in acute ischemic stroke using continuous arterial spin labeling. *Stroke* 2000; 31: 680–687.

40 Detre JA, Alsop DC, Vives LR, Maccotta L, Teener JW, Raps EC. Noninvasive MRI evaluation of cerebral blood flow in cerebrovascular disease. *Neurology* 1998; 50: 633–641.

41 Caplan LR, Hennerici M. Impaired clearance of emboli (washout) is an important link between hypoperfusion, embolism, and ischemic stroke. *Arch Neurol* 1998; 55: 1475–1482.

42 Detre JA, Samuels OB, Alsop DC, Gonzalez-At JB, Kasner SE, Raps EC. Noninvasive magnetic resonance imaging evaluation of cerebral blood flow with acetazolamide challenge in patients with cerebrovascular stenosis. *J Magn Reson Imaging* 1999; 10: 870–875.

43 Bronner LL, Kanter DS, Manson JE. Primary prevention of stroke. *N Engl J Med* 1995; 333: 1392–1400.

44 Rempp KA, Brix G, Wenz F, Becker CR, Guckel F, Lorenz WJ. Quantification of regional cerebral blood-flow and volume with dynamic susceptibility contrast-enhanced MR-imaging. *Radiology* 1994; 193: 637–641.

45 Norris DG, Schwarzbauer C. Velocity selective radio-frequency pulse trains. *J Magn Reson* 1999; 137: 231–236.

Clinical role of echoplanar MRI in stroke

Stephen Davis and Mark Parsons

Department of Neurology, Royal Melbourne Hospital and University of Melbourne, Victoria, Australia

Introduction

Stroke is a leading cause of death in Western countries, with a case mortality rate of 24% within the first month, higher than most forms of cancer.[1] It is the commonest cause of long-term adult disability.[2] Recent important advances in acute stroke therapy include the established benefits of stroke units, and the introduction of the first proven interventional therapies. These include intravenous t-PA within 3 hours,[3] acute use of aspirin[4,5] and administration of intra-arterial thrombolysis within 6 hours of stroke onset.[6] A range of new strategies are being investigated, which generally involve either rapid reperfusion with thrombolytic agents, or neuroprotection from the damaging neurotoxic cascade that follows ischemia.[7]

Both strategies focus on treatment of the ischemic penumbra.[8–10] An understanding of the pathophysiologic basis of brain ischemia and the penumbra is important in interpreting the magnetic resonance (MR) changes imaged in acute stroke. The penumbra is a variable region of critically underperfused but still viable tissue surrounding the infarcted core. Despite symptomatic hypoperfusion, essential energy-requiring processes such as the Na–K ATPase system, are still able to maintain ionic gradients, and hence membrane and neuronal integrity.[9,10] The penumbra represents a therapeutic window for intervention. However, the duration of this interval is uncertain and is likely to vary considerably from person to person. Rapid identification of the penumbra can allow rational therapeutic decisions to be made based on assessment of pathophysiology in the individual patient, rather than relying on the arbitrary time windows used in clinical trials.[11,12]

Echoplanar magnetic resonance imaging (EPI) enables rapid, non-invasive imaging and analysis of cerebral pathophysiology in acute stroke. Echoplanar techniques include diffusion-weighted imaging (DWI), a measure of tissue water diffusion, perfusion-weighted imaging (PWI), which measures various indices of cerebral perfusion, and magnetic resonance spectroscopy (MRS), allowing analysis of in vivo biochemistry. Because DWI can rapidly detect ischemic cerebral tissue, which is usually destined to infarct, and distinguish acute from chronic infarction, it represents an important clinical advance over computed tomography (CT) and conventional magnetic resonance (MR) scanning. Both of these modalities are relatively insensitive to early brain ischemia.

In addition, combined use of DWI and PWI can allow assessment of at-risk or threatened brain tissue in the ischemic penumbra. The presence of penumbral tissue is estimated as the difference, or mismatch, between the perfusion rim on PWI and the ischemic core, defined by DWI.[13] Rapid evaluation of the presence and extent of the penumbra is likely to be valuable in the selection of patients for acute therapy. For example, thrombolysis can reperfuse and hence rescue threatened penumbral tissue, with reduction in eventual infarct size and improved outcome.[14] Although tissue plasminogen activator (t-PA) improves outcome in ischemic

Table 14.1. Comparison of CT, SPECT, PET, conventional MRI, EPI modalities in acute stroke

Technique	CT	SPECT	PET	Conventional MRI	EPI DWI/PWI
Current use in stroke	Standard diagnostic technique	Restricted role, chiefly in research centres	Research technique	Alternative technique to CT, but less used as screening method	Increasing use (particularly DWI)
Advantages	Widely available. Sensitively excludes hemorrhage	Perfusion information. Complementary to CT, MRI	Measures perfusion, metabolism, 'at risk' penumbral tissue	Lack of bone artefacts; better imaging brain-stem	Highly sensitive diagnosis early ischemia. Potential to image penumbral tissue
Disadvantages	Insensitive for early ischemia, 'at risk' tissue	Cannot replace structural imaging techniques. Does not allow measurement of metabolism, 'at risk' tissue	Expensive, logistically difficult. Very limited availability	Cost. Relatively insensitive in first 6 hours. Previous concerns about exclusion of hemorrhage	Availability. PWI requires post-processing
Future clinical role in stroke	May be replaced by EPI	Diminishing	Research only	EPI applications	Might become investigative modality of choice

stroke within 3 hours of onset, not all patients treated benefit, *as* there is a significant risk of hemorrhage. Furthermore, the time window for benefit may well exceed 3 hours in some patients. Because of the heterogeneity of human stroke and the cerebral circulation, it is recognized that there is no universal time window for acute treatments. Combined DWI/PWI, with rapid diagnosis of cerebral pathophysiology, is likely to facilitate acute therapeutic decisions.

The high sensitivity and specificity of EPI in stroke together with its potential to guide therapy have led to the widespread view that DWI/PWI, combined with magnetic resonance angiography (MRA), is likely to replace CT as the primary modality in stroke investigation. Others are more cautious,[15] emphasizing that more clinical correlations are needed, particularly in confirming its accuracy compared with CT scanning.

Imaging techniques in brain ischemia (Table 14.1)

Computed tomographic scanning (CT) has been the investigation of choice for acute stroke evaluation for the past three decades. It sensitively excludes hemorrhage, but ischemic changes can be subtle. In the first 6 hours of stroke onset, CT is often normal. Major ischemic changes can be identified in some cases within about 2 hours of onset,[16–18] but CT remains a relatively blunt instrument in the evaluation of hyperacute brain ischemia (Table 14.1). Various functional imaging methods have been used in the evaluation of acute stroke. Positron emission tomography (PET) enables imaging and measurement of both perfusion and metabolism. While important information about cerebral pathophysiology in acute brain ischemia has been obtained from PET studies,

Table 14.2. Echoplanar MR techniques in stroke

Techniques	DWI	PWI	MRS
Measures	Translational movement of water (ADC values)	Cerebral perfusion indices (mean transit time, cerebral blood volume, cerebral blood flow)	NAA, lactate – Chemical shift imaging
Acute stroke	'Light bulb' signal due to attenuated water diffusion	Reduced blood flow	Reduced NAA, increased lactate
Clinical role	Highly sensitive diagnosis of acute ischemia – Differentiation from chronic ischemia	Hypoperfusion in acute stroke. DWI/PWI mismatch allows estimation of 'at risk' penumbral tissue	Early chemical derangements may complement DWI/PWI information

acute stroke studies are logistically difficult, the technique is expensive and not widely available. Single photon emission computed tomography (SPECT) is more suited to acute studies, is widely available and can give information about cerebral blood flow abnormalities. Acute hypoperfusion in stroke correlates with outcome and repeat imaging allows assessment of reperfusion, also shown to correlate with functional recovery.[12,19–22] Although SPECT can be used to retrospectively evaluate the effects of acute therapies,[21–24] it cannot delineate metabolism or identify the irreversibly damaged and hence non-viable infarct core. Therefore, the inability of SPECT to define the critical penumbral region has limited its role in stroke management.

Conventional magnetic resonance imaging (MRI) reveals the structure of the brain with excellent spatial resolution. However, standard MRI with T_2-weighted imaging does not reliably show changes in the brain within 6 hours of stroke onset. This is likely to be the time window for most acute stroke therapies.

In contrast, echoplanar imaging (EPI) of the brain's diffusion of water (DWI), perfusion (PWI) or metabolite concentrations on magnetic resonance spectroscopy (MRS) can reveal abnormalities within 1–2 minutes of the onset of ischemia.[13,25,26] It is an increasingly available technology and far more useful than T_2-weighted MRI within the first 48 hours of acute stroke.[26,27] The major clinical applications that have been defined by EPI research and clinical experience include the sensitive diagnosis of acute ischemia, the differentiation of acute from chronic infarcts, the prognostic value of acute DWI and PWI lesions, insights into infarct topography and pathophysiology, use as a surrogate endpoint in drug trials and the potential of combined DWI/PWI as a powerful tool in providing a template for acute therapy (Table 14.2).

There is a view in experienced centres that multimodality MRI can be used as the sole diagnostic modality in acute stroke.[28] In contrast, others[29] have argued for more studies to demonstrate the evidence for the replacement of CT. There has nonetheless been a debate in the recent literature as to whether EPI is ready for 'prime time' in acute stroke evaluation.[30,31] We and others certainly believe that it is.[12,28,32,33]

Clinical applications of EPI in acute stroke

Diagnosis of acute and chronic ischemia

Diffusion-weighted imaging (DWI) involves measurement of alterations in the diffusion of water molecules. At present, DWI is the most used of the EPI parameters in clinical practice. With acute ischemia, there is a marked reduction in the apparent diffusion coefficient of water (ADC), reflecting

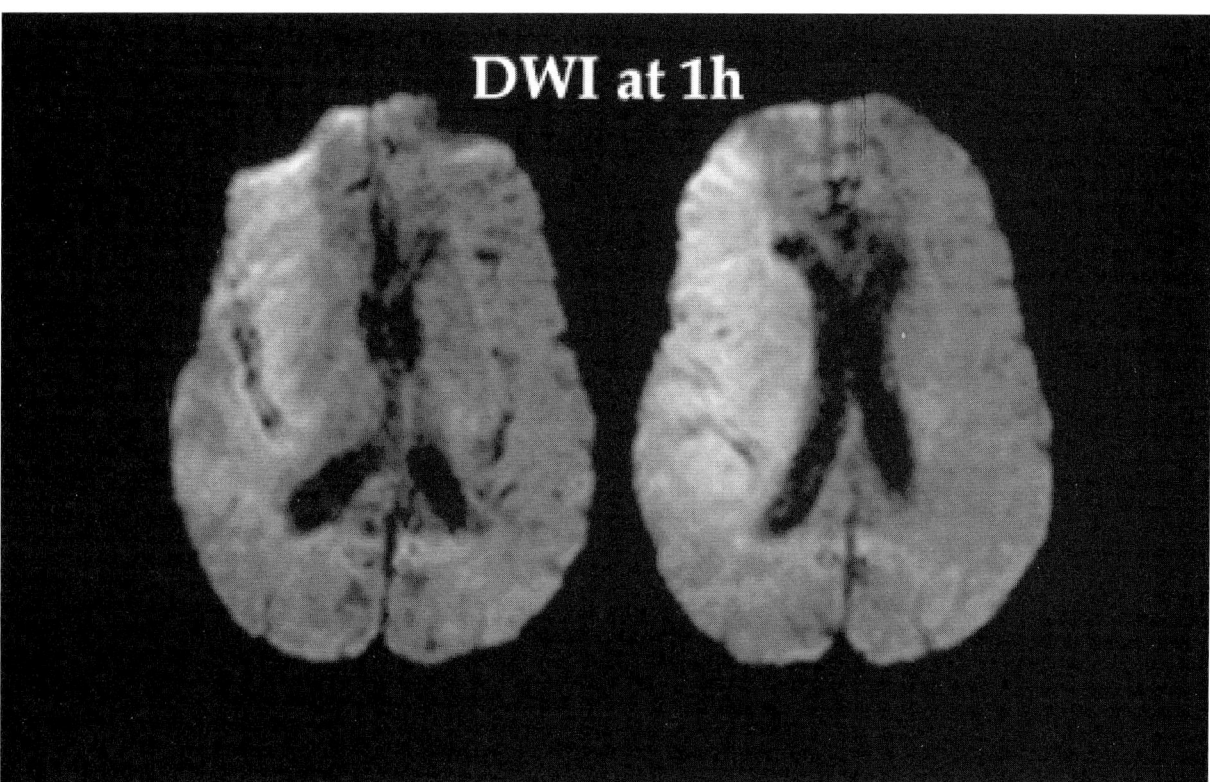

Fig. 14.1. Patient scanned at 1 hour after symptom onset. There is an extensive diffusion lesion in the right middle cerebral artery territory.

early disruption of high-energy metabolism, with failure of ion pumps and cytotoxic edema. Ischemic lesions appear hyperintense on DWI, termed the 'lightbulb sign' and are apparent within minutes of onset (Fig. 14.1). These brain regions represent the irreversibly damaged infarct core, and the minimal extent of the final infarct size in most cases. Very early reperfusion has been shown to reverse small DWI lesions in animal models and occasional human cases,[34,35] as will be seen below.

Within the first few days after stroke onset, there is typically expansion of the non-viable infarct core, demonstrated by serial DWI scans.[12,36,37] Eventually, the ADC values in the infarcted tissue increase, related to a breakdown in cell membranes with resultant increase in extracellular space and increased diffusional movement of water molecules. Hence, older infarcts appear hypointense on DWI scans compared with normal brain. This change is called 'pseudonormalization' and occurs about 7–10 days after stroke onset, although earlier in some cases.[38] This phenomenon is clinically useful in distinguishing acute from chronic infarcts, often difficult with CT or conventional MR scanning.[32,33,38]

DWI is both highly sensitive and specific for acute stroke. In 194 cases studied within 24 hours of stroke onset, Lovblad et al. reported 88% sensitivity and 95% specificity. In the first 6 hours, the sensitivity rose to 94% with 100% specificity. We found 100% sensitivity and 100% specificity in patients with a clinical diagnosis of acute stroke, imaged within 6 hours of onset.[39] In one patient with a normal DWI scan, further investigations led to the diagnosis of an acute brachial plexopathy. However, DWI-negative stroke has been reported by many groups, particularly with small, deep lesions in the brainstem.[33,40]

The high-intensity 'lightbulb sign' is of great clinical value in differentiating acute from chronic

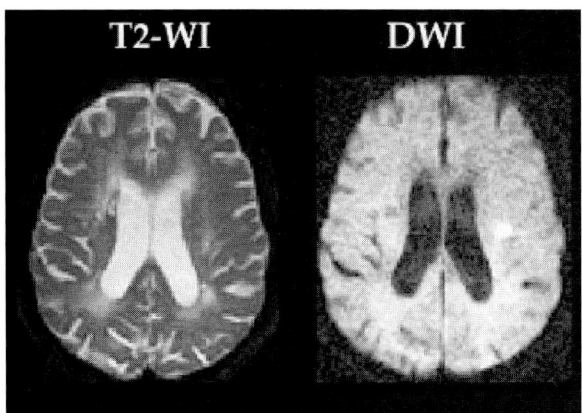

Fig. 14.2. Patient imaged at 12 hours after onset of right hemiparesis. There is marked white matter ischemic change on T_2-weighted imaging, but the culprit lesion for acute symptoms is not apparent. DWI shows an acute lesion in the left internal capsule.

infarcts, particularly in patients with multiple ischemic lesions of different ages (Fig. 14.2). A number of studies have compared the clinical utility of DWI with conventional MRI. The Albers group[41,42] showed that DWI could sometimes identify the stroke lesion at a site other than clinically thought, show multiple lesions and demonstrated that lesions considered acute on conventional MRI were actually old. They also confirmed the superiority of DWI over CT within the first few hours after stroke onset, as shown by others.[43] DWI has also provided insight into the pathophysiology of patients with transient ischemic attacks. DWI abnormalities are present in nearly 50% of patients, with full reversibility in about half of these.[44] Persisting DWI lesions were particularly common in patients with symptoms lasting greater than 1 hour.

Echoplanar imaging has also allowed rapid gradient echo susceptibility-weighted sequences that can sensitively exclude acute hemorrhage.[45] In a small series of patients with hemorrhage within 2 hours of symptom onset, all patients were identified with MRI.[46] Because of the slight uncertainty about the accuracy of MRI in acute cerebral hemorrhage, a large trial, involving randomization of acute stroke patients to either CT or MRI, is being mounted to address this question.

Perfusion-weighted imaging (PWI) is currently less used in routine practice than DWI, but provides invaluable complementary information in acute stroke, particularly in measurement of acute pathophysiology and at-risk tissue in the ischemic penumbra, as will be seen below. PWI involves the acquisition of whole brain T_2^*-weighted perfusion scans every 2 seconds following paramagnetic contrast injection (Gadolinium-DTPA) and makes use of the signal loss that occurs during the dynamic tracking of the first pass of the contrast agent.[47,48] A signal intensity-time curve allows measurements of relative cerebral blood volume (CBV), mean transit time (MTT) and an estimation of regional cerebral blood flow (CBF), where $CBF = CBV/MTT$ (Fig. 14.3, see colour plate section). Because the MTT is hyperintense in regions of impaired perfusion, most groups have used the MTT as an index of CBF. However, work in our laboratory has shown that CBF is likely to be a better correlate of neurological impairment and functional outcome.[14]

Magnetic resonance angiography complements PWI and DWI by allowing determination of middle cerebral artery (MCA) stem and major branch patency [37,49]. The table time for the performance of DWI, PWI and MRA is approximately 20 minutes, a practical duration for most stroke patients. In summary, combined DWI and PWI allow hyperacute, sensitive and specific diagnosis of ischemia, distinction of older strokes, measurement of at-risk tissue in the ischemic penumbra and concurrent visualization of arterial pathology such as stenosis or occlusion.

Stroke prognosis

Lovblad et al.[50] pointed out the acute prognostic potential of DWI lesions in ischemic stroke. Large acute DWI lesions usually predict poor outcome. We and others have emphasized the prognostic value of combined DWI and PWI lesion volumes.[11,12,51] Both DWI and PWI lesion volumes obtained within 6 hours of stroke onset have been correlated with the neurological impairment scores at 24 hours and infarct size at 7 days on T_2-weighted MRI.[51] Our group reported that the volume of both the DWI and PWI lesions correlated with acute clinical impairment scores, the eventual infarct size at

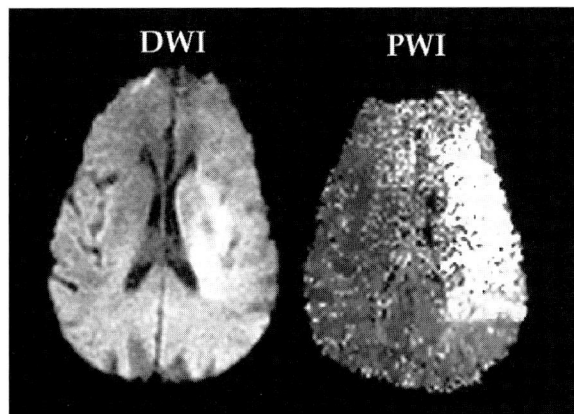

Fig. 14.4. PWI > DWI mismatch pattern. Patient imaged at 3 hours after onset of aphasia and right hemiparesis. The PWI lesion is extensive and involves the entire MCA territory. The DWI lesion is much smaller, in the striatocapsular region.

the chronic 90-day stage, as well as the outcome functional status of the patient.[12] However, these relationships dynamically evolve over the first few days after stroke onset, which helps explain the differences in the volume of the acute parameters measured within hours of stroke onset, compared with the final infarct size.[12,36]

Relationship between DWI and PWI : imaging tissue at-risk in the ischemic penumbra

Baird et al. first explored the different patterns of match and mismatch between DWI and PWI in acute stroke.[36] Our group[12] reported that 6 patterns could be identified in acute ischemia, which we found predicted the evolution of ischemic deficits, and outcome. The most common of these is the putative penumbral pattern, defined by a PWI lesion of greater volume than a DWI lesion (Fig. 14.4). Warach et al. first proposed that PWI > DWI mismatch represented the ischemic penumbra, brain tissue at risk of infarction that might be potentially rescued by acute therapy such as thrombolysis.[11,13]

We found that a penumbral pattern was present in 75% of stroke patients imaged within 6 hours and that the probability of a penumbral pattern decreased with time over the first 24 hours after stroke.[12,52] In untreated patients, an acute penumbral pattern generally predicts expansion of the infarcted DWI core into the surrounding hypoper-

fused brain. However, some patients have spontaneous reperfusion of penumbral tissue between acute and subacute studies, associated with significantly improved clinical outcome. The final infarct size is usually intermediate between the DWI core and perfusion boundary in patients with a demonstrable penumbra, and the patient's neurological course typically correlates with this evolution.

It should be emphasised that PWI > DWI mismatch patterns are, at best, an approximation of the 'true' ischemic penumbra. PWI may overestimate the mismatch region, as current bolus-tracking techniques may not reliably distinguish between critically hypoperfused tissue at risk and oligemic regions with lesser degrees of hypoperfusion, not destined to infarct.[53–55] The recent use of thresholded PWI maps, which identify differing severities of contrast bolus delay, might circumvent this problem.[56–59] In addition, DWI lesions may overestimate irreversibly damaged tissue, as rapid reperfusion with thrombolysis has been shown to lead to permanent reversal of some DWI lesions.[35] In the future, sophisticated statistical algorithms may be able to predict tissue fate on a voxel-by-voxel basis using DWI and PWI parameters rather than the currently used volumetric techniques.[60] Nonetheless, the presence of a PWI > DWI mismatch pattern is at present, the most practical definition of at-risk tissue for the clinician, and this group of patients are likely to have the greatest potential to benefit from thrombolytic therapy.[35,53,61,62]

We have also identified patients with hypoperfusion yet normal DWI, typical of transient ischemic attacks, where there is tissue at risk, but without frank infarction. However, as previously noted, a significant proportion of TIA patients have DWI abnormalities.[44] We and others have explored the relationships between MRA findings and DWI/PWI patterns. In acute stroke, MCA stem occlusion on MRA studies is usually associated with a penumbral pattern (Fig. 14.5).[37,49] Untreated, these patients show typically greater expansion of the ischemic core, larger final infarct size and worse clinical outcome than penumbral patients with a patent artery.[37] However, the penumbral pattern can also be seen with normal MRA. These patients are likely

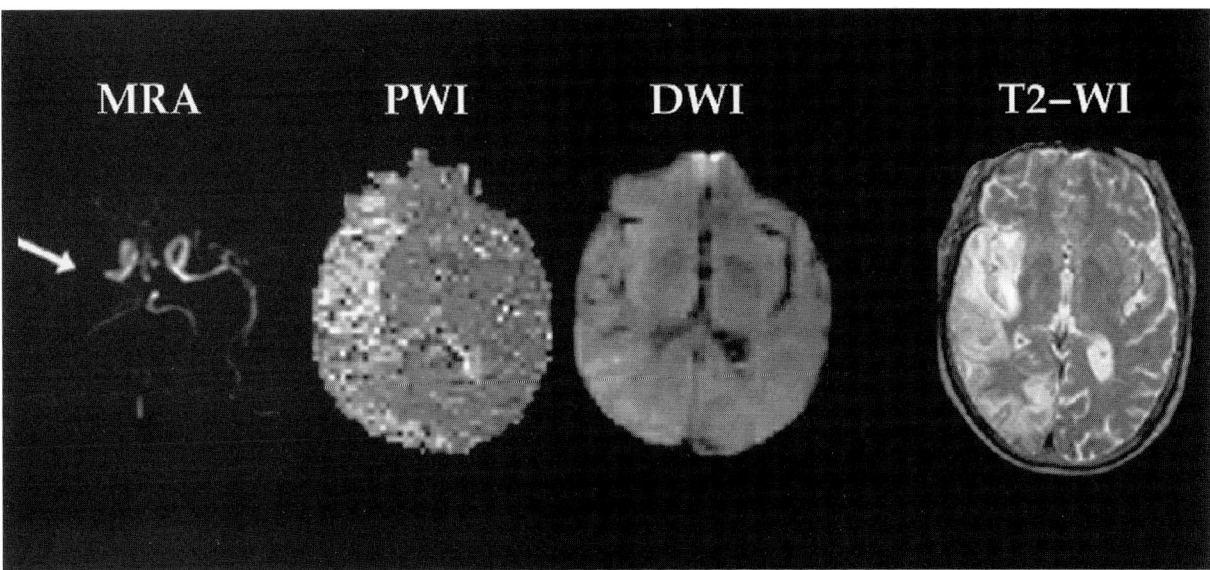

Fig. 14.5. Typical picture of right MCA occlusion at 4 hours (arrow). There is associated PWI>DWI mismatch, with subsequent expansion of the ischemic core at day 90 T_2-weighted imaging (right).

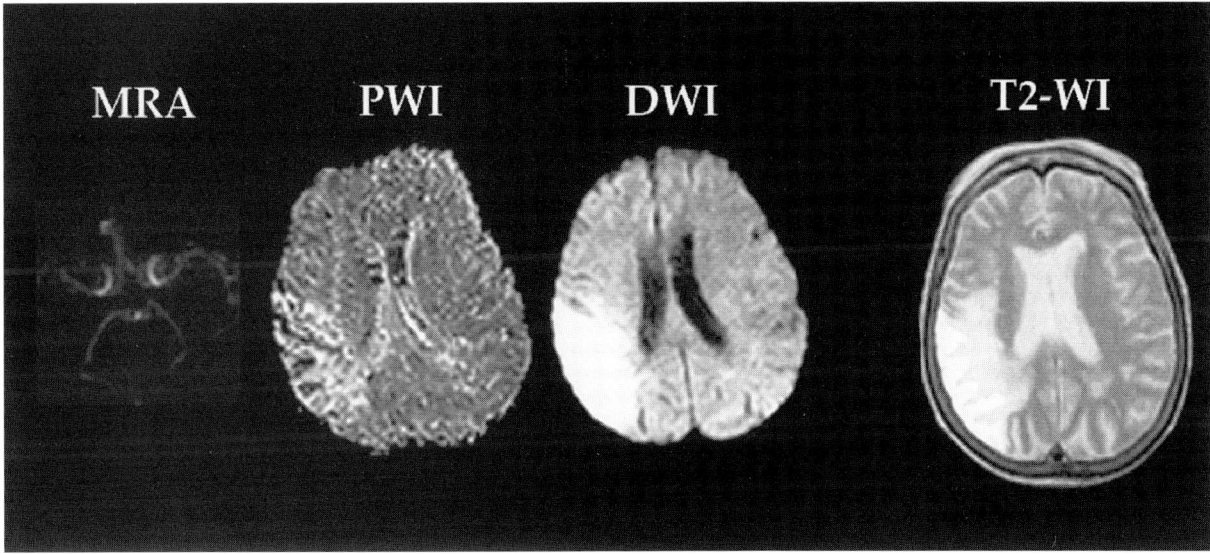

Fig. 14.6. Non-mismatch (non-penumbral) pattern. At 15 hours after symptom onset this patient had no visible vessel occlusion on MRA, and the acute DWI lesion is equal in size to the acute PWI lesion. There is no expansion of the ischemic core at 3 month T_2-weighted imaging.

to have occlusion of more distal second and third order arterial branches, beyond the spatial resolution of MRA.[37]

Non-mismatch patterns are those in which PWI lesions are smaller or absent compared with DWI. In these patients, there is usually no expansion of the ischemic core between acute, subacute and outcome studies,[37] and final infarct size is similar to the size of the acute DWI lesion (Fig. 14.6). Therefore, it is generally considered that patients with such non-mismatch patterns are unlikely to have penumbral tissue present.

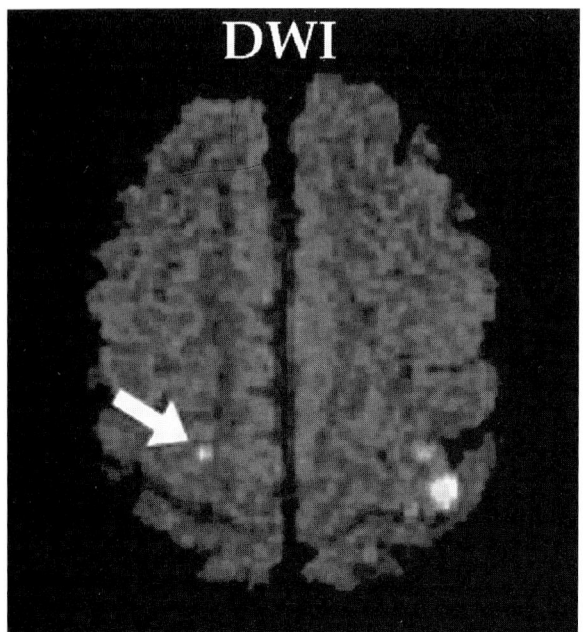

Fig. 14.7. Cardio-embolic infarction. DWI at 23 hours after presentation with a right cortical hand, shows the culprit lesion, but also an occult acute diffusion lesion (arrow).

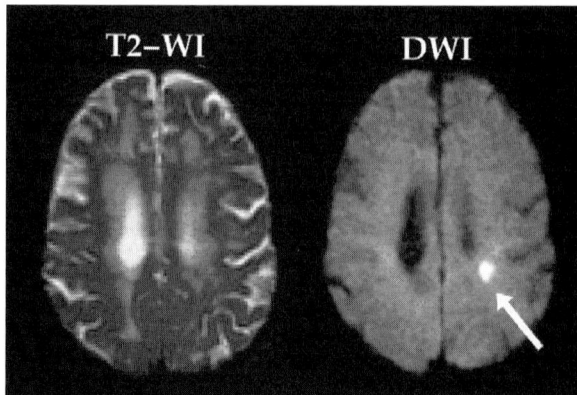

Fig. 14.8. Patient scanned 13 hours after onset of right sensorimotor hemiparesis. DWI highlights acute infarction in the posterior limb of the left internal capsule that is indistinguishable from chronic ischemic change on concomitant T_2-weighted imaging.

Infarct topography and pathogenesis

Our studies of acute infarct topography have shown that the proximal MCA territory in the insular region is particularly susceptible to infarction.[52] However, the range of MCA subcortical and cortical infarct types are readily identified including lacunar lesions, striatocapsular and branch arterial infarcts. An increasing number of studies have indicated that the combined use of DWI and PWI can help determine the likely pathophysiology of acute stroke. The Los Angeles group showed that multimodal MRI (DWI and MRA) within 24 hours substantially improved the diagnosis of stroke subtype, using the TOAST and Oxfordshire classifications.[63]

A pattern of a proximal DWI lesion with separate, distal PWI lesions in the MCA territory suggests an embolic pathogenesis.[52] Cardiac emboli are suggested by a cluster of acute DWI lesions in different arterial territories (Fig. 14.7). One group reported that acute, multiple brain infarcts were detected in 29% of a large series studied with DWI, due to either large-vessel disease or cardiogenic embolism.[64]

In subcortical infarction, conventional imaging with MRI or CT is often of limited clinical utility in the acute setting. In contrast, Singer et al.[65] reported a 94.6% accuracy with DWI in acute subcortical infarction. Lacunar infarcts are often multiple. The high intensity 'lightbulb' signature on DWI allows delineation of acute lacunar infarction from chronic white matter lesions (Fig. 14.8). Singer et al. noted that in 10% of cases, the acute infarction was not detected on conventional MRI. Delineation of the acute lesion with DWI was possible in all cases of multiple lacunes, corresponding to the acute clinical symptomatology. Similarly, Noguchi et al.[66] used DWI in patients with lacunar infarcts and were also able to identify acute small infarcts and separate these from chronic lesions. In 3 of 35 patients, small hyperacute brain stem infarcts, within 6 hours of onset were seen only with DWI and in 5 patients, fresh small infarcts adjacent to multiple old infarcts could only be distinguished with DWI. Other reports have shown the superiority of DWI over conventional MRI for the diagnosis of clinically relevant, penetrating artery infarcts.[67] A recent study used DWI to determine whether clinical lacunar syndromes predicted lacunar infarcts.[68] Twenty-three patients with clinical lacunar syndromes had DWI within 3 days of onset. In most cases, acute lacunar syndromes correlated with small subcortical infarcts compatible with single-

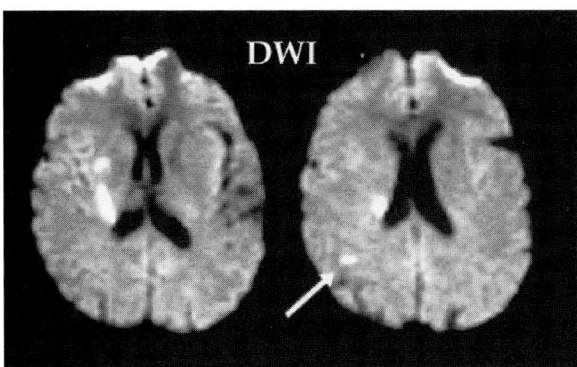

Fig. 14.9. Patient presenting with left pure motor hemiparesis. DWI at 9 hours reveals right striatocapsular infarction, and a small region of infarction in the right parietal cortex (arrow). Despite having a classical clinical syndrome, a proximal embolic source must be the pathogenic mechanism for the stroke.

penetrator occlusion. However, a small number had cortical involvement.

These newer MRI techniques may contribute to a modification of the lacunar hypothesis, namely that they are small vessel infarcts due to in situ lipohyalinosis and microatheroma, rather than embolic pathology. There is accumulating evidence that acute DWI identifies a subset of patients presenting with typical lacunar syndromes with a pattern of ischemic lesions suggesting an embolic pathogenesis[68–70] (Fig. 14.9). In a study of 62 patients with classical lacunar syndromes studied with DWI within 3 days, 16% had multiple regions of increased signal intensity. The index lesion could be identified in the hemisphere or brainstem, while these 'subsidiary infarcts' usually occurred in leptomeningeal artery territories and were more often associated with an embolic stroke source.[69] Our group recently found that in 16 patients with clinical presentations of subcortical infarcts, 10 had some evidence to suggest an embolic etiology, with a pattern of multiple, acute lesions in more than one single small-vessel territory.[70] Schonewille et al. used DWI to study 43 patients presenting acutely with classical lacunar syndromes. They confirmed that lacunar syndromes could be caused by deep ischemic infarcts, but also by superficial infarction and hemorrhage. Furthermore, lesions in the same location could give rise to a variety of clinical lacunar syndromes.[71] Conversely, Lindgren et al.[68] found a good correlation between lacunar syndromes and subcortical lesions using DWI.

Use of DWI/PWI as surrogate endpoints in investigational drug trials

With the lengthy list of failed neuroprotective strategies in Phase III trials, it has been suggested that DWI/PWI studies could be used to test proof of concept in early human studies.[37,72] Because DWI lesions correlate with acute and outcome clinical scores and infarct size, they can be used as valid surrogate measures of stroke outcome in acute investigational drug trials.[12,50] Attenuation of the typical expansion of acute DWI lesions has been used as a surrogate endpoint of drug efficacy. Fisher's group used DWI in a rat stroke model to evaluate a putative neuroprotective NMDA antagonist.[73] They correlated drug efficacy with the imaging results and reduced histological infarct size. The neuroprotective agent citicholine was evaluated in an MR substudy, measuring lesion growth between the acute stage and 12 weeks.[72] Although no difference was found in the primary endpoint, lesion volume reduction correlated with measured neurological improvement and lesion volume attenuation was correlated with the drug between weeks 1 and 12.[72] Similar proof of concept studies with PWI and DWI have been performed or are currently under way with other neuroprotective agents.[74] Such studies can be performed with 50–100 patients per treatment arm and are likely to indicate the probability of success in large and expensive phase III studies.[72]

Selection of patients for acute therapies

As discussed earlier, patients with an acute penumbral (PWI > DWI mismatch) pattern should be ideal candidates for thrombolysis.[11,12] The pivotal NINDS trial established the efficacy of t-PA in the treatment of acute ischemic stroke, and led to its licensing as the first acute stroke therapy in the USA, for selected patients within 3 hours of stroke onset.[3,75] Trials with a 6-hour window have been negative and only indicated a trend towards clinical efficacy.[76]

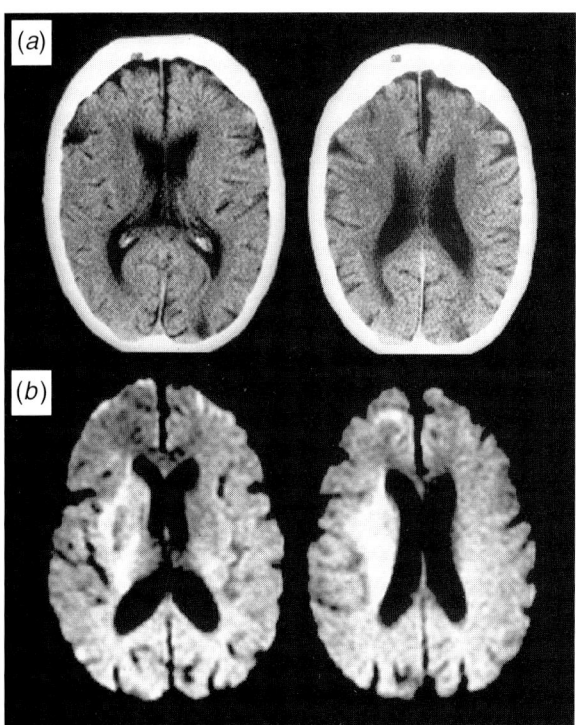

Fig. 14.10. (*a*) CT at 2.5 hours after onset of left hemiparesis. There is perhaps some subtle reduced density in the deep white matter. (*b*) DWI performed prior to CT highlights the greater sensitivity of this technique for acute ischemia.

It is clear that not all patients treated within 3 hours of ischemic stroke onset benefit from thrombolytic therapy. In addition, a therapeutic window of 3 hours significantly limits the number of stroke patients who can be treated. Ideally, stroke physicians would like to be able to identify patients with the greatest potential to benefit from, and the lowest risk of induced hemorrhage as a result of thrombolysis and to extend the current therapeutic window beyond three hours in selected patients. This would involve a strategy to individualize the therapeutic time window in acute stroke patients.

There is also speculation that use of combined DWI/PWI might improve patient selection in terms of safety. Early major ischemic changes on CT scan, defined by the ECASS Investigators as change involving more than one-third of the middle cerebral artery (MCA) territory, appear to predict a higher risk of hemorrhagic transformation and worse outcome.[77] However, these acute CT changes are subtle, and different interpretations can be made by skilled observers.[78] We compared the size of the DWI lesions with the extent of early ischemia on acute CT scan (Fig. 14.10). Ischemic lesions greater than one third of the MCA territory were identified by DWI in all cases, while DWI showed more extensive lesions than CT in some cases.[39] Large acute DWI lesions may predict an unacceptably high rate of hemorrhage with thrombolytic therapy.

We, and collaborating centres in Australia, have used PWI and DWI techniques to study 20 patients before and after treatment with t-PA within 6 hours of stroke onset[14] (Fig. 14.11). Most patients had a penumbra. Reperfusion occurred in most patients, with attenuation of infarct expansion, in contrast with our matched, historical controls who did not receive thrombolysis. These results support the hypothesis that t-PA facilitates reperfusion and attenuates infarct expansion in penumbral patients. These results are consistent with data from other groups.[61,62,79] Marks et al.[62] studied a small group of patients, although only after t-PA, and found early reperfusion compared with untreated subjects. The UCLA group studied patients before and after intra-arterial thrombolysis and found resolution of perfusion deficits and indeed some shrinkage of the initial DWI lesion volume.[35] The Heidelberg group[61] concluded that MRI was an effective and comprehensive tool in evaluating stroke patients for thrombolysis. They also indicated that PWI/DWI represented the target group for thrombolysis and that reperfusion in the penumbra followed recanalization.

Trials are now under way in Australia and North America to prospectively evaluate the hypothesis that the presence and extent of the ischemic penumbra using EPI will predict patients most likely to respond to thrombolytic therapy. In Australia, the EPITHET trial involves a double-blind, randomized, multicentre controlled trial of t-PA vs. placebo in 100 eligible patients with hemispheric infarction 3–6 hours after stroke onset.[80] In the USA, the DEFUSE trial involves patients openly treated with t-PA up to 6 hours, to determine which DWI/PWI parameters best predict response to t-PA.[79] In Germany, centres are already selecting

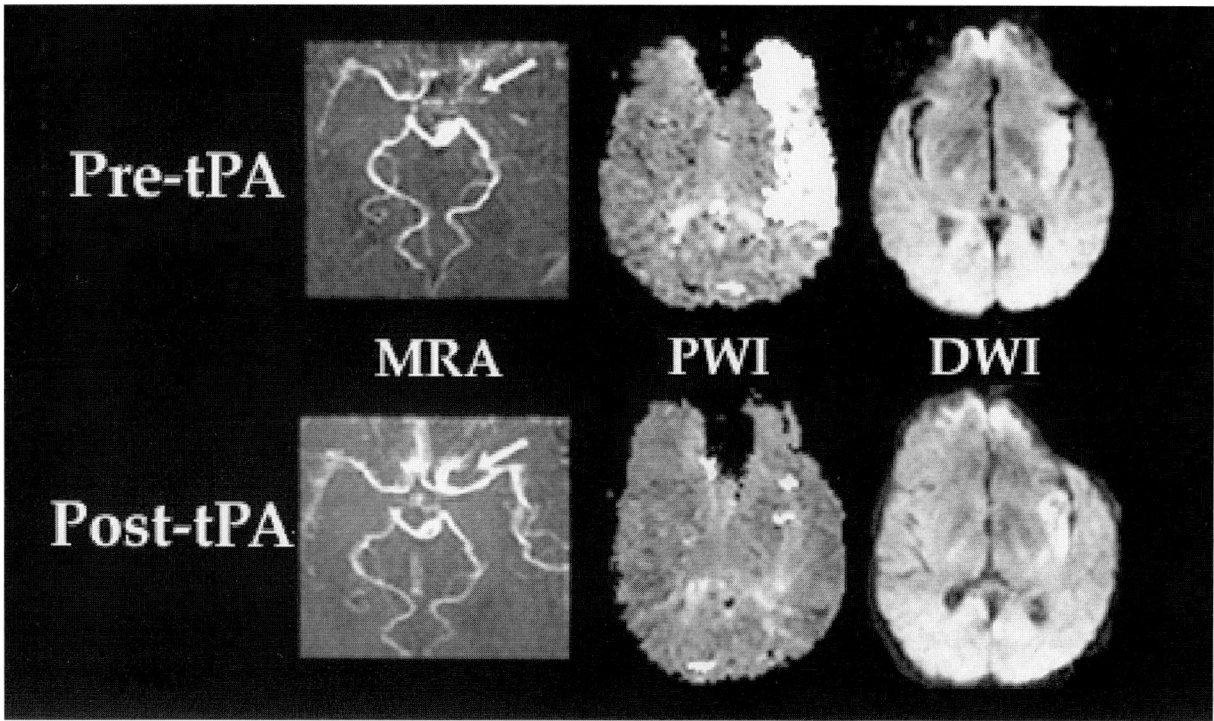

Fig. 14.11. Patient with acute right MCA occlusion at 2.5 hours and associated PWI > DWI mismatch. Following intravenous thrombolysis, recanalization of the occluded vessel has occurred, with complete reperfusion (lower PWI map) and no infarct expansion.

patients for thrombolysis beyond 3 hours, using evidence of PWI/DWI mismatch on MRI.[61]

MR spectroscopy in clinical practice

Magnetic resonance spectroscopy (MRS) allows the non-invasive assessment of metabolic changes during stroke.[81] This information can be obtained in conjunction with other MRI sequences so that correlations between anatomical and physiological changes can be made with changes in the biochemical processes occurring in cerebral ischemia.[82] Lactate and N-acetylaspartate (NAA) are two metabolites that can be measured by ^{1}H MRS, which are of major relevance in stroke (Fig. 14.12).[83–85] Lactate, which is not detectable in non-ischemic brain, is elevated almost immediately after the onset of cerebral ischemia,[86,87] and indicates a switch from oxidative metabolism to anerobic glycolysis.[88] We have found that lactate levels in the acute ischemic region provide independent predictive information when combined with DWI, highlighting the complementary nature of MRS and MRI. NAA begins to decline within several hours of acute infarction,[81,83–85] and is thought to indicate a loss of neuronal viability.[89] Several groups have found a correlation between NAA levels and stroke outcome that is independent of infarct size, emphasizing the potential clinical utility of this technique.[90,91]

A number of studies have suggested that MRS may herald the presence of hypoperfused but still viable neural cells within or surrounding infarcted tissue, as these cells continue to produce lactate.[86,92,93] Therefore, lactate levels measured within the penumbra may be a marker of tissue that ultimately progresses to infarction. This clearly has implications for acute stroke management. Furthermore, our group has recently demonstrated that acute hyperglycemia leads to elevated lactate production, which in turn leads to increased conversion of penumbral tissue to infarction.[94] The more widespread availability, along with shorter imaging times of multivoxel MRS, or chemical shift

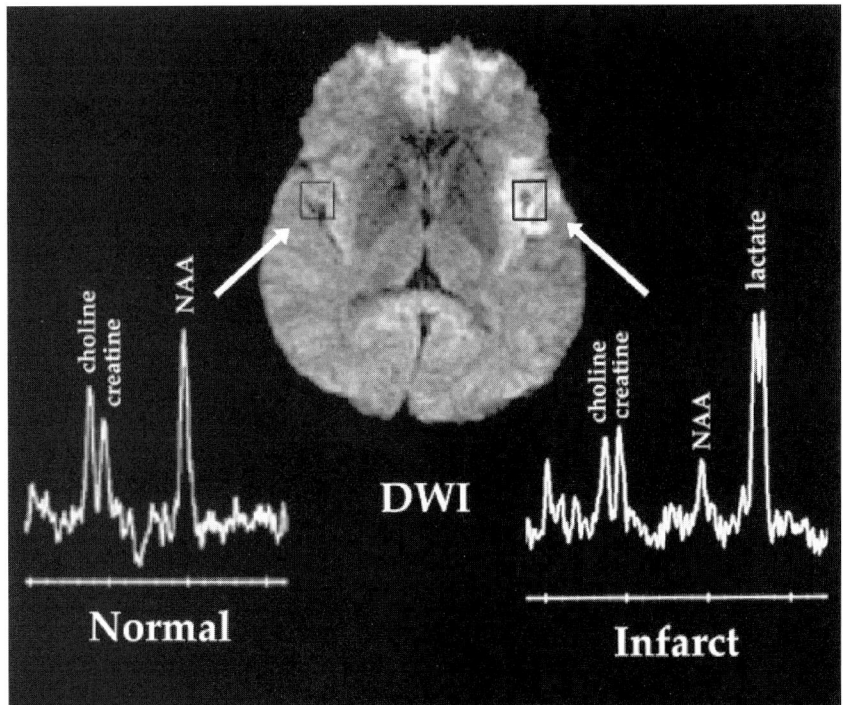

Fig. 14.12. Acute left MCA branch diffusion lesion imaged at 14 hours after symptom onset in which proton magnetic resonance spectroscopy (MRS) with a single voxel in the core of the infarct shows reduced NAA to choline ratio and a large lactate peak. A voxel placed in the homologous region on the left for comparison shows a normal spectrum, there is no lactate peak.

imaging (CSI), may enable assessment of metabolic changes occurring within the full extent of the penumbra (Fig. 14.13, see colour plate section).[85,93,95] The addition of CSI to a multimodal acute stroke MRI examination may confer additional accuracy to the identification of at-risk ischemic tissue.

Conclusions and future directions

We conclude that EPI with DWI, PWI and MRS offers unique insights into acute brain ischemia. These techniques have now moved from the research arena into routine clinical use. Given the highly sensitive detection of ischemia and the potential for rational selection of acute therapies, we predict that EPI will replace CT as the method of choice for acute stroke evaluation, particularly in patients being considered for acute interventional stroke therapy.

REFERENCES

1 Anderson CS, Jamrozik KD, Burvill PW, Chakera TM, Johnson GA, Stewart-Wynne EG. Ascertaining the true incidence of stroke: experience from the Perth Community Stroke Study, 1989–1990. *Med J Aust* 1993; 158: 80–84.

2 Bennett SA, Magnus P. Trends in cardiovascular risk factors in Australia. Results from the National Heart Foundation's Risk Factor Prevalence Study, 1980–1989. *Med J Aust* 1994; 161: 519–527.

3 Tissue plasminogen activator for acute ischemic stroke. The National Institute of Neurological Disorders and Stroke rt-PA Stroke Study Group. *N Engl J Med* 1995; 333: 1581–1587.

4 The International Stroke Trial (IST): a randomised trial of aspirin, subcutaneous heparin, both, or neither among 19435 patients with acute ischaemic stroke. International Stroke Trial Collaborative Group. *Lancet* 1997; 349: 1569–1581.

5 CAST: randomised placebo-controlled trial of early aspirin use in 20,000 patients with acute ischaemic stroke. CAST (Chinese Acute Stroke Trial) Collaborative Group. *Lancet* 1997; 349: 1641–1649.

6 Furlan A, Higashida R, Wechsler L et al. Intra-arterial prourokinase for acute ischemic stroke. The PROACT II study: a randomized controlled trial. Prolyse in acute cerebral thromboembolism. *J Am Med Assoc* 1999; 282: 2003–2011.
7 Davis SM. Tissue rescue therapy for ischaemic stroke. *J Clin Neurosci* 1995; 2: 7–15.
8 Astrup J, Siesjo BK, Symon L. Thresholds in cerebral ischemia – the ischemic penumbra. *Stroke* 1981; 12: 723–725.
9 Ginsberg MD, Pulsinelli WA. The ischemic penumbra, injury thresholds, and the therapeutic window for acute stroke [editorial; comment]. *Ann Neurol* 1994; 36: 553–554.
10 Hossmann KA. Viability thresholds and the penumbra of focal ischemia [see comments]. *Ann Neurol* 1994; 36: 557–565.
11 Warach S, Dashe JF, Edelman RR. Clinical outcome in ischemic stroke predicted by early diffusion-weighted and perfusion magnetic resonance imaging: a preliminary analysis. *J Cereb Blood Flow Metab* 1996; 16: 53–59.
12 Barber PA, Darby DG, Desmond PM et al. Prediction of stroke outcome with echoplanar perfusion- and diffusion-weighted MRI. *Neurology* 1998; 51: 418–426.
13 Warach S, Gaa J, Siewert B, Wielopolski P, Edelman RR. Acute human stroke studied by whole brain echo planar diffusion-weighted magnetic resonance imaging. *Ann Neurol* 1995; 37: 231–241.
14 Parsons MW, Barber PA, Darby DG, Tress BM, Donnan GA, Davis SM. Hyperacute diffusion- and perfusion-weighted MRI identified t-PA responders in stroke. *Ann Neurol* 2002; 51: 28–37.
15 Wardlaw JM, Sandercock PA, Warlow CP, Lindley RI. Trials of thrombolysis in acute ischemic stroke: does the choice of primary outcome measure really matter? *Stroke* 2000; 31: 1133–1135.
16 Barber PA, Demchuk AM, Zhang J, Buchan AM. Validity and reliability of a quantitative computed tomography score in predicting outcome of hyperacute stroke before thrombolytic therapy. ASPECTS Study Group. Alberta Stroke Programme Early CT Score. *Lancet* 2000; 355: 1670–1674.
17 Moulin T, Cattin F, Crepin-Leblond T et al. Early CT signs in acute middle cerebral artery infarction: predictive value for subsequent infarct locations and outcome. *Neurology* 1996; 47: 366–375.
18 Wardlaw JM, Lewis SC, Dennis MS, Counsell C, McDowall M. Is visible infarction on computed tomography associated with an adverse prognosis in acute ischemic stroke? *Stroke* 1998; 29: 1315–1319.
19 Davis SM, Chua MG, Lichtenstein M, Rossiter SC, Binns D, Hopper JL. Cerebral hypoperfusion in stroke prognosis and brain recovery. *Stroke* 1993; 24: 1691–1696.
20 Baird AE, Donnan GA, Austin MC, Fitt GJ, Davis SM, McKay WJ. Reperfusion after thrombolytic therapy in ischemic stroke measured by single-photon emission computed tomography. *Stroke* 1994; 25: 79–85.
21 Infeld B, Davis SM, Donnan GA et al. Streptokinase increases luxury perfusion after stroke. *Stroke* 1996; 27: 1524–1529.
22 Yasaka M, O'Keefe GJ, Chambers BR et al. Streptokinase in acute stroke: effect on reperfusion and recanalization. Australian Streptokinase Trial Study Group. *Neurology* 1998; 50: 626–632.
23 Barber PA, Davis SM, Infeld B et al. Spontaneous reperfusion after ischemic stroke is associated with improved outcome. *Stroke* 1998; 29: 2522–2528.
24 Infeld B, Davis SM, Donnan GA et al. Nimodipine and perfusion changes after stroke. *Stroke* 1999; 30: 1417–1423.
25 Edelman RR, Wielopolski P, Schmitt F. Echo-planar MR imaging. *Radiology* 1994; 192: 600–612.
26 Sorensen AG, Buonanno FS, Gonzalez RG et al. Hyperacute stroke: evaluation with combined multi-section diffusion-weighted and hemodynamically weighted echo-planar MR imaging. *Radiology* 1996; 199: 391–401.
27 Lutsep HL, Albers GW, DeCrespigny A, Kamat GN, Marks MP, Moseley ME. Clinical utility of diffusion-weighted magnetic resonance imaging in the assessment of ischemic stroke. *Ann Neurol* 1997; 41: 574–580.
28 Baird AE, Warach S. Magnetic resonance imaging of acute stroke. *J Cereb Blood Flow Metab* 1998; 18: 583–609.
29 Keir SL, Wardlaw JM. Systematic review of diffusion and perfusion imaging in acute ischemic stroke. *Stroke* 2000; 31: 2723–2731.
30 Powers WJ, Zivin J. Magnetic resonance imaging in acute stroke: not ready for prime time [editorial; comment]. *Neurology* 1998; 50: 842–843.
31 Bryan RN. Diffusion-weighted imaging: to treat or not to treat? That is the question. *Am J Neuroradiol* 1998; 19: 396–397.
32 Warach S, Boska M, Welch KM. Pitfalls and potential of clinical diffusion-weighted MR imaging in acute stroke. *Stroke* 1997; 28: 481–482.
33 Lovblad KO, Laubach HJ, Baird AE et al. Clinical experience with diffusion-weighted MR in patients with acute stroke [see comments]. *Am J Neuroradiol* 1998; 19: 1061–1066.

34 Minematsu K, Li L, Sotak CH, Davis MA, Fisher M. Reversible focal ischemic injury demonstrated by diffusion-weighted magnetic resonance imaging in rats. *Stroke* 1992; 23: 1304–1310; discussion 1310–1311.

35 Kidwell CS, Saver JL, Mattiello J et al. Thrombolytic reversal of acute human cerebral ischemic injury shown by diffusion/perfusion magnetic resonance imaging. *Ann Neurol* 2000; 47: 462–469.

36 Baird AE, Benfield A, Schlaug G et al. Enlargement of human cerebral ischemic lesion volumes measured by diffusion-weighted magnetic resonance imaging [see comments]. *Ann Neurol* 1997; 41: 581–589.

37 Barber PA, Davis SM, Darby DG et al. Absent middle cerebral artery flow predicts the presence and evolution of the ischemic penumbra. *Neurology* 1999; 52: 1125–1132.

38 Warach S, Mosley M, Sorensen AG, Koroshetz W. Time course of diffusion imaging abnormalities in human stroke [letter; comment]. *Stroke* 1996; 27: 1254–1256.

39 Barber PA, Davis SM, Darby DG et al. Screening for thrombolytic therapy in acute stroke: diffusion-weighted imaging vs. computed tomography. (Abstract). *Cerebrovasc Dis* 1999; 9: 73.

40 Wang PY, Barker PB, Wityk RJ, Ulug AM, van Zijl PC, Beauchamp NJ. Diffusion-negative stroke: a report of two cases. *Am J Neuroradiol* 1999; 20: 1876–1880.

41 Albers GW, Lansberg MG, Norbash AM et al. Yield of diffusion-weighted MRI for detection of potentially relevant findings in stroke patients. *Neurology* 2000; 54: 1562–1567.

42 Lansberg MG, Albers GW, Beaulieu C, Marks MP. Comparison of diffusion-weighted MRI and CT in acute stroke. *Neurology* 2000; 54: 1557–1561.

43 Lansberg MG, Norbash AM, Marks MP, Tong DC, Moseley ME, Albers GW. Advantages of adding diffusion-weighted magnetic resonance imaging to conventional magnetic resonance imaging for evaluating acute stroke. *Arch Neurol* 2000; 57: 1311–1316.

44 Kidwell CS, Alger JR, Di Salle F et al. Diffusion MRI in patients with transient ischemic attacks. *Stroke* 1999; 30: 1174–1180.

45 Patel MR, Edelman RR, Warach S. Detection of hyperacute primary intraparenchymal hemorrhage by magnetic resonance imaging. *Stroke* 1996; 27: 2321–2324.

46 Linfante I, Llinas RH, Caplan LR, Warach S. MRI features of intracerebral hemorrhage within 2 hours from symptom onset. *Stroke* 1999; 30: 2263–2267.

47 Kucharczyk J, Vexler ZS, Roberts TP et al. Echo-planar perfusion-sensitive MR imaging of acute cerebral ischemia. *Radiology* 1993; 188: 711–717.

48 Edelman RR, Siewert B, Darby DG et al. Qualitative mapping of cerebral blood flow and functional localization with echo-planar MR imaging and signal targeting with alternating radio frequency. *Radiology* 1994; 192: 513–520.

49 Rordorf G, Koroshetz WJ, Copen WA et al. Regional ischemia and ischemic injury in patients with acute middle cerebral artery stroke as defined by early diffusion-weighted and perfusion-weighted MRI. *Stroke* 1998; 29: 939–943.

50 Lovblad KO, Baird AE, Schlaug G et al. Ischemic lesion volumes in acute stroke by diffusion-weighted magnetic resonance imaging correlate with clinical outcome. *Ann Neurol* 1997; 42: 164–170.

51 Tong DC, Yenari MA, Albers GW, O'Brien M, Marks MP, Moseley ME. Correlation of perfusion- and diffusion-weighted MRI with NIHSS score in acute (6.5 hour) ischemic stroke [see comments]. *Neurology* 1998; 50: 864–870.

52 Darby DG, Barber PA, Gerraty RP et al. Pathophysiological topography of acute ischemia by combined diffusion-weighted and perfusion MRI. *Stroke* 1999; 30: 2043–2052.

53 Fisher M. Diffusion and perfusion imaging for acute stroke. *Surg Neurol* 1995; 43: 606–609.

54 Beaulieu C, de Crespigny A, Tong DC, Moseley ME, Albers GW, Marks MP. Longitudinal magnetic resonance imaging study of perfusion and diffusion in stroke: evolution of lesion volume and correlation with clinical outcome. *Ann Neurol* 1999; 46: 568–578.

55 Barber PA, Consolo HK, Yang Q et al. Comparison of MRI perfusion imaging and single photon emission computed tomography in chronic stroke. *Cerebrovasc Dis* 2001; 11: 128–136.

56 Neumann-Haefelin T, Wittsack HJ, Wenserski F et al. Diffusion- and perfusion-weighted MRI. The DWI/PWI mismatch region in acute stroke. *Stroke* 1999; 30: 1591–1597.

57 Ostergaard L, Sorensen AG, Kwong KK, Weisskoff RM, Gyldensted C, Rosen BR. High resolution measurement of cerebral blood flow using intravascular tracer bolus passages. Part II: Experimental comparison and preliminary results. *Magn Reson Med* 1996; 36: 726–736.

58 Neumann-Haefelin T, Wittsack HJ, Fink GR et al. Diffusion- and perfusion-weighted MRI: influence of severe carotid artery stenosis on the DWI/PWI mismatch in acute stroke. *Stroke* 2000; 31: 1311–1317.

59 Parsons MW, Yang Q, Barber PA et al. Perfusion magnetic resonance imaging maps in hyperacute stroke: relative cerebral blood flow most accurately identifies tissue destined to infarct. *Stroke* 2001; 32: 1581–1587.

60 Wu O, Koroshetz WJ, Ostergaard L et al. Predicting tissue outcome in acute human cerebral ischemia using combined diffusion- and perfusion-weighted MR imaging. *Stroke* 2001; 32: 933–942.

61 Schellinger PD, Jansen O, Fiebach JB et al. Monitoring intravenous recombinant tissue plasminogen activator thrombolysis for acute ischemic stroke with diffusion and perfusion MRI. *Stroke* 2000; 31: 1318–1328.

62 Marks MP, Tong DC, Beaulieu C, Albers GW, de Crespigny A, Moseley ME. Evaluation of early reperfusion and i.v. tPA therapy using diffusion- and perfusion-weighted MRI [see comments]. *Neurology* 1999; 52: 1792–1798.

63 Lee LJ, Kidwell CS, Alger J, Starkman S, Saver JL. Impact on stroke subtype diagnosis of early diffusion-weighted magnetic resonance imaging and magnetic resonance angiography. *Stroke* 2000; 31: 1081–1089.

64 Roh JK, Kang DW, Lee SH, Yoon BW, Chang KH. Significance of acute multiple brain infarction on diffusion-weighted imaging. *Stroke* 2000; 31: 688–694.

65 Singer MB, Chong J, Lu D, Schonewille WJ, Tuhrim S, Atlas SW. Diffusion-weighted MRI in acute subcortical infarction [published erratum appears in *Stroke* 1998 Mar; 29(3): 731]. *Stroke* 1998; 29: 133–136.

66 Noguchi K, Nagayoshi T, Watanabe N et al. Diffusion-weighted echo-planar MRI of lacunar infarcts. *Neuroradiology* 1998; 40: 448–451.

67 Oliveira-Filho J, Ay H, Schaefer PW et al. Diffusion-weighted magnetic resonance imaging identifies the 'clinically relevant' small-penetrator infarcts. *Arch Neurol* 2000; 57: 1009–1014.

68 Lindgren A, Staaf G, Geijer B et al. Clinical lacunar syndromes as predictors of lacunar infarcts. A comparison of acute clinical lacunar syndromes and findings on diffusion-weighted MRI. *Acta Neurol Scand* 2000; 2000: 2.

69 Ay H, Oliveira-Filho J, Buonanno FS et al. Diffusion-weighted imaging identifies a subset of lacunar infarction associated with embolic source. *Stroke* 1999; 30: 2644–2650.

70 Gerraty RP, Parsons M, Barber PA et al. Acute echoplanar diffusion and perfusion MRI improves diagnostic accuracy in subcortical cerebral infarction (Abstract). *Stroke* 2000; Accepted for Publication.

71 Schonewille WJ, Tuhrim S, Singer MB, Atlas SW. Diffusion-weighted MRI in acute lacunar syndromes. A clinical-radiological correlation study. *Stroke* 1999; 30: 2066–2069.

72 Warach S, Pettigrew LC, Dashe JF et al. Effect of citicoline on ischemic lesions as measured by diffusion-weighted magnetic resonance imaging. Citicoline 010 Investigators. *Ann Neurol* 2000; 48: 713–722.

73 Meadows ME, Fisher M, Minematsu K. Delayed treatment with a non-competitive NMDA antagonist, CNS-1102, reduces infarct size in rats. *Cerebrovasc Dis* 1994; 4: 26–31.

74 Fisher M, Albers GW. Applications of diffusion-perfusion magnetic resonance imaging in acute ischemic stroke. *Neurology* 1999; 52: 1750–1756.

75 Adams HP, Jr., Brott TG, Furlan AJ et al. Guidelines for Thrombolytic Therapy for Acute Stroke: a Supplement to the Guidelines for the Management of Patients with Acute Ischemic Stroke. A statement for healthcare professionals from a Special Writing Group of the Stroke Council, American Heart Association. *Stroke* 1996; 27: 1711–1718.

76 Hacke W, Kaste M, Fieschi C et al. Randomised double-blind placebo-controlled trial of thrombolytic therapy with intravenous alteplase in acute ischaemic stroke (ECASS II). Second European–Australasian Acute Stroke Study Investigators [see comments]. *Lancet* 1998; 352: 1245–1251.

77 Hacke W, Kaste M, Fieschi C et al. Intravenous thrombolysis with recombinant tissue plasminogen activator for acute hemispheric stroke. The European Cooperative Acute Stroke Study (ECASS) [see comments]. *J Am Med Assoc* 1995; 274: 1017–1025.

78 Grotta JC, Chiu D, Lu M et al. Agreement and variability in the interpretation of early CT changes in stroke patients qualifying for intravenous rtPA therapy. *Stroke* 1999; 30: 1528–1533.

79 Albers GW. Expanding the window for thrombolytic therapy in acute stroke. The potential role of acute MRI for patient selection. *Stroke* 1999; 30: 2230–2237.

80 Davis SM, Tress B, Barber PA et al. Echoplanar magnetic resonance imaging in acute stroke. *J Clin Neurosci* 2000; 7: 3–8.

81 Graham GD, Kalvach P, Blamire AM, Brass LM, Fayad PB, Prichard JW. Clinical correlates of proton magnetic resonance spectroscopy findings after acute cerebral infarction. *Stroke* 1995; 26: 225–229.

82 Moonen CT, van Zijl PC, Frank JA, Le Bihan D, Becker ED. Functional magnetic resonance imaging in medicine and physiology. *Science* 1990; 250: 53–61.

83 Graham GD, Blamire AM, Howseman AM et al. Proton magnetic resonance spectroscopy of cerebral lactate and other metabolites in stroke patients. *Stroke* 1992; 23: 333–340.

84 Gideon P, Henriksen O, Sperling B et al. Early time course of N-acetylaspartate, creatine and phosphocreatine, and compounds containing choline in the brain after acute stroke. A proton magnetic resonance spectroscopy study. *Stroke* 1992; 23: 1566–1572.

85 Barker PB, Gillard JH, van Zijl PC et al. Acute stroke: evaluation with serial proton MR spectroscopic imaging. *Radiology* 1994; 192: 723–732.

86 Higuchi T, Fernandez EJ, Maudsley AA, Shimizu H, Weiner MW, Weinstein PR. Mapping of lactate and N-acetyl-L-aspartate predicts infarction during acute focal ischemia: in vivo 1H magnetic resonance spectroscopy in rats. *Neurosurgery* 1996; 38: 121–129; discussion 129–130.

87 Petroff OA, Ogino T, Alger JR. High-resolution proton magnetic resonance spectroscopy of rabbit brain: regional metabolite levels and postmortem changes. *J Neurochem* 1988; 51: 163–171.

88 Petroff OA, Prichard JW, Ogino T, Shulman RG. Proton magnetic resonance spectroscopic studies of agonal carbohydrate metabolism in rabbit brain. *Neurology* 1988; 38: 1569–1574.

89 Prichard JW. The ischemic penumbra in stroke: prospects for analysis by nuclear magnetic resonance spectroscopy. *Res Publ Assoc Res Nerv Ment Dis* 1993; 71: 153–174.

90 Pereira AC, Saunders DE, Doyle VL et al. Measurement of initial N-acetyl aspartate concentration by magnetic resonance spectroscopy and initial infarct volume by MRI predicts outcome in patients with middle cerebral artery territory infarction. *Stroke* 1999; 30: 1577–1582.

91 Wardlaw JM, Marshall I, Wild J, Dennis MS, Cannon J, Lewis SC. Studies of acute ischemic stroke with proton magnetic resonance spectroscopy: relation between time from onset, neurological deficit, metabolite abnormalities in the infarct, blood flow, and clinical outcome. *Stroke* 1998; 29: 1618–1624.

92 Petroff OA, Graham GD, Blamire AM et al. Spectroscopic imaging of stroke in humans: histopathology correlates of spectral changes. *Neurology* 1992; 42: 1349–1354.

93 Gillard JH, Barker PB, van Zijl PC, Bryan RN, Oppenheimer SM. Proton MR spectroscopy in acute middle cerebral artery stroke. *Am J Neuroradiol* 1996; 17: 873–886.

94 Parsons MW, Barber PA, Yang Q et al. Acute hyperglycemia adversely affects stroke outcome: an MRI imaging and spectroscopy study. *Ann Neurol* 2002; 52: 20–28.

95 Wild JM, Wardlaw JM, Marshall I, Warlow CP. N-acetylaspartate distribution in proton spectroscopic images of ischemic stroke: relationship to infarct appearance on T_2-weighted magnetic resonance imaging. *Stroke* 2000; 31: 3008–3014.

The ischemic penumbra: the evolution of a concept

Geoffrey A. Donnan, Peter M. Wright, Romesh Markus, Thanh Phan and David C. Reutens

National Stroke Research Institute, Heidelberg, Victoria, Australia

Definition

In human ischemic stroke the affected brain tissue has metabolic requirements that can no longer be supported by a sudden interruption, or at least reduction, in nutrient supply and waste disposal resulting from disease in a proximal artery. The underlying pathophysiological changes immediately following arterial occlusion include an initial loss of neuronal electrical activity followed by depletion of cellular energy stores and the loss of the transmembrane ion pumps which maintain water, sodium, chloride and potassium balance. Cellular necrosis will follow these changes if the cell's minimum energy requirements are not met.[1–3] The tissue supplied by the artery is not affected homogeneously by this process, and critical blood flow thresholds associated with irreversible tissue infarction, functional tissue impairment, or benign oligemia can be identified. Several methods of threshold detection using modern imaging techniques lead to differing interpretations of this in vivo, and the extensive molecular and biochemical mechanisms in the penumbra can only partially be evaluated in human stroke patients. The region of incomplete ischemia in stroke usually adjacent to the area of profound ischemia has been termed the ischemic penumbra. A useful functional definition of the penumbra is that region of under-perfused brain tissue that is metabolically impaired, classically showing electrical inactivity, but with cellular morphology intact. In humans, this region is closely associated with established critical thresholds for blood flow rates using positron emission tomography (PET).

Importance

The fundamental importance of the concept of the ischemic penumbra is the recognition that ischemic processes may be reversible. In theory, this zone of functionally inactive but structurally intact tissue may, at any time point, be restored to functional normality. The best clinical validation of this principal is the observed correlation between the volume of surviving penumbra and clinical outcome.[4,5] The recognition of this relationship has stimulated research efforts to develop therapeutic approaches to increase the proportion of salvageable tissue. Since clinicians can now detect penumbral tissue very early after stroke onset with a variety of neuroimaging modalities, particularly magnetic resonance imaging, there is great clinical potential for individualized patient selection for therapy. The ability to identify critical thresholds for cerebral blood flow rates offers important potential advantages: reperfusion into penumbral tissue following the use of thrombolysis in stroke is associated with improved clinical outcome, compared with a failure to reperfuse;[6–9] those thresholds which predict hemorrhagic risk, or lack of thrombolysis may be identified;[8] and the lack of penumbral tissue due to early reperfusion may obviate the need for therapy. Hence, this proven treatment may potentially be enhanced using this model. The ischemic penumbra may also be useful as a surrogate target for clinical research into new therapies. This issue has become more important since many large phase III trials of neuroprotection in acute ischemic stroke have been negative, in spite of good evidence for efficacy in animal models.

Table 15.1. Flow thresholds in ml/100 g per min (% of reference) for irreversible damage and penumbra from functional neuroimaging studies in acute stroke[12]

Modality	Authors	Damage		Penumbra	
PET	Baron et al. (1984)[13]	12			
	Powers et al. (1985)[14]	12		22	
	Hakim et al. (1989)[15]	12		18	
	Furlan et al. (1996)[16]	7			
	Marchal et al. (1996)[17]			22	
	Heiss et al. (2000)[12]	4.8	(22)	14.1	(54)
MRI	Schlaug et al (1999)[18]	6	(12)	18.5	(37)
SPECT	Giubilei et al. (1990)[19]		(60)		(70)
	Shimosegawa et al. (1994)[20]		(48)		(75)
	Ezura et al. (1996)[8]		(35)		(70)
	Berrouschot et al. (1998)[21]		(0)		(70)
	Hatazawa et al. (1999)[22]		(39)		(69)
	Ueda et al. (1999)[23]		(35)		(55)
Xe-CT	Firlik et al. (1998)[24]	17.3		35.4	
	Kaufmann et al. (1999)[25]	6		20	

Notes:
PET, positron emission tomography; MRI, magnetic resonance imaging; SPECT, single photo emission computed tomography; Xe-CT, Xenon-enhanced X-ray computed tomography.

Flow thresholds for the ischemic penumbra

The concept of the ischemic penumbra was pioneered in baboon models of focal ischemia using occluded middle cerebral arteries by Astrup, Siesjo and Symons.[10,11] They identified three distinct regions of blood flow disruption. Regions of severely hypoperfused tissue (the ischemic core) with cerebral blood flow less than 6–10 ml/100 g per min were usually irreversibly damaged and exhibited features of cellular necrosis, such as an efflux of intracellular potassium. This region was usually within the basal ganglia and anterior temporal region. Less profoundly hypoperfused penumbral tissue, usually more cortically located, had a CBF <20 ml/100 g per min, and demonstrated functional electrical impairment with an isoelectric electroencephalograph and absent evoked potentials but could potentially be salvaged if the middle cerebral artery occlusion was transient. This region was not associated with early evidence of cellular necrosis.[2] A third, peripheral region of benign oligemia (mildly reduced blood flow) was not usually at risk of infarction. The accumulated experience from functional imaging studies in human stroke over the subsequent three decades has identified estimates of the upper and lower critical flow thresholds to define penumbral regions. These are shown in Table 15.1.

The dynamic and time-related nature of the penumbra

Ischemia will inevitably occur in tissues dependent on an acutely occluded large artery. Heiss and colleagues demonstrated in a primate model that a CBF of up to 14 ml/100 g/min for more than 45 minutes was associated with necrosis, but that even profound flow disturbances could be associated with neuronal survival if reperfused within 20 minutes.[26] In another model Morawetz and colleagues have demonstrated that blood flow below 10–12 ml/100 g/min for more than 2 hours was

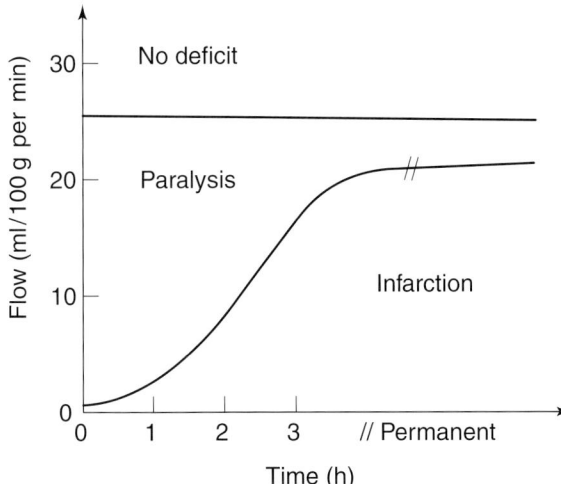

Fig. 15.1. Developed from Jones et al.[28] A monkey model of the relationship between the cerebral blood flow in ml/100 g/min (y-axis), and the duration of ischemia in causing signs, and tissue infarction. Reversible paralysis develops if the CBF falls below 23 ml/100 g/min. Even profound ischemia is tolerable for very brief periods, and if CBF is below 10 ml/100 g per min for >2 hours, or below 18 ml/100 g/min in the setting of permanent occlusion, then irreversible tissue infarction occurs.

consistently associated with tissue infarction,[27] and tissue with a CBF of 15 ml/100 g per min could be supported for about 3 hours without infarction, whilst tissue with a CBF of 5 ml/100 g/min only remained viable for 2 hours. The area of irreversibly damaged tissue expanded at the expense of the penumbral region over time, leaving only a small region of penumbral tissue at 3 hours.[28] Flow thresholds appear to differ between animal species, with rats needing over 25 ml/100 g per min,[29] and cats 15 ml/100 g per min for tissue viability.[30] Figure 15.1 demonstrates the relationship between the severity and duration of flow reduction and the ultimate fate of the tissue affected.

Heiss and colleagues studied ten human patients with positron emission tomography within 3 hours of stroke. In these, penumbral tissue consisted of only about 18% of the total tissue with reduced CBF, while 12% was oligemic, and the remaining 70% was critically hypoperfused tissue at these early time points.[31] This would imply that there is a low likelihood of significant clinical recovery after 3 hours. However, accumulating evidence that some patients benefit from intra-arterial, and possibly intravenous reperfusion treatments for up to 6 hours have limited the acceptance of this view.[31–33] In addition, Baron and colleagues studied eight patients between 7–17 hours from stroke onset using positron emission tomography (PET), who had both acute misery perfusion (see section on PET), and a final infarction of more than 16 mm diameter. Eventually infarcted tissue with preserved early $CMRO_2$ values above the threshold for irreversible infarction were found in each of these eight cases. This pattern constituted 10% to 52% of the final infarct volume. Several patients still had penumbra at 13–16 hours after stroke, and this late penumbral tissue made up on average 35% of the final infarct volume.[34] Read and colleagues studied 24 patients up to 51 hours after ischemic stroke using ^{18}F-fluoromisonidazole (FMISO) as a ligand that labels hypoxic but viable tissue in positron emission tomography. Penumbral tissue, labelled with FMISO, was found in 15 patients and the proportion of patients with penumbra, and penumbral volume, decreased with time. On average, 45% of the tissue that trapped FMISO survived. Up to 68% (mean, 17.5%) of the infarct volume was initially hypoxic. Most of the tissue initially affected proceeded to infarction.[4] Darby and colleagues have also shown the penumbra, as defined by a mismatch between diffusion-weighted, and perfusion-imaging lesion volumes using MRI, gradually declines with time up to about 18 hours following stroke onset. This is shown in Fig. 15.2.

In addition to the severity and duration of arterial occlusion, the availability of an alternate blood supply from collateral vessels,[36] and environmental stressors such as hyperglycemia, arterial hypoxia and hyperthermia may play important roles in determining the duration of tissue viability. Misery perfusion, recurrent spreading depression, excitotoxin release and acidosis all contribute to this dynamic state in the penumbra.[37,38] Microvessel plugging by platelets, fibrin or neutrophils has been found in baboon models and will affect the dynamic process of tissue reperfusion. This may also occur even in the presence of early reopening of the diseased artery.[12,34,39–41]

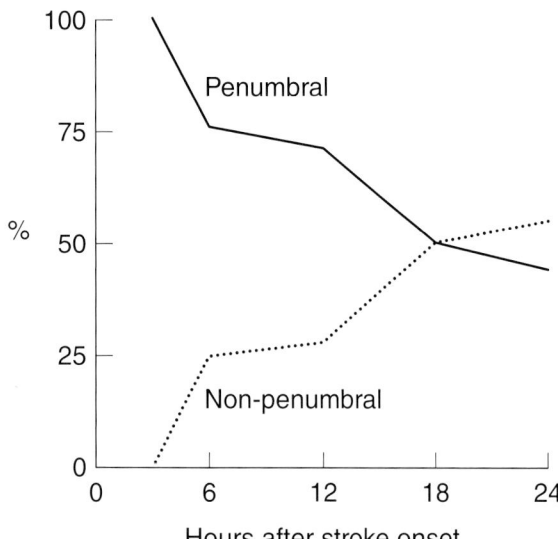

Fig. 15.2. Plot of penumbral or non-penumbral patterns as a percentage of total number of patients scanned within each period (0–3 hours, 0–6 hours, 6–12 hours, 12–18 hours, >18 hours).[35]

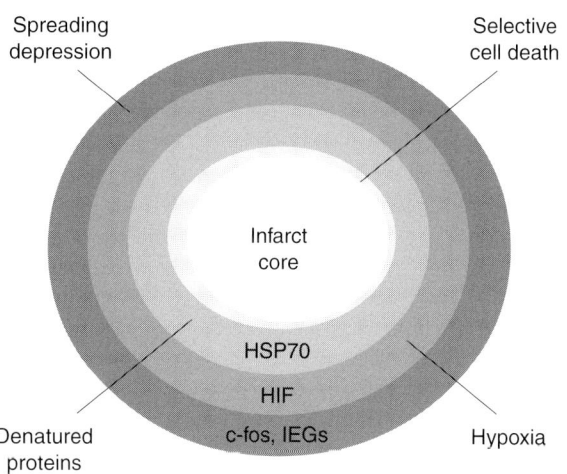

Fig. 15.3. Schematic of multiple molecular penumbras after a stroke. A zone of selective neuronal cell death borders the infarct. The zone of protein denaturation extends outside of this and is demarcated by heat shock protein 70 (HSP70) expression in injured neurons. Hypoxia inducible factor (HIF) is exposed in areas where blood flow is persistently decreased and oxygen delivery is impaired. This may be coincident with HSP 70 or extend over more widespread regions depending on collaterals. Ischemia-induced spreading depression induces c-fos and many other immediate early genes (IEGs) at some distances from the infarct, including the ipsilateral rat occipital and frontal lobes, contralateral cortex and many subcortical structures. Derived from Sharp et al.[42]

The ischemic penumbra: a molecular view

Although founded on the concept of critical changes of blood flow, the ischemic penumbra can also be described in molecular terms. While this concept is based on animal models of cerebral ischemia, and no means of imaging molecular changes are yet available in vivo, there are important implications for therapy in humans. Sharp and colleagues described no less than five distinct regions associated with focal cerebral ischemia based on the molecular changes being exhibited.[42]

Defining the ischemic core in molecular terms

Protein synthesis is inhibited by the release of glutamate, and energy depletion in ischemia, decreasing by about 50% at a CBF of 55 ml/100 g per min and ceasing almost completely below 35 ml/100 g/min.[42,43] A molecular delineation of the ischemic core employs analyses of appropriate proteins, many of which have a short half-life, and hence rapid reductions in concentration. These include intercellular adhesion molecule-1 (ICAM-1 or CD54),[44] matrix metalloproteases (MMPs),[45] tumour necrosis factor (TNF) alpha and TNF receptors,[46,47] transcription regulatory nuclear factor kB (NFkB), and the targets for NFkB which include manganese (Mn^{2+}), superoxide dismutase, inducible nitric oxide synthetase (iNOS), matrix metalloprotease-9 (MMP-9) and cyclo-oxygenase-2 (COX-2).[42] In addition, the expression of the anti-apoptotic genes *Bcl-2* and *Bcl-x*$_L$ is decreased among neurons lethally injured, whereas they are increased in mildly compromised neurons within the penumbral region.

Defining the ischemic penumbra in molecular terms

Outside the core of the infarct, a series of four further regions can be defined in molecular terms. Given that there is potential reversibility of neuronal impairment in each zone, the term 'penumbra' is applicable for each. As can be seen in Fig. 15.3, the first topographical area is immediately adjacent to the core of the infarct, and extends for no more than one centimetre. Histologically, selective neuronal death has been documented.[48]

The next zone is an area of protein denaturation, and is manifest by the continued expression of the heat shock protein 70 (HSP70). Induction of the *HSP70* gene, together with other heat shock chaperones, acts to renature the affected proteins. While these changes may be expressed on blood vessels, it is their neuronal expression which is important in this potentially viable area surrounding an infarct.[42] The next zone is demarcated by the presence of the transcription factor, hypoxia inducible factor 1 (HIF-I). This is induced by changes in molecular oxygen levels in tissue.[49] It has been suggested that this region may represent an area of chronically depleted blood flow and, hence, hypoxia surrounding infarcts.[42] Although it has been shown that HIF-I and related transcription factors may increase blood flow, glucose delivery and energy maintenance under hypoxic conditions, their role is still unclear.[42] The final zone (not penumbral by standard blood flow definitions) is far more widespread, and represents areas affected by spreading depression. This phenomenon induces a number of intermediate early genes (IEGs), particularly c-fos, over the entire hemisphere, and some may play a role in protecting the brain against ischemic insults.[50] The delineation of these five zones (one core, and four penumbral) is extremely useful, since many of these molecular changes represent potential targets for therapy. It should be said that many of these 'multiple penumbras' are still poorly understood in molecular terms and further research may reveal further avenues for penumbral salvage, or neuroprotection.

Ischemic penumbra: operational definitions in humans

As outlined earlier, there are many concurrent vascular, environmental and molecular processes occurring in early stroke. Of the several imaging modalities that offer potential for the assessment of the penumbra in human patients, each assesses only a portion of these events. None of the available modalities offers an exact definition of the functional ischemic penumbra for every patient. An operational definition requires information which will allow identification of the upper and lower tissue CBF thresholds for penumbra. These must correctly identify the ischemic core, the potentially viable tissue, and exclude the benign oligemic tissue, by ensuring the tissue involved is clinically functionally impaired. In humans, this definition is difficult to achieve and alternative means of validation of penumbral imaging techniques are needed. A pragmatic approach adopted by a number of investigators is to establish a positive correlation between the amount of putative penumbral tissue that survives and an improved clinical outcome.[4,5] Another approach is to regard the PET analysis of cerebral blood flow (CBF), regional cerebral metabolic rate of oxygen ($CMRO_2$), oxygen extraction fractions (OEF), as the current 'gold standard', and performing comparative studies against newer techniques. However, this approach is logistically difficult and is yet to be implemented satisfactorily.

Positron emission tomography (PET)

^{15}O PET

Multitracer PET imaging with ^{15}O allows generation of quantitative brain maps for CBF, $CMRO_2$, OEF, cerebral blood volume (CBV), and regional cerebral metabolic rate of glucose. Analysis of data from several small human stroke studies performed at 5–48 h after onset of symptoms allows estimation of thresholds of flow and metabolic activity that can reasonably differentiate the tissue subtypes of ischemia, penumbra, oligemia and unaffected tissue at the time of the study. The penumbra is described by reduced CBF and increased OEF but with a relatively preserved $rCMRO_2$, indicating stressed but viable tissue, a state described by Baron as 'miserly perfusion'.[51] While regions with $CMRO_2$ of less than 65 μmol/100 g/min predict infarction,[13] those with an increased OEF >70%, with $CMRO_2$ relatively preserved despite reduction in CBF are penumbral. Where the CBF is between 12 and 22 ml/100 g per min, the tissue outcome depends on the duration of ischemia, and other undetermined factors,[15] although the outcome is often infarction unless the $CMRO_2$ derangements are particularly mild.[16,52] Heiss and colleagues found that 95% of regions with CBF <4.8 ml/100 g per min became infarcted, but 95% of regions with CBF >14.1 ml/100 g/min escaped infarction.[12] The most profound drops in $CMRO_2$ occur in the deep MCA territory, consistent with relative preservation of cortical tissue at follow-up.[53–56] Baron reported for the first time in humans a well validated operational model of the ischemic penumbra. Using 30 patients imaged 5–18 hours after stroke onset, they identified the ischemic core as tissue with $CMRO_2$ of metabolic thresholds with multitracer PET studies or MRI have not been established. Limited validation has been reported correlating surviving penumbral tissue with outcome.[4]

Single photon emission computed tomography (SPECT)

Areas of relatively reduced CBF can be determined using ^{99m}Technetium-hexamethylpropylene-aminooxime (HMPAO), or ^{99m}Technetium-ethyl-cysteinate dimer (ECD). The latter also contribute limited metabolic information regarding the tissue. Volumes of reduced, and profoundly reduced CBF in acute stroke can be demonstrated using SPECT. It can be compared with a 'normal' population, or a region of interest from the contralateral hemisphere, but an accurate description of penumbra is difficult, as the regions of ischemic core, and of oligemia are not identified well. A number of investigators have demonstrated that severe, large regions of reduction in uptake of these radioactive labels is associated with poor clinical outcome,[19,57–59] and normal or increased uptake is predictive of good outcome.[57,21,60] The relative CBF reductions that predicted the region of infarction at follow-up ranged from no flow up to 60% flow as shown in Table 15.2. The range of flow reduction, as represented by reduced tissue label uptake, found to represent tissue that, although ischemic, has a moderate chance of escaping infarction is between 40 and 70%.[8,9,19,21,57,60,61]

Computerized tomography (CT) perfusion radiography

This new modality has become practicable with helical CT scanners, which are able to track intravenous contrast to generate angiographic images, then in the tissue phase of contrast passage to determine semiquantitative cerebral blood volume analysis.[62] The quantitated CBF rates generated do not correlate well with CBF values determined by PET and thresholds for defining the ischemic penumbra have not been identified. Koenig and colleagues analysed the relative comparison to the contralateral hemisphere, semiquantitate CBF, CBV, and time to peak perfusion maps in stroke. They found CBF values of around 34% compared with 62%, and CBV values of 43% and 62% respectively, for areas of infarction and areas suffering from reversible ischemia. 'Reversible ischemia' was not operationally defined to be consistent with ischemic penumbra in this study. While perfusion CT is still restricted to a single slice, multislice technology is currently being developed.[63]

Xenon-enhanced CT

This uses stable xenon gas and has not been taken up widely, probably due to difficulties managing the gas itself, and to its side effects when used. Quantitative CBF analysis has been possible in a baboon stroke model, essentially validating it as a technique, but finding lower CBF values than are usually documented with PET studies.[64] Studies in acute human stroke within 6 hours of onset have correlated permanent tissue infarction with CBF values below 20 ml/100 g per min. The most profound middle cerebral artery strokes had a mean CBF of 8.6 ml/100 g per min in contrast to a mean of 18 ml/100 g per min in those with milder strokes. Profound reductions in CBF to 6 ml/100 g/min closely predicted tissue infarction, and were associated with a small rim of tissue with CBF values of 7–20 ml/100 g/min.[25] Stroke patients had a mean CBF in areas of ischemia of 17.3 ml/100 g/min compared with 35.4 ml/100 g/min for those with reversible ischemic events.[24]

Magnetic resonance diffusion-weighted and perfusion imaging of the penumbra

Evolving MRI techniques are useful for assessment of penumbral tissue in acute stroke. The blood flow

Table 15.2. Operational definitions of the ischemic penumbra in humans: clinically validated definitions of tissue at risk of infarction but not in the ischemic core. For definitions of the penumbra, evidence is required that the tissue is functionally impaired due to hypoperfusion, but has not already been recruited into the irreversibly damaged ischemic core

Imaging	Definition penumbra	Definition core	Advantages	Disadvantages
SPECT	Relative CBF 40–70%	Relative CBF 0–60%	Cheap Available	Poorly defines core Poor agreement about thresholds Time delays
PET FMZ	15-O PET CBF/FMZ mismatch or 2 minute FMZ binding	<3.5 times contralateral FMZ binding	Not time dependent	Not clinically validated No FMZ penumbra definition No subcortical data
PET F-MISO	18-F MISO trapping	Central void uptake	Biochemical definition Direct, simple measure	Poor validation Not clinically applicable
PET (15-O)	CBF 7–22 ml[a] $CMRO_2$ >54 picoM[a] Grey $CMRO_2$ >1.4 ml[a] OEF > 70%	CBF <12 ml[a] $CMRO_2$ <65 picoM[a] Grey $CMRO_2$ <1.4 ml[a] Lower OEF	Reproducible Clinically validated	Limited availability High cost Slow technique
CT perfusion	Relative CBF 34–62%	Relative CBF <34%	Cheap, available, fast	Poor PET correlation Not quantified Not operationally valid
Xe-CT	7–20ml[a]	CBF <6 ml[a]	Increasingly available Quantitation	Poor validation Technically problematic Anesthetic side effects
MRI DWI/PI	PW/DWI mismatch with: Relative CBV to 137% Relative CBF to 37% Relative ADC to 56% Relative MTT to 165%	Relative CBV to 76% Relative CBF to 11% Relative ADC to 91%	Increasingly available Fast Clinically feasible	Validation retrospective No external validation Not quantitated Oligemia not excluded Reversible DWI include

Notes:
SPECT = single photon emission computed tomography; CBF = cerebral blood flow; PET = positron emission tomography; FMZ = [11]C flumazenil ligand; F-MISO = [18]Fluoromisonidazole ligand; $CMRO_2$ = cerebral metabolic rate of oxygen; OEF = oxygen extraction fraction; CT = computed tomography; Xe-CT = stable xenon CT; MRI = magnetic resonance imaging; DWI = diffusion-weighted imaging; PI = perfusion imaging.
[a] = ml/100 g tissue per minute

and metabolic imaging methods have the advantages of higher spatial resolution and speed, when compared to the other imaging modalities that can assess the ischemic penumbra, and can easily be combined with high resolution anatomic, and arterial imaging in a single imaging session. The rapid and clinically available assessment of mismatch between diffusion-weighted imaging lesion volume, and the often larger perfusion abnormality is a marker of the ischemic penumbra.[12] The diffusion-weighted lesion loosely represents the ischemic core, and the various potential measures of relative or semiquantitative cerebral blood flow mark the disturbance in perfusion of the tissue. Commonly, in the early stroke setting the flow disturbance is contiguous to the diffusion lesion, and the area of mismatch between these two tissue volumes is taken to represent the ischemic penumbra.

Diffusion-weighted MRI (DWI)

DWI is increasingly available in the setting of acute stroke, and for rapid acquisition is performed using echoplanar magnetic resonance imaging methods. This technique is able to detect changes in tissue water motion shortly after a focal ischemic insult as mentioned in an earlier chapter. These changes are thought to reflect intracellular water accumulation (cytotoxic edema) related to high-energy metabolism failure, hence accumulation of osmotically significant byproducts, and loss of ion homeostatic mechanisms.[65] This allows very early and sensitive imaging of the damaged tissue in stroke. There are, however, regions where these DW images are contaminated by significant susceptibility artefacts causing anatomic distortions to the image that are most severe in the posterior fossa, the anterior and inferior temporal lobes, and the paranasal sinuses. In addition, these regions often appear bright due to artefact, making interpretation of similarly bright adjacent areas of tissue damage difficult. The apparent diffusion coefficient (ADC) map is a quantitated measure of water molecule diffusion, and is able to take into account errors in detecting ischemic damage, particularly eliminating any unwanted T_2 signal which may be visible in the DW images (T_2 shine-through effect).

A number of investigators using animal models of cerebral ischemia, have shown close relationships between the tissue with reduced apparent diffusion coefficient, tissue with abnormal pH, ATP, and glucose[66] and tissue that later is found to have histopathological damage.[66,67] There is also an evolution in the ADC during prolonged tissue ischemia that plays a role in tissue outcome.[68] A reduction in ADC values has been demonstrated within minutes of arterial occlusion in animal models. The severity of reduction in ADC tends to increase over the next 24–48 hours, during which time tissue water content begins to increase and is detected on T_2-weighted images.[69] The ADC value will then increase through a phase of 'pseudo-normalization' to the increased levels seen in later cellular necrosis. A pattern of increasing size of the ADC lesion over 24 hours may be due to both cytotoxic edema and to vasogenic edema from as early as 6 hours from stroke onset.[70] There is also a correlation between the ADC value and cerebral blood flow during aterial occlusion.[71] The mean acute relative ADC reduction in a visible DWI lesion is 58% when compared to the contralateral hemisphere. In animal models this should correspond to a CBF of 10–15 ml/100 g per min together with energy failure.[18] It has also been found that ADC abnormalities may be seen at the periphery of a lesion even before ATP energy stores have been fully depleted, which suggests that some of the ADC-detected lesion may be penumbral rather than representing the infarct core.[65] In addition, the reduction of ADC values correlate with the severity of ischemia,[65] and are more profoundly decreased toward the core of the ADC lesion than in the periphery.[72] They become more severe with longer duration of ischemia, are less intense in reversible than in irreversible areas,[73] and after transient arterial occlusion diffusion changes only predict infarction if severely decreased.[74] Kidwell and colleagues also found that the MRI of patients with transient ischemic attacks typically shows less severely reduced ADC values than patients with strokes, even though all ADC values identified were moderate–severely reduced (less than 545 $\mu m^2/s$).[75] Hasegawa and colleagues found that potential ADC thresholds exist that may separate reversible from irreversible abnormalities.[76] A schematic representation of this penumbral component of the diffusion lesion is shown in Fig. 15.4. If the ischemic insult is short lived, even severe ADC reductions are known to be potentially reversible in humans. Doege and colleagues reported six patients with small subcortical grey matter ischemia in whom a large portion of the ADC lesion was reversible, as judged from the lesion size on final T_2 image.[77] Recovery of tissue showing DWI changes has also been reported by others,[78] and was found in nearly half of patients with TIA who initially presented with DWI changes.[75] Ueda and colleagues also found that in the first 72 hours of ischemic stroke the ADC map overestimated the final infarction size by 182%, although this subacute assessment has little bearing on the acute management of stroke.[79] ADC values are continuous rather than simply normal or abnormal, and further research is required to identify more precise thresholds of ADC abnormality that predict the ischemic core and perhaps the penumbra, and how these values interact with the duration of regional ischemia.

Perfusion MRI

The use of MRI to detect cerebral perfusion at the capillary level in acute stroke is an evolving technology, and at present has the best spatial resolution of any imaging technique for this purpose. An injection-free arterial spin labelling technique is in early stages of development and has been discussed in an earlier chapter. The most commonly used technique employs the injection of a paramagnetic contrast agent intravenously that will cause T_2 shortening, and dynamically tracking the signal changes as the contrast passes through the brain. A T_2-weighted echoplanar imaging sequence is best suited as it is fast, and allows serial scans every 1–2 seconds.[80,81] This technique allows generation of time-contrast concentration curves based on the assumption that contrast concentration is proportional to the amount of signal loss in the tissue over the range of concentrations being observed.

Using this approximation of tissue gadolinium concentration in brain tissue, a pixel by pixel analysis of blood flow, blood volume and mean transit time can be determined wherever the signal to noise characteristics are satisfactory. It has been estimated that in an acute stroke, tissue that has a 73% increase in the tissue mean transit time (MTT), and a 29% increase in CBV as compared to the contralateral hemisphere is at risk of infarction.[82] It has also been shown that MTT and CBF brain maps are larger than cerebral blood volume (CBV) maps typically, and that these markers of abnormal blood flow are usually more extensive than the diffusion image abnormality.[83] The pathophysiological responses to obstructed blood supply to a tissue are complex, and the ability to use MRI markers of blood flow disturbance are limited by a lack of absolute quantitation, and hence the severity of abnormality is measured as a relative disturbance as compared to the patient's contralateral (presumed normal) hemisphere. On this basis, a reduction of relative CBF (rCBF) to 37%, and rCBV to 47% have identified at-risk tissue, and a reduction to less than 12% of rCBF, or 19% of rCBV identified the core of tissue infarction.[18] The severity of clinical presentation[84] and later outcome of stroke has been found to correlate with the volume of tissue with abnormal perfusion acutely. In Fig. 15.5 it can be seen how relatively more straightforward, and sensitive it is to measure volumes based on the MTT and 'time-to-peak' (TTP) maps compared with the CBV and CBF maps when assessing the penumbra.

An important issue to consider when using perfusion MRI is that the exact critical penumbral thresholds of hypoperfusion are not reliably identified in any one patient.[85] Contributing to errors in assessment is the difficulty with identifying and deconvolving an arterial input function from the tissue signal, delay and dispersion of the tissue impulse function, limitations to the correlation between gadolinium concentration and the perfusion-weighted signal intensity, anatomic warping and susceptibility artefact using the echoplanar MRI techniques, and abnormalities in perfusion in the patient's contralateral hemisphere due to prior strokes or diaschisis. Attempts to correlate the MRI determined blood flow indices with the more established PET methods are ongoing. Absolute quantitation of CBF for MRI, independent of the PET 'gold standard', and validating the results by operationally defining the tissue compartments have not yet been possible. It is known that vasoregulatory mechanisms are important in compensation for acute reductions in perfusion pressures, and that flow heterogeneity is reduced in ischemic areas, thus increasing the mean capillary concentrations of vital energy and nutrient substances. In humans, there has been some preliminary work to show that areas of prolonged MTT can be further analysed to determine areas where the heterogeneity of MTTs is reduced. This implies a maximal capillary dilatation response to ischemic stress and may identify areas at greater risk of infarction.[86] Similarly, the CBV is initially increased in ischemic stroke.[18] These findings are in agreement with PET evidence of an early compensatory vasodilatory response to reduced perfusion pressures which results in a relatively maintained CBF despite prolongation of MTT.[14,87]

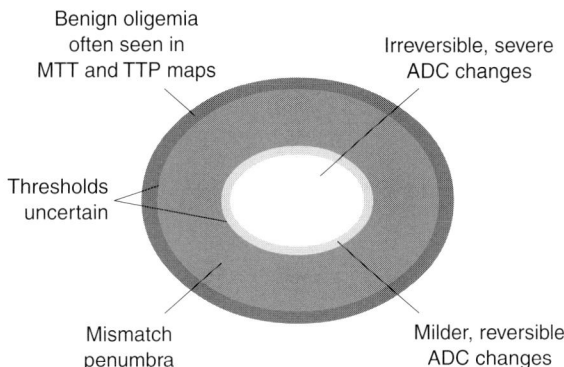

Fig. 15.4. Proposed schematic of the layers that are present within the region of focal cerebral ischemia, as identified using a diffusion/perfusion mismatch in MR imaging in humans. If standard imaging techniques are used these layers are not yet readily identifiable in patients with acute ischemic stroke.

The most sensitive MRI measure of abnormal blood flow, is the 'time-to-peak' (TTP) contrast concentration. This is known to routinely identify tissue that is not at risk of infarction, because it includes tissue that is merely oligemic, rather than truly penumbral in the functional sense. This is represented as benign oligemia in Fig. 15.4, and it can be seen in Fig. 15.5 that the TTP and MTT lesion size is greater than the CBF and CBV lesions. However, even using this sensitive marker the appearance of a mismatch between the usually irreversibly damaged DWI lesion core and a larger surrounding 'time-to-peak' perfusion abnormality has been found to correlate with enlargement of the infarction over time.[88] In addition, spontaneous early reperfusion of the hypoperfused area of mismatch is a clinically favourable finding.[89] It is not yet clear what combinations of CBV, CBF, MTT and ADC abnormalities should be used for each individual patient to correctly define the ischemic penumbra using MRI.

Imaging the ischemic penumbra is hoped to refine the patient selection for the use of thrombolysis in acute stroke. In theory, the physician might look for patterns where significant amounts of penumbral tissue exist, where the ADC values are normal, yet perfusion is significantly reduced. Kidwell and colleagues have recently reported in abstract form their evaluation of perfusion and diffusion MRI for predicting hemorrhagic transformation after intra-arterial rt-PA thrombolysis.[90] They found that mean ADC values of 583 $\mu m^2/s$ (in the typical range for irreversible infarction), and MTT values of 38 were statistically correlated with hemorrhagic transformation, and 746 $\mu m^2/s$ and 25 predicted infarction, whereas 874 $\mu m^2/s$ and 17 were correlated with salvage. Therefore, this describes a model wherein the most sluggish blood supply, and most damaged tissue is that most likely to hemorrhage following thrombolysis, and the least sluggish flow, and least impaired tissue was potentially salvageable. It is of interest to note that ADC values of 746 $\mu m^2/s$ are only mildly abnormal, largely invisible to the eye, and only a little below the 874 $\mu m^2/s$ mean value for tissue that survived. Using serial MRI around intra-arterial thrombolysis they found that of the tissue showing initial DWI changes 41% remained injured at 4 hours after thrombolytic treatment (mean ADC was 624 $\mu m^2/s$), 18% showed early reversal of DWI changes but recurrence at 7 days (mean ADC was 641 $\mu m^2/s$), and 33% showed sustained reversal of the DWI lesion (mean ADC was 677 $\mu m^2/s$).

Magnetic resonance imaging: proton spectroscopy

Proton magnetic resonance spectroscopy

This evolving technique allows the measurement of several brain metabolites, either with single or multiple voxel studies (chemical shift imaging).[91,92] N-acetyl aspartate (NAA) is a putative marker of neuronal viability and reduces with neuronal loss.[93] Hyperacute changes in NAA concentration may even occur within 30–60 minutes of experimental infarction.[94] Lactate, a metabolite that is not usually detectable in brain tissue, is a byproduct of anaerobic metabolism, particularly in ischemia.[95] Data from animal studies are consistent with a CBF threshold of 20 ml/100 g per minute required for the production of lactate, and that this occurs

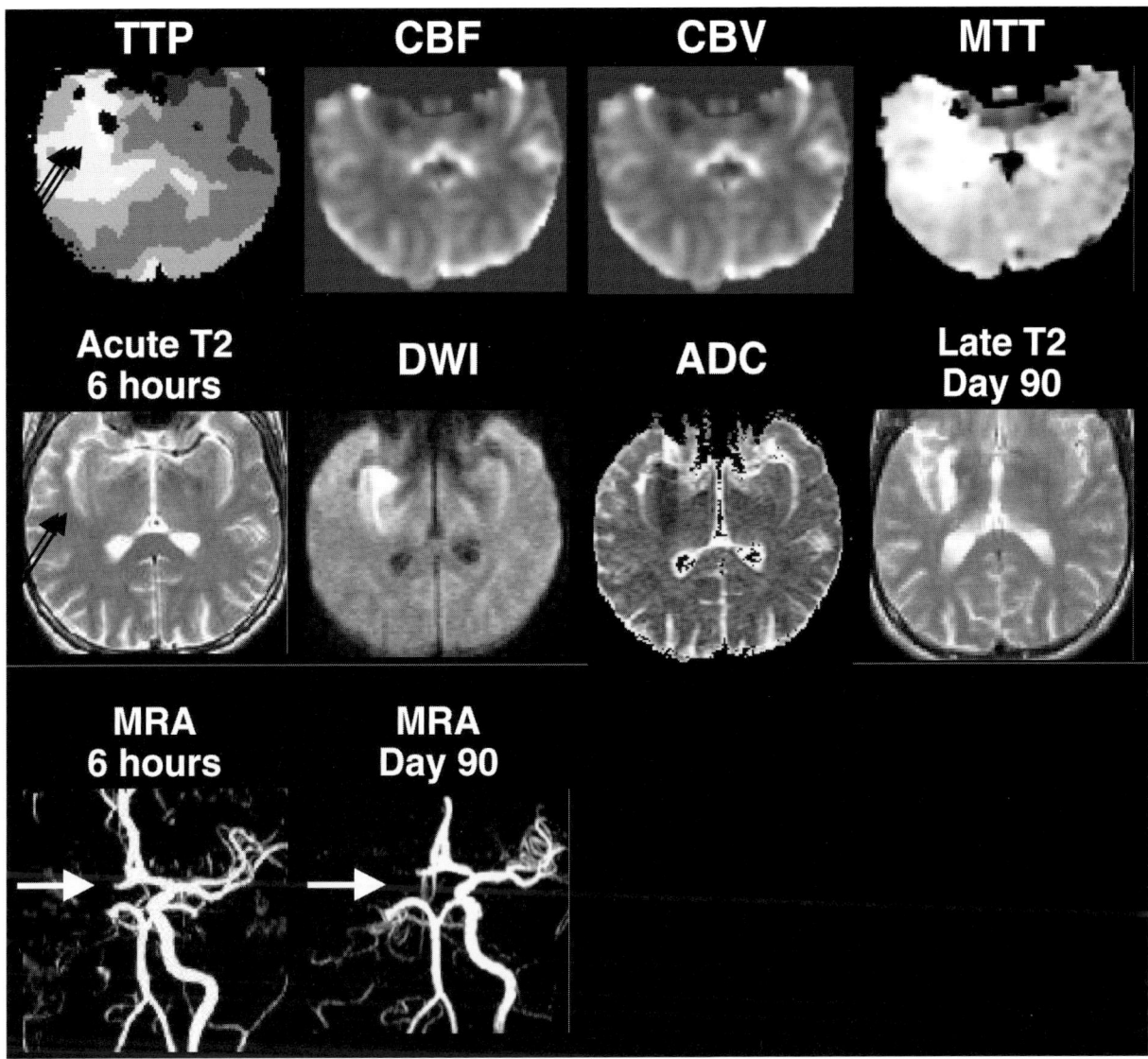

Fig. 15.5. Example from a 36-year-old female with complete absence of flow signal in the right middle cerebral artery (MCA) and internal carotid artery (ICA) occlusion. The mean transit time (MTT), and 'time-to-peak' (TTP) maps show perfusion abnormality that is far more extensive than the apparent diffusion coefficient of water map (ADC) lesion and the final infarct size. Cerebral blood volume (CBV) and cerebral blood flow (CBF), whilst harder to visualize, are intermediate in size. Acute T_2-weighted, diffusion weighted (DWI), and ADC images, with the follow-up T_2 imaging are shown in the second row. Acute and follow-up magnetic resonance angiography (MRA) show absent flow in the right ICA and MCA. White arrows indicate absent middle cerebral arteries. Black arrows indicate relevant ischemic changes.

within minutes of such a compromised state.[96] It has been postulated that lactate elevation may be a marker of the ischemic penumbra in stroke, and in animal studies high levels of lactate have been correlated with worse outcome, and with greater reductions in NAA.[92]

Future directions

The combination of diffusion-weighted imaging and perfusion imaging represent the future of penumbral imaging as it is readily available in most centres and can be applied along with other hemorrhage sensitive sequences as a first line tool in the evaluation of patients with sudden neurological deficits. The addition of proton/phosphorus/sodium multivoxel MR spectroscopy can help with further delineation of the ischemic core and penumbra. However, the prolonged imaging time for multivoxel MR spectroscopy even for a single slice acquisition, substantial postprocessing, and lack of availability makes this tool likely to be limited to research units and not yet applicable for phase II proof of concept studies unless advances in time efficiency occur. Emerging MR imaging techniques in ischemic stroke evaluation is the use of blood oxygen level dependent (BOLD) contrast, which up until now has been used mainly for anatomical localization, neurocognitive research and mechanism of recovery from ischemic stroke.[97] This technique depends on generation of contrast by deoxyhemoglobin, which possesses paramagnetic properties compared to oxyhemoglobin which is diamagnetic. The BOLD technique has been used to differentiate perfused and non-perfused tissues (decreased BOLD signal) during experimental ischemia in cats.[98] Additionally, the use of acetazolamide challenge or breath holding with BOLD techniques can be used to assess vascular reactivity to determine autoregulatory reserve capacity such as in patients with occluded carotid arteries.[90,100] The recent description of quantitative assessment of cerebral blood flow, cerebral blood volume and tissue oxygen extraction suggests some potential for this technique in evaluating regions, together along with diffusion-weighted and perfusion imaging.[101]

REFERENCES

1. Astrup J, Blennov G, Nilsson B. Effects of reduced cerebral blood flow upon EEG pattern, cerebral extracellular potassium, and energy metabolism in the rat cortex during biculline-induced seizures. *Brain Res* 1979; 177: 115–126.
2. Astrup J, Symon L, Branston NM, Lassen NA. Cortical evoked potential and extracellular K$^+$ and H$^+$ at critical levels of brain ischemia. *Stroke* 1977; 8: 51–57.
3. Branston N, Strong A, Symon L. Extracellular potassium activity, evoked potential and tissue blood flow. Relationships during progressive ischemia in baboon cerebral cortex. *J Neurol Sci* 1977; 32: 305–321.
4. Read S, Hirano T, Abbott D et al. The fate of hypoxic tissue on ^{18}F-fluoromisonidazole positron emission tomography after ischemic stroke. *Ann Neurol* 2000; 48: 228–235.
5. Marchal G, Benali K, Iglesias S, Viader F, Derlon JM, Baron JC. Voxel-based mapping of irreversible ischemic damage with PET in acute stroke. *Brain* 1999; 122: 2387–2400.
6. Herderschee D, Limburg M, van Royen EA, Hijdra A, Buller HR, Koster PA. Thrombolysis with recombinant tissue plasminogen activator in acute ischemic stroke: evaluation with rCBF-SPECT. *Acta Neurol Scand* 1991; 83: 317–322.
7. Baird AE, Donnan GA, Austin MC, Fitt GJ, Davis SM, McKay WJ. Reperfusion after thrombolytic therapy in ischemic stroke measured by single-photon emission computed tomography. *Stroke* 1994; 25: 79–85.
8. Ezura M, Takahashi A, Yoshimoto T. Evaluation of regional cerebral blood flow using single photon emission tomography for the selection of patients for local fibrinolytic therapy of acute cerebral embolism. *Neurosurg Rev* 1996; 19: 231–236.
9. Ryu YH, Chung TS, Yoon PH et al. Evaluation of reperfusion and recovery of brain function before and after intracarotid arterial urokinase therapy in acute cerebral infarction with brain SPECT. *Clin Nucl Med* 1999; 24: 566–571.
10. Astrup J, Siesjo BK, Symon L. Thresholds in cerebral ischemia – the ischemic penumbra. *Stroke* 1981; 12: 723–725.
11. Symon L, Branston NM, Strong AJ, Hope TD. The concepts of thresholds of ischemia in relation to brain structure and function. *J Clin Pathol Suppl (R Coll Pathol)* 1977; 11: 149–154.
12. Heiss WD. Ischemic penumbra: evidence from functional imaging in man. *J Cereb Blood Flow Metab* 2000; 20: 1276–1293.
13. Baron JC, Rougemont D, Soussaline F et al. Local interrelationships of cerebral oxygen consumption and glucose utilization in normal subjects and in ischemic stroke patients: a positron tomography study. *J Cereb Blood Flow Metab* 1984; 4: 140–149.
14. Powers WJ, Grubb RL, Jr., Darriet D, Raichle ME. Cerebral blood flow and cerebral metabolic rate of oxygen requirements for cerebral function and viability in humans. *J Cereb Blood Flow Metab* 1985; 5: 600–608.

15 Hakim AM, Evans AC, Berger L et al. The effect of nimodipine on the evolution of human cerebral infarction studied by PET. *J Cereb Blood Flow Metab* 1989; 9: 523–534.

16 Furlan M, Marchal G, Viader F, Derlon JM, Baron JC. Spontaneous neurological recovery after stroke and the fate of the ischemic penumbra. *Ann Neurol* 1996; 40: 216–226.

17 Marchal G, Beaudouin V, Rioux P et al. Prolonged persistence of substantial volumes of potentially viable brain tissue after stroke: a correlative PET–CT study with voxel-based data analysis. *Stroke* 1996; 27: 599–606.

18 Schlaug G, Benfield A, Baird AE et al. The ischemic penumbra: operationally defined by diffusion and perfusion MRI. *Neurology* 1999; 53: 1528–1537.

19 Giubilei F, Lenzi GL, Di Piero V et al. Predictive value of brain perfusion single-photon emission computed tomography in acute ischemic stroke. *Stroke* 1990; 21: 895–900.

20 Shimosegawa E, Hatazawa J, Inugami A et al. Cerebral infarction within six hours of onset: prediction of completed infarction with technetium-99m-HMPAO SPECT. *J Nucl Med* 1994; 35: 1097–1103.

21 Berrouschot J, Barthel H, Hesse S, Koster J, Knapp WH, Schneider D. Differentiation between transient ischemic attack and ischemic stroke within the first six hours after onset of symptoms by using 99mTc-ECD-SPECT. *J Cereb Blood Flow Metab* 1998; 18: 921–929.

22 Hatazawa J, Shimosegawa E, Toyoshima H et al. Cerebral blood volume in acute brain infarction: a combined study with dynamic susceptibility contrast MRI and 99mTc-HMPAO-SPECT. *Stroke* 1999; 30: 800–806.

23 Ueda T, Sakaki S, Yuh WT, Nochide I, Ohta S. Outcome in acute stroke with successful intra-arterial thrombolysis and predictive value of initial single-photon emission-computed tomography. *J Cereb Blood Flow Metab* 1999; 19: 99–108.

24 Firlik AD, Rubin G, Yonas H, Wechsler LR. Relation between cerebral blood flow and neurologic deficit resolution in acute ischemic stroke. *Neurology* 1998; 51: 177–182.

25 Kaufmann AM, Firlik AD, Fukui MB, Wechsler LR, Jungries CA, Yonas H. Ischemic core and penumbra in human stroke. *Stroke* 1999; 30: 93–99.

26 Heiss WD, Rosner G. Functional recovery of cortical neurons as related to degree and duration of ischemia. *Ann Neurol* 1983; 14: 294–301.

27 Morawetz RB, DeGirolami U, Ojemann RG, Marcoux FW, Crowell RM. Cerebral blood flow determined by hydrogen clearance during middle cerebral artery occlusion in unanesthetized monkeys. *Stroke* 1978; 9: 143–149.

28 Jones TH, Morawetz RB, Crowell RM et al. Thresholds of focal cerebral ischemia in awake monkeys. *J Neurosurg* 1981; 54: 773–782.

29 Tyson GW, Teasdale GM, Graham DI, McCulloch J. Focal cerebral ischemia in the rat: topography of hemodynamic and histopathological changes. *Ann Neurol* 1984; 15: 559–567.

30 Strong AJ, Venables GS, Gibson G. The cortical ischemic penumbra associated with occlusion of the middle cerebral artery in the cat: 1. Topography of changes in blood flow, potassium ion activity, and EEG. *J Cereb Blood Flow Metab* 1983; 3: 86–96.

31 Heiss WD, Thiel A, Grond M, Graf R. Which targets are relevant for therapy of acute ischemic stroke? *Stroke* 1999; 30: 1486–1489.

32 Furlan A, Higashida R, Wechsler L et al. Intra-arterial prourokinase for acute ischemic stroke. The PROACT II study: a randomized controlled trial. Prolyse in Acute Cerebral Thromboembolism. *J Am Med Assoc* 1999; 282: 2003–2011.

33 Fisher M, Baron JC. Which targets are relevant for therapy of acute ischemic stroke? *Stroke* 2000; 31: 984–986.

34 Baron J. Mapping the ischemic penumbra with PET: implications for acute stroke treatment. *Cerebrovasc Dis* 1999; 9: 193–201.

35 Darby DG, Barber PA, Gerraty RP et al. Pathophysiological topography of acute ischemia by combined diffusion-weighted and perfusion MRI. *Stroke* 1999; 30: 2043–2052.

36 Jacewicz M, Tanabe J, Pulsinelli WA. The CBF threshold and dynamics for focal cerebral infarction in spontaneously hypertensive rats. *J Cereb Blood Flow Metab* 1992; 12: 359–370.

37 Fisher M, Garcia JH. Evolving stroke and the ischemic penumbra. *Neurology* 1996; 47: 884–888.

38 Takano K, Latour LL, Formato JE et al. The role of spreading depression in focal ischemia evaluated by diffusion mapping. *Ann Neurol* 1996; 39: 308–318.

39 Garcia JH, Liu KF, Yoshida Y, Chen S, Lian J. Brain microvessels: factors altering their patency after the occlusion of a middle cerebral artery (Wistar rat). *Am J Pathol* 1994; 145: 728–740.

40 Abumiya T, Fitridge R, Mazur C et al. Integrin alpha(IIb)beta(3) inhibitor preserves microvascular patency in experimental acute focal cerebral ischemia. *Stroke* 2000; 31: 1402–1409; discussion 1409–1410.

41 Mori E, del Zoppo GJ, Chambers JD, Copeland BR, Arfors KE. Inhibition of polymorphonuclear leukocyte adherence suppresses no-reflow after focal cerebral ischemia in baboons. *Stroke* 1992; 23: 712–718.

42 Sharp FR, Lu A, Tang Y, Millhorn DE. Multiple molecular penumbras after focal cerebral ischemia. *J Cereb Blood Flow Metab* 2000; 20: 1011–1032.

43 Mies G, Ishimaru S, Xie Y, Seo K, Hossmann KA. Ischemic thresholds of cerebral protein synthesis and energy state following middle cerebral artery occlusion in rat. *J Cereb Blood Flow Metab* 1991; 11: 753–761.

44 Mabuchi T, Kitagawa K, Ohtsuki T et al. Contribution of microglia/macrophages to expansion of infarction and response of oligodendrocytes after focal cerebral ischemia in rats. *Stroke* 2000; 31: 1735–1743.

45 Heo JH, Lucero J, Abumiya T, Koziol JA, Copeland BR, del Zoppo GJ. Matrix metalloproteinases increase very early during experimental focal cerebral ischemia. *J Cereb Blood Flow Metab* 1999; 19: 624–633.

46 Zhai QH, Futrell N, Chen FJ. Gene expression of IL-10 in relationship to TNF-alpha, IL-beta and IL-2 in the rat brain following middle cerebral artery occlusion. *J Neurol Sci* 1997; 152: 119–124.

47 Feuerstein GZ, Wang X, Barone FC. Inflammatory gene expression in cerebral ischemia and trauma. Potential new therapeutic targets. *Ann NY Acad Sci* 1997; 825: 179–193.

48 Nedergaard M. Neuronal injury in the infarct border: a neuropathological study in the rat. *Acta Neuropathol* 1987; 73: 267–274.

49 Wang GL, Jiang BH, Rue EA, Semenza GL. Hypoxia-inducible factor 1 is a basic-helix–loop–helix-PAS heterodimer regulated by cellular O_2 tension. *Proc Natl Acad Sci USA* 1995; 92: 5510–5514.

50 Matsushima K, Schmidt-Kastner R, Hogan MJ, Hakim AM. Cortical spreading depression activates trophic factor expression in neurons and astrocytes and protects against subsequent focal brain ischemia. *Brain Res* 1998; 807: 47–60.

51 Baron JC, Bousser MG, Rey A, Guillard A, Comar D, Castaigne P. Reversal of focal 'misery-perfusion syndrome' by extra-intracranial arterial bypass in hemodynamic cerebral ischemia. A case study with ^{15}O positron emission tomography. *Stroke* 1981; 12: 454–459.

52 Heiss WD, Fink GR, Herolz K, Pietrzyk U, Wagner R, Wienhard K. Progressive derangement of periinfarct viable tissue in ischemic stroke. *J Cereb Blood Flow Metab* 1992; 12: 193–203.

53 Touzani O, Yound AR, Derlon JM et al. Sequential studies of severely hypometabolic tissue volumes after permanent middle cerebral artery occlusion. A positron emission tomographic investigation in anesthetized baboons. *Stroke* 1995; 26: 2112–2119.

54 Heiss W, Graf R, Fujita T et al. Early detection of irreversible damaged ischemic tissue by flumazenil positron emission tomography in cats. *Stroke* 1997; 28: 2045–2051; discussion 2051–2052.

55 Heiss W, Grond M, Thiel A et al. Permanent cortical damage detected by flumazenil positron emission tomography in acute stroke. *Stroke* 1998; 29: 454–461.

56 Heiss WD, Kracht LW, Thiel A, Grond M, Pawlik G. Penumbral probability thresholds of cortical flumazenil binding and blood flow predicting tissue outcome in patients with cerebral ischemia. *Brain* 2001; 124: 20–29.

57 Hanson S, Grotta J, Rhoades H et al. Value of single-photon emission-computed tomography in acute stroke therapeutic trials. *Stroke* 1993; 24: 1322–1329.

58 Laloux P, Richelle F, Jamart J, De Coster P, Laterre C. Comparative correlations of HMPAO SPECT indices, neurological score, and stroke subtypes with clinical outcome in acute carotid infarcts. *Stroke* 1995; 26: 816–821.

59 Berrouschot J, Barthel H, von Kummer R, Knapp WH, Hesse S, Schneider D. 99m technetium-ethyl-cysteinate-dimer single-photon emission CT can predict fatal ischemic brain edema. *Stroke* 1998; 29: 2556–2562.

60 Marchal G, Bouvard G, Iglesias S et al. Predictive value of (99m) Tc-HMPAO-SPECT for neurological outcome/recovery at the acute stage of stroke. *Cerebrovasc Dis* 2000; 10: 8–17.

61 Hartmann A. Prolonged disturbances of regional cerebral blood flow in transient ischemic attacks. *Stroke* 1985; 16: 932–939.

62 Hunter GJ, Hamberg LM, Ponzo JA et al. Assessment of cerebral perfusion and arterial anatomy in hyperacute stroke with three-dimensional functional CT: early clinical results. *Am J Neuroradiol* 1998; 19: 29–37.

63 Koenig M, Kraus M, Theek C, Klotz E, Gehlen W, Heuser L. Quantitative assessment of the ischemic brain by means of perfusion-related parameters derived from perfusion CT. *Stroke* 2001; 32: 431–437.

64 Yonas H, Gur D, Claassen D, Wolfson SK, Jr., Moossy J. Stable xenon-enhanced CT measurement of cerebral blood flow in reversible focal ischemia in baboons. *J Neurosurg* 1990; 73: 266–273.

65 Hoehn-Berlage M, Eis M, Back T, Kohno K, Yamashita K. Changes of relaxation times (T1, T2) and apparent diffusion coefficient after permanent middle cerebral artery occlusion in the rat: temporal evolution regional extent, and comparison with histology. *Magn Reson Med* 1995; 34: 824–834.

66 Kucharczyk J, Mintorovitch J, Asgari H, Moseley M. Diffusion/perfusion MR imaging of acute cerebral ischemia. *Magn Reson Med* 1991; 19: 311–315.

67 Back T, Hoehn-Berlage M, Kohno K, Hossmann K. Diffusion nuclear magnetic resonance imaging in experimental stroke. Correlation with cerebral metabolites. *Stroke* 1994; 25: 494–500.

68 Jiang Q, Zhang Z, Chopp M et al. Temporal evolution and spatial distribution of the diffusion constant of water in rat brain after transient middle cerebral artery occlusion. *Neurol Sci* 1993; 120: 123–130.

69 Moseley ME, Cohen Y, Mintorovitch J et al. Early detection of regional cerebral ischemia in cats: comparison of diffusion- and T_2-weighted MRI and spectroscopy. *Magn Reson Med* 1990; 14: 330–346.

70 Loubinoux I, Volk A, Borredon J et al. Spreading of vasogenic edema and cytotoxic edema assessed by quantitative diffusion and T2 magnetic resonance imaging. *Stroke* 1997; 28: 419–426; discussion 426–427.

71 Miyabe M, Mori S, van Zijl PC et al. Correlation of the average water diffusion constant with cerebral blood flow and ischemic damage after transient middle cerebral artery occlusion in cats. *J Cereb Blood Flow Metab* 1996; 16: 881–891.

72 Rother J, de Crespigny AJ, D'Arceuil H, Iwai K, Moseley ME. Recovery of apparent diffusion coefficient after ischemia-induced spreading depression relates to cerebral perfusion gradient. *Stroke* 1996; 27: 980–986; discussion 986–987.

73 Minematsu K, Li L, Sotak C, Davis M, Fisher M. Reversible focal ischemic injury demonstrated by diffusion-weighted magnetic resonance imaging in rats. *Stroke* 1992; 23: 1304–1310.

74 Mintorovitch J, Moseley ME, Chileuitt L, Shimizu H, Cohen Y, Weinstein PR. Comparison of diffusion- and T_2-weighted MRI for the early detection of cerebral ischemia and reperfusion in rats. *Magn Reson Med* 1991; 18: 39–50.

75 Kidwell CS, Alger JR, Di Salle F et al. Diffusion MRI in patients with transient ischemic attacks. *Stroke* 1999; 30: 1174–1180.

76 Hasegawa Y, Fisher M, Latour LL, Dardzinski BJ, Sotak CH. MRI diffusion mapping of reversible and irreversible ischemic injury in focal brain ischemia. *Neurology* 1994; 44: 1484–1490.

77 Doege C, Kerskens C, Romero B et al. MRI of small human stroke shows reversible diffusion changes in subcortical gray matter. *Neuroreport* 2000; 11: 2021–2024.

78 Marks MP, de Crespigny A, Lentz D, Enzmann DR, Albers GW, Moseley ME. Acute and chronic stroke: navigated spin-echo diffusion-weighted MR imaging. *Radiology* 1996; 199: 403–408.

79 Ueda T, Yuh W, Maley J, Quets J, Hahn P, Magnotta V. Outcome of acute ischemic lesions evaluated by diffusion and perfusion MR imaging. *Am J Neuroradiol* 1999; 20: 983–989.

80 Sorensen AG, Buonanno FS, Gonzalez RG et al. Hyperacute stroke: evaluation with combined multi-section diffusion-weighted and hemodynamically weighted echo-planar MR imaging. *Radiology* 1996; 199: 391–402.

81 Warach S, Chien D, Li W, Ronthal M, Edelman RR. Fast magnetic resonance diffusion-weighted imaging of acute human stroke. *Neurology* 1992; 42: 1717–1723.

82 Sorensen A, Gonzalez R, Copen W et al. Quantitation of diffusion/perfusion MRI mismatch in acute human cerebral infarction. *Stroke* 1997; 28: 252.

83 Sorensen AG, Copen WA, Ostergaard L et al. Hyperacute stroke: simultaneous measurement of relative cerebral blood volume, relative cerebral blood flow, and mean tissue transit time. *Radiology* 1999; 210: 519–527.

84 Tong D, Yenari M, Albers G, O'Brien M, Marks M, Moseley M. Correlation of perfusion- and diffusion-weighted MRI with NIHSS score in acute (<6.5 hour) ischemic stroke. *Neurology* 1998; 50: 864–870.

85 Calamante F, Thomas DL, Pell GS, Wiersma J, Turner R. Measuring cerebral blood flow using magnetic resonance imaging techniques. *J Cereb Blood Flow Metab* 1999; 19: 701–735.

86 Ostergaard L, Sorensen AG, Chesler DA et al. Combined diffusion-weighted and perfusion-weighted flow heterogeneity magnetic resonance imaging in acute stroke. *Stroke* 2000; 31: 1097–1103.

87 Baron JC, Frackowiack RS, Herholz K et al. Use of PET methods for measurement of cerebral energy metabolism and hemodynamics in cerebrovascular disease. *J Cereb Blood Flow Metab* 1989; 9: 723–742.

88 Barber P, Darby D, Desmond P et al. Prediction of stroke outcome with echoplanar perfusion and diffusion weighted MRI. *Neurology* 1998; 51: 418–426.

89 Barber P, Davis S, Infeld B et al. Spontaneous reperfusion after ischemic stroke is associated with improved outcome. *Stroke* 1998; 29: 2522–2528.

90 Saver J, Kidwell C, Liebeskind D, Starkman S. (Abstr) Acute ischemic stroke trials. *Stroke* 2001; 32: 275–278.

91 Beauchamp NJ, Jr., Barker PB, Wang PY, van Zijl PC. Imaging of acute cerebral ischemia. *Radiology* 1999; 212: 307–324.

92 Gillard JH, Barker PB, van Zijl PC, Bryan RN, Oppenheimer SM. Proton MR spectroscopy in acute middle cerebral artery stroke. *Am J Neuroradiol* 1996; 17: 873–886.

93 Saunders DE, Howe FA, van den Boogaart A, McLean MA, Griffiths JR, Brown MM. Continuing ischemic damage after acute middle cerebral artery infarction in humans demonstrated by short-echo proton spectroscopy. *Stroke* 1995; 26: 1007–1013.

94 Penrice J, Cady EB, Lorek A et al. Proton magnetic resonance spectroscopy of the brain in normal preterm and term infants, and early changes after perinatal hypoxia-ischemia. *Pediatr Res* 1996; 40: 6–14.

95 Barker PB, Gillard JH, van Zijl PC et al. Acute stroke: evaluation with serial proton MR spectroscopic imaging. *Radiology* 1994; 192: 723–732.

96 Allen K, Busza AL, Crockard HA et al. Acute cerebral ischemia: concurrent changes in cerebral blood flow, energy metabolites, pH, and lactate measured with hydrogen clearance and ^{31}P and ^{1}H nuclear magnetic resonance spectroscopy. III. Changes following ischemia. *J Cereb Blood Flow Metab* 1988; 8: 816–821.

97 Neumann-Haefelin T, Moseley ME, Albers GW. New magnetic resonance imaging methods for cerebrovascular disease: emerging clinical applications. *Ann Neurol* 2000; 47: 559–570.

98 de Crespigny AJ, Wendland MF, Derugin N, Vexler ZS, Moseley ME. Rapid MR imaging of a vascular challenge to focal ischemia in cat brain. *J Magn Reson Imaging* 1993; 3: 475–481.

99 Kleinschmidt A, Steinmetz H, Sitzer M, Merboldt KD, Frahm J. Magnetic resonance imaging of regional cerebral blood oxygenation changes under acetazolamide in carotid occlusive disease. *Stroke* 1995; 26: 106–110.

100 Kastrup A, Li TQ, Glover GH, Moseley ME. Cerebral blood flow-related signal changes during breath-holding. *Am J Neuroradiol* 1999; 20: 1233–1238.

101 van Zijl PC, Eleff SM, Ulatowski JA et al. Quantitative assessment of blood flow, blood volume and blood oxygenation effects in functional magnetic resonance imaging. *Nat Med* 1998; 4: 159–167.

16

New MR techniques to select patients for thrombolysis in acute stroke

Vincent N. Thijs[1], and Gregory W. Albers[2]

[1] Department of Neurology, UZ Gasthuisberg, Leuven, Belgium
[2] Stanford Stroke Center, Stanford University Medical Center, Palo Alto, CA 94304, USA

Introduction

The landmark NINDS IV tPA trial showed that treatment with tPA within 3 hours of symptom onset improved neurologic impairment and functional outcome.[1] Despite an increase in symptomatic hemorrhages from 0.6% in the placebo treated group to 6.4% in the active treatment group, mortality was not increased and functional outcome improved, even among patients with the most severe strokes.[2]

The NINDS trial was subsequently criticized because it subjected some patient groups who were assumed to be unlikely to benefit from thrombolytic agents to a potentially harmful treatment.[3,4] For instance, patients with proximal ICA-occlusions are unlikely to benefit from IV-tPA.[5–7] Similarly, it has been suggested that patients with small, deep infarcts should not receive thrombolytics because of the generally favourable outcome and the presumed different pathological processes underlying small vessel occlusions.[8]

In the NINDS trial, no patient subgroups could be identified that appeared not to benefit from tPA. However, in this trial stroke subtype was established based on clinical impression. Many studies suggest that the identification of stroke subtypes cannot be made reliably on clinical criteria and early CT alone.[9–13]

In the NINDS trial, the only factor that appeared to improve the favourable response to tPA was the time between symptom onset and treatment. In the initial publication of the trial results, the authors reported that the benefit of tPA was not different between the patients treated within 0–90 minutes and the patients treated between 90 and 180 minutes,[1] although no adjustment for differences in baseline stroke severity between the early and late treated patients was performed. A subsequent report by the same investigators found that, after adjustment for baseline stroke severity, favourable outcomes were more frequently observed in the patients who were enrolled earlier and that treatment during the last portion of the 3-hour time window was associated with a confidence interval that crossed,[14] suggesting that the benefit might be reduced during this time period.

In North America, thrombolytic therapy with IV-tPA is currently used in only about 1–6% of all ischemic stroke patients, despite major endorsements from the American Academy of Neurology, the American Heart Association and the Canadian Stroke Consortium.[15–17] The low treatment rate is related to both the perceived risks associated with treatment and the small fraction of eligible patients presenting to the hospital within the 3-hour time window.[18–21] A greater number of patients could be treated with tPA if the time window could be expanded to 6 hours after symptom onset. In recent surveys, about 60% of stroke patients arrived in the emergency department within 6 hours of symptom onset.[22,23]

Trials that have attempted to expand the time window of treatment with IV tPA to five or 6 hours have not been successful.[24–26] Both the PROACT II trial, that compared intra-arterial pro-urokinase with placebo and a recent meta-analysis of all IV thrombolytic stroke trials provided proof of the principle that stroke can be treated up to 6 hours after symptom onset.[27–29] Several explanations have been proposed to account for the failure of some of the individual IV thrombolytic trials beyond 3 hours. ECASS I suffered from protocol violations due to the erroneous inclusion of patients with large regions of early infarction evident on the baseline CT scan, and the trial showed a positive effect if these patients were excluded. If ECASS II had chosen the endpoint of independence (modified Rankin Score 0–2) instead of recovery (modified Rankin 0–1), possibly a more realistic target given the longer time window for inclusion, the trial would have been positive.[25,30] However, despite the promising results of posthoc analyses of ECASS and ECASS II, ATLANTIS did not find a benefit for IV tPA thrombolysis, even when different endpoints were considered.[26]

There are additional theoretical reasons to explain why these trials failed. The presumed target of acute stroke therapy is the ischemic penumbra. Yet, none of the clinical trials of new therapeutic agents has attempted to use the existence or size of the penumbra as a selection criterion for entry. Only CT technology was used to exclude patients with intracerebral hemorrhage or to exclude patients with early extensive cerebral edema. The inclusion of patients without substantial regions of reversible brain injury in trials of new therapeutic agents for stroke may have allowed entry of patients in whom treatment was likely to be futile or even harmful. We believe that the ability of trials to distinguish effective from ineffective therapeutic agents in stroke can be maximized by using techniques to image the ischemic penumbra.[31]

Imaging the ischemic penumbra: the gold standard(s)

A theoretical benefit of imaging in acute stroke is to non-invasively and rapidly identify the presence of tissue that is at risk of infarction but can still be salvaged by an effective therapy. Other goals are to identify the etiology and location of the ischemic lesions and to provide an estimate of the prognosis of these lesions if left untreated. Ideally, imaging may also be able to detect patients in whom treatment is harmful or unnecessary.

The penumbra can be defined as hypoperfused brain tissue that is not yet irreversibly damaged but at risk of infarction. The penumbra can be defined in various ways depending on the modality used to identify it.[32–40]

Biochemically the penumbra can be defined as the area in which protein synthesis is suppressed as a result of hypoperfusion, but ATP depletion, and therefore energy failure, has not yet occurred.[41–46] The penumbra can be identified as existing between two levels of metabolic dysfunction. A lower level exists beyond which ATP depletion and irreversible damage occurs. The higher level distinguishes between hypoperfused tissue without a suppression in protein synthesis which is therefore not at risk of infarction, from tissue that demonstrates suppression of protein synthesis. Animal experiments indicate that with persisting vascular occlusion brain regions beneath the threshold of ATP-depletion gradually expand and within hours equal the size of the regions at the threshold of reduced protein synthesis.[34,42,47] This suggests that tissue salvage can only occur early before this process is complete. Unfortunately, thresholds of ATP depletion and reduced protein synthesis can not be evaluated in humans using currently available technology. Estimations of these regions using PET, SPECT, Xenon CT and diffusion and perfusion MRI, and recently CT-perfusion have been proposed.[37,48–60]

PET with ^{15}O-labelled oxygen and water is the only established method for identifying the ischemic penumbra in humans.[61–65] Using this approach the penumbra can be defined as tissue with a critical flow decrease but preserved oxygen consumption as reflected in a high oxygen extraction fraction or a preserved metabolic rate of oxygen.[66] The studies of Baron and coworkers indicate that tissue fulfilling these requirements is present up to 24 hours after occlusion in the border areas of the ischemic region and that survival of these areas can occur spontaneously or following administration of tPA.[67–70] These quantitative PET measurements require arterial sampling and are cumbersome to obtain.

Recently novel, semiquantitative PET measurements have been proposed to study the penumbra in humans that partially overcome the complexity of quantitative PET measurements. Fluoromisonidazole is a marker of hypoxic yet viable tissue. Read et al. found large areas of increased tracer on FMISO-PET studies up to 43 hours after symptom onset.[71,72] This technique is not suitable as a clinical tool since it requires a delay between tracer injection and imaging of at least 2 hours. No distinction can be made between irreversible and reversible injury. Flumazenil, a tracer that binds to GABA-receptors in grey matter can be used to identify morphologically intact tissue.[73,74] The penumbra can be defined with this technique as the area with a critical flow decrease but with preserved radioactively labelled flumazenil binding.[75] This technique permits imaging of the penumbra within a few hours after symptom onset and does not require arterial sampling which is contraindicated if thrombolysis is given. Heiss et al. estimated the amount of salvageable tissue within the entire volume of hypoperfused tissue using this technique. In patients studied within 12 hours after symptom onset about 50% of the initial ischemic lesion is composed of already irreversibly damaged tissue and therefore represents the ischemic core. A substantial variability was noted: in some patients the core regions measured only 15.5% of the initial ischemic lesion while in others 94% of the ischemic lesion was beyond reversibility. Overall, the penumbra measured about 20% of the hypoperfused lesion volume, ranging from 0.3% to 55.9%.[76] The complex logistics involved in maintaining a PET facility prohibit widespread use of PET imaging in clinical practice.

Diffusion- and perfusion-weighted imaging to study the ischemic penumbra.

Diffusion-weighted imaging can assess the mobility of water protons within the brain parenchyma.[77,78] Extensive animal and human experimental data show that diffusion of water protons is restricted after ischemic stroke.[79–82] This reduction of water movement is probably due to cytotoxic edema associated with energy failure caused by reductions in cerebral blood flow. The apparent diffusion coefficient (ADC) is a quantitative parameter that reflects the degree of mobility of water within the brain parenchyma.

PWI is an evolving MR technology to study cerebral hemodynamics.[82,83] Hemodynamic maps of cerebral blood flow (CBF), cerebral blood volume (CBV) and mean transit time (MTT) or time to bolus peak (TTP) can be created by mathematical analysis of the evolution of the intensity of the T_2^*-weighted gradient or spin echo images after a Gadolinium bolus (Fig. 16.1). The advantages of these perfusion-weighted imaging techniques (PWI) are their high resolution and non-invasive nature compared to positron emission tomography. PWI can easily be combined with other MR techniques like magnetic resonance angiography (MRA) to assess vessel patency and diffusion weighted imaging (DWI) to assess injury to brain parenchyma.[79,84,85] Current controversies regarding PWI include the determination of the most accurate and cost-effective MR method to acquire perfusion images (gradient-echo or spin-echo), the most precise postprocessing method (single value decomposition, maximum likelihood approach, gamma-variate) to determine hemodynamics quantitatively and the most predictive parameters to identify tissue at risk (MTT, CBF or CBV).[86–94]

It has been proposed that a combination of perfusion- and diffusion-weighted MR might be able to identify the ischemic penumbra.[95,96] In this initial hypothesis the lesion identified on the diffusion-weighted imaging was thought to represent the core of the infarct and the component of lesion on the perfusion-weighted image that extends beyond the DWI lesion represents the penumbra.[97] This 'mismatch' hypothesis has been challenged by both animal and human experiments.

DWI and ADC lesions are reversible

Animal ischemia experiments have demonstrated that the lesion identified on diffusion-weighted

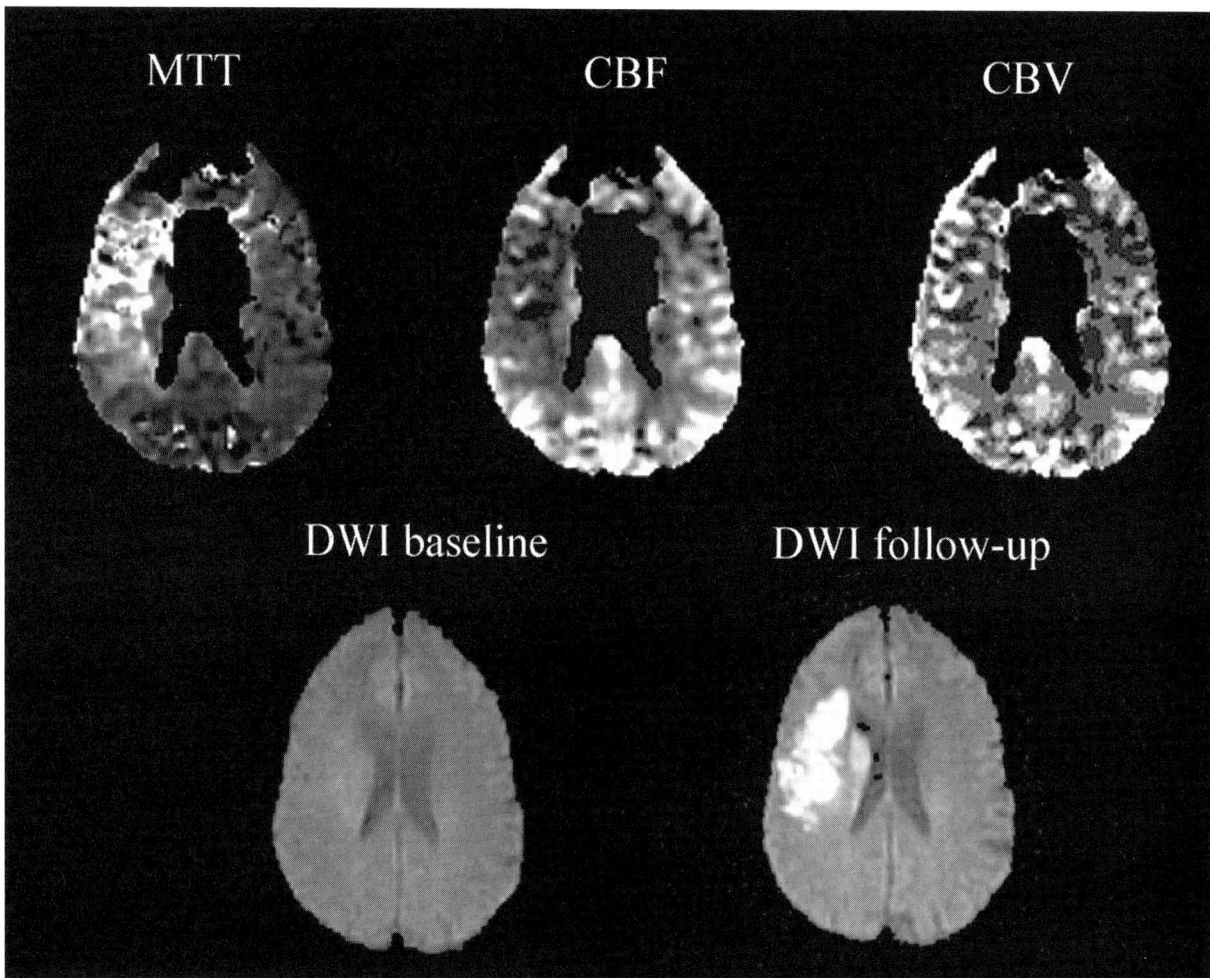

Fig. 16.1. DWI and PWI images from a patient imaged 6.8 hours after symptom onset with a baseline NIHSS of 13. The baseline DWI lesion expands dramatically to almost equal the size of the baseline perfusion deficit.

imaging is larger than the area where ATP depletion has occurred, indicating that only part of the DWI lesion represents the ischemic core.[98–100] Studies using ADC mapping to provide a quantitative estimate of the degree of cytotoxic edema show that lesions with mild ADC usually normalize after reperfusion while lesions with more severe ADC reduction go on to infarction.[101] Interestingly, ADC lesions can disappear entirely after early successful reperfusion but reappear later.[102,103] This delayed re-emergence of ADC lesions together with T_2 and DWI hyperintensities occurs following longer durations of hypoperfusion and is associated with the presence of tissue necrosis on pathological examination. This resolution and re-emergence of DWI lesions is not associated with neurologic improvement followed by worsening.[104]

Permanent reversal of early DWI lesions has also been demonstrated in humans following early reperfusion confirming that early DWI lesions do not represent the ischemic core in stroke patients.[105–109] Kidwell et al. showed the resolution of diffusion lesions among patients with TIAs.[110] The same group demonstrated that after recanalization with intra-arterial (i.a.) t-PA therapy or combined i.v./i.a. t-PA treatment, DWI lesion volumes regressed from baseline to follow-up.[111] In 50% of these patients, this reversal of DWI lesions was temporary with the development of recurrent lesions within one week. This pattern of disappearance and re-emergence of diffusion lesions appears very similar to the animal observations discussed above. Again, this pattern appears not to be associated with early clinical improvement and subsequent neurological deterioration.[112,113]

Although these data suggest that early diffusion lesions do not represent the ischemic core, accurate determination of the core might be achieved by a quantitative analysis of the ADC map together with parameters derived from PWI. Preliminary multi-parametric analyses suggest that very low ADC values represent irreversibly damaged tissue and are also at higher risk of hemorrhagic transformation.[113-115]

Visual analysis of the PWI lesion does not accurately identify tissue at risk of infarction

The goal of hemodynamic imaging is to rapidly and accurately identify the area of hypoperfusion. Within this lesion, tissue at risk of infarction should be distinguished from tissue that is mildly hypoperfused, but not at risk of infarction. This is especially important in the design of clinical trials of new thrombolytic agents as the inclusion of patients who have large areas of hypoperfused tissue that is not at risk of infarction could lead to bias if these patients are overrepresented in either the active treatment or the control group.

Recent evidence indicates that visual analysis of the perfusion lesion volume may substantially overestimate the final infarction volume and critically hypoperfused tissue can be identified by grading the degree of hypoperfusion. Neumann-Haefelin et al. reported that hypoperfused lesions with a time to peak delay (a measure of the degree of hypoperfusion) of more than 6 seconds were at risk of subsequent lesion enlargement in stroke patients studied within 24 hours.[116] Schlaug et al. studied 15 patients within 6 hours after symptom onset and found that tissue that was at risk of infarction had rCBF values < than 37% of the contralateral side and mean transit time (MTT) increases of more than 165% of the contralateral side.[117] We recently reported that mean MTT increases of >4 or >6 seconds identified tissue at risk of infarction in patients studied within 7 hours after symptom onset (Fig. 16.2, see colour plate section).[118]

Therefore, it now appears that the ischemic penumbra can be estimated by using a graded, quantitative analysis of the perfusion lesion and the ADC map. Lesions with early ADC values below a yet to be determined threshold represent the ischemic core. Mild, non-critical hypoperfusion can probably be distinguished from tissue at risk of infarction using a semiquantitative analysis of the hypoperfused tissue volume. Tissue with ADC values above the threshold for the ischemic core and PWI evidence of critical hypoperfusion will correspond to the penumbra (Fig. 16.3).

Factors influencing DWI and PWI lesion evolution

In untreated stroke patients, DWI lesions typically enlarge during the first week after symptom onset.[95,96,119-122] In a randomized placebo-controlled trial of the putative neuroprotective agent citicholine, an MR substudy showed that in untreated patients studied within 24 hours after symptom onset the follow-up lesion volume was 180% the size of the baseline lesion volume, although there was substantial variability.[123] Factors that were associated with more impressive lesion growth were the presence of a large hypoperfusion lesion on PWI, evidence of occlusion on MRA and larger size of the baseline diffusion lesion. Patients studied within 12 hours also had more substantial lesion growth. These findings confirm previous observations using DWI and PWI in acute stroke patients.[92,95,120]

Darby et al. studied the presence of a PWI/DWI mismatch over time and found that a PWI/DWI mismatch was present in 75% of stroke patients scanned within 6 hours of symptom onset, 70% of patients studied at 12 hours and 44% of the patients scanned at 18 hours after symptom onset.[84] The same group studied the evolution of patients who had isolated hypoperfusion lesions (normal DWI) at baseline. Subsequent infarction occurred in 6/11 patients within the PI abnormality. The remaining five showed no later infarction. The volume of the

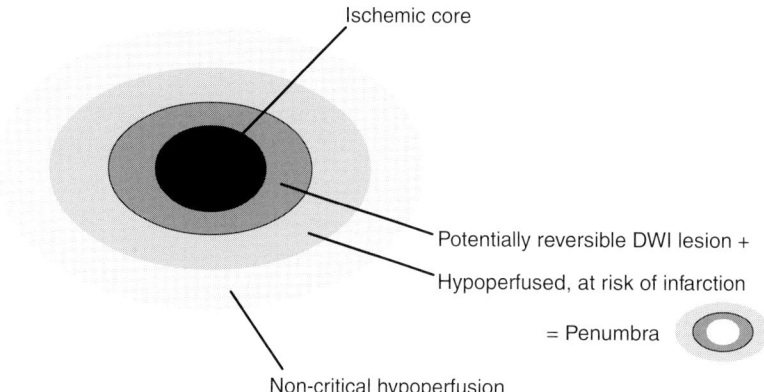

Fig. 16.3. Current concept of the ischemic penumbra as imaged using DWI and PWI. The baseline DWI lesion consists of tissue that is salvageable and tissue that is irreversibly damaged. These compartments can probably be distinguished by quantifying the ADC. Regions with ADC values below $300-350 \times 10^{-6}$ mm^2/s have a low likelihood of recovery. The hypoperfusion lesion contains both tissue at risk of infarction and mild, non-critical hypoperfusion. These compartments can probably be distinguished by quantifying the PWI lesion. For instance, regions with MTT increase of less than 4 seconds appear to be at minimal risk of infarction. The ischemic penumbra consists of both the potentially reversible area of the early diffusion lesion and tissue with critical levels of hypoperfusion identified within the entire baseline hypoperfusion lesion (pale area).

PWI lesion did not predict recovery. The degree of the hypoperfusion deficit at baseline was not studied. It is unclear if these patients had mild, non-critical hypoperfusion or if spontaneous early reperfusion prevented the development of infarction.[124]

Karonen performed serial studies in 49 stroke patients. Imaging was performed during the first day after symptom onset, at day 2 and at 1 week. Eighty per cent of the patients had a PWI/DWI mismatch at baseline. The mismatch volumes correlated significantly with the presence of lesion growth between day 1 and day 2 and day 1 and 1 week on diffusion-weighted imaging.[122]

The presence of a PWI/DWI mismatch is associated with the presence of a major vessel occlusion, although exceptions occur. Rordorf et al. studied 17 patients within 12 hours after symptom onset and found a PWI/DWI mismatch in 9/10 patients with M1-occlusion. Six out of seven patients without M1-occlusion did not have a PWI/DWI mismatch.[125] Barber et al. found MRA-identified vessel occlusion in 9 of 14 patients studied within 24 hours after symptom onset with a PWI/DWI mismatch. None of the patients without a mismatch had major vessel occlusion.[126] The absence of an MRA identified vessel occlusion in patients with a PWI/DWI mismatch might be related to the insensitivity of MRA to identify cortical branch vessel occlusion or to the existence of a no reflow phenomenon following recanalization or to the latency for PWI lesions to disappear following spontaneous or treatment induced reperfusion.[127] Diffusion lesions have been shown to exhibit substantially more growth in patients with a major vessel occlusion compared to patients without a vessel occlusion. These observations support the hypothesis that patients with occluded vessels still have more tissue at risk of infarction compared to patients who have likely experienced spontaneous reperfusion.[125,126]

Monitoring thrombolysis using DWI and PWI

The rationale of thrombolysis in acute stroke is to open occluded vessels and therefore provide beneficial reperfusion. Both the NINDS trial and the PROACT trials suggest that reperfusion is the most promising strategy for acute stroke therapy to date, as none of the putative neuroprotective agents have yet proven beneficial in acute stroke patients.[128–130] The frequency of finding occluded vessels within

6 hours of stroke onset is high. When examined by angiography within 6 hours of acute onset, approximately 10–20% of patients do not show a major vessel occlusion.[5,27,131–133] Most patients with moderate to severe stroke who are enrolled in acute intervention trials have either an M1 occlusion (30% of patients), or an M2 occlusion (25% of patients). The remaining patients have either a carotid 'T' occlusion (10%), a proximal occlusion or severe stenosis of the internal carotid artery or a vertebrobasilar occlusion (5–10%).[7,132]

Only a few serial DWI and PWI studies have compared the lesion evolution of patients who had evidence of early reperfusion (either spontaneous or with thrombolytic therapy) with patients without reperfusion. Compared to patients with other PWI/DWI profiles, patients with a PWI/DWI mismatch are thought to be the ideal candidates for thrombolysis as they are the most likely to have salvageable brain tissue.

Barber et al. studied 28 untreated patients with MCA territory stroke within 12 hours of stroke onset. Major spontaneous reperfusion defined as a >90% reduction in PWI lesion by day 3 occurred in 45% of patients and was associated with better clinical outcome and smaller final infarct size. In patients with major reperfusion the expansion of the baseline DWI lesion was reduced by 67%.[134]

We recently studied 21 patients within 7 hours after symptom onset with serial diffusion and perfusion-weighted MR. All 21 patients had a measurable DWI lesion on the initial scan compared to only 10% who had a visible lesion on the initial FLAIR image. Abnormal regions of marked delay in contrast arrival times (PWI lesions) were seen on time-to-peak maps in 16/18 patients. DWI lesion volumes grew substantially during the first week, reaching a mean of 320% at 5–7 days. Lesion volumes typically decreased between the 5–7-day scan and the 30-day scan, however, the final infarct size was nearly twice as large as the early DWI lesion. Patients with DWI/PWI mismatch experienced larger increases in early DWI lesion growth than patients without this pattern. In patients without a mismatch, the average lesion growth between baseline and 30-day follow-up was 120%, compared to 250% in patients with a PWI/DWI mismatch. Early resolution of PWI abnormalities occurred frequently in patients treated with IV t-PA and may be a predictor of a favourable clinical response and a reduction in the expansion of the early DWI lesion. The initial MRI scan (typically performed about 2 hours after the initiation of t-PA therapy) revealed a PWI lesion that was smaller than the initial DWI lesion in 5/6 t-PA-treated patients. In contrast, this pattern was only seen in one of the six non-t-PA-treated patients. This suggests that most of the t-PA-treated patients had already begun to experience reperfusion before the first MRI scan was obtained. Furthermore, 83% of the t-PA-treated patients showed a substantial decrease in PWI volume between baseline and the first repeat MR scan whereas none of the non-t-PA patients showed this degree of improvement.[120,135,136]

Schellinger and Jansen studied 24 patients treated with t-PA within 6 hours after onset. Most (66%) were scanned prior to t-PA treatment and others were scanned during or immediately after tPA infusion. Vessel occlusion was present in 20/24 patients and in 11/20 recanalization occurred. Nineteen of 20 patients with vessel occlusions had a PWI/DWI mismatch. In patients with early recanalization, functional and radiological outcomes were significantly better than in patients who did not have recanalization. Patients with a PWI/DWI mismatch who had early reperfusion had significantly greater improvements in NIH Stroke Scale scores and smaller final lesion volumes than patients who had a PWI/DWI mismatch but in whom no reperfusion occurred.[137,138]

Parsons et al. recently described 14 patients in whom DWI and PWI were performed within 3 hours after symptom onset. Eighty per cent of patients with a PWI/DWI mismatch who were treated with t-PA had no significant expansion of the early DWI lesion, whereas all untreated patients with a mismatch had final infarcts that were considerably larger than the early DWI lesions.[139]

These small, non-randomized studies suggest that DWI and PWI could be used to monitor thrombolytic therapy and indicate that specific MR patterns can be identified among patients who are likely to respond favorably to thrombolytic therapy.

Use of DWI and PWI as surrogate markers in acute stroke trials

In animal stroke models, primary evidence of the efficacy of therapeutic intervention is established by a reduction in ischemic lesion volume compared to non-treated animals. A surrogate end point in a clinical trial is a laboratory measurement that is used as a substitute for a clinically meaningful endpoint.[140] Changes induced by a therapy on a surrogate endpoint are expected to reflect changes in the clinically meaningful endpoint. To be used as an endpoint, the surrogate marker should be tightly linked to the outcome characteristic. Several studies using DWI and PWI in humans have reported moderate correlations between the volume of the early DWI and PWI lesion and functional outcome scales like the Barthel index.[120,141–145] We reported that, along with the NIHSS and patient age, DWI lesion volume was an independent prognostic marker.[146] The modest correlations between lesion volume on DWI and functional outcome scales can probably be attributed to both the numerous additional factors that influence functional outcome and the relative inadequacy of stroke outcome scales. In addition, lesions of similar volume in different brain regions are likely to have variable influences on functional outcome. Most of the available data support the idea that DWI lesion volumes could be used as a surrogate marker for functional outcome.

Although we do not advocate to rely solely on measurements of lesion volumes in phase III trials, we believe there is a role for DWI and PWI in the selection and development of new therapeutic agents in phase II trials. This technology can dramatically reduce the sample size necessary to show meaningful effects by using the patient as his own control. We calculated that to demonstrate the effect of a drug that is able to reduce lesion expansion by 25% between day 1 and day 3, a sample size of only 80 patients per treatment group would be necessary.[147]

In evaluating the effects of thrombolytic agents, the use of DWI, PWI and MRA can provide accurate, non-invasive measurements of the rates of reperfusion achieved. Finally, an objective analysis of lesion volumes early after stroke onset is not affected by factors that can influence functional outcome, such as social circumstances or the quality of rehabilitative treatment. These factors are very difficult to control in small samples and can bias the results of a small trial. An objective measurement, such as a reduction in the early growth of the ischemic lesion size, could demonstrate a proof of the principle on which the experimental treatment was based.[128,130,148]

Future prospects

We have designed a clinical trial that will test the hypothesis that stroke patients with a PWI/DWI mismatch and early successful recanalization have a more favourable clinical and radiological response to tPA than patients without these features in patients treated with i.v. t-PA within 3 to 6 hours after symptom onset. This non-randomized, prospective multicentre study of 80 patients will provide the necessary pilot data to plan a placebo controlled randomized trial using MRI selection criteria to include patients most likely to respond favourably to tPA.

If the primary hypothesis of this study is correct, a future placebo-controlled efficacy trial will be designed to include only patients who have evidence of an ischemic penumbra of significant size based on PWI/DWI parameters. The pilot trial will provide accurate sample size calculations and address safety issues (e.g. exclusion of patients with DWI lesions above a certain size to exclude hemorrhage or herniation). It is possible that MRI profiles, other than a PWI/DWI mismatch, will predict a favourable clinical response to t-PA. In addition, certain MRI or MRA profiles (perhaps an extremely large baseline PWI lesion or proximal or distal carotid occlusions) might be associated with a very low rate of early reperfusion and an unfavourable clinical response. In addition, contrary to our hypothesis, this pilot study might demonstrate that MRA findings are equally or more predictive of the clinical response to t-PA than DWI/PWI profiles. If this is the case, then it may be justified to base the inclusion/exclusion criteria for the future efficacy trial on MRA or MRA plus DWI criteria, eliminating the requirement for PWI studies in a future trial.

In conclusion, we suspect that DWI and PWI will revolutionize clinical trial design in acute stroke and will be shown to provide an accurate and non-invasive approximation of the ischemic penumbra.

ACKNOWLEDGEMENTS

This study was supported in part by National Institutes of Health grants NS-34088–03, NS35959, NS-39324–01.

REFERENCES

1. The National Institute of Neurological Disorders and Stroke rt-PA Stroke Study Group. Tissue plasminogen activator for acute ischemic stroke. *N Engl J Med* 1995; 333: 1581–1587.
2. Subgroup analysis of the NINDS t-PA Stroke Trial. Generalized efficacy of t-PA for acute stroke. *Stroke* 1997; 28: 2119–2125.
3. Caplan LR, Mohr JP, Kistler JP, Koroshetz W. Should thrombolytic therapy be the first-line treatment for acute ischemic stroke? Thrombolysis–not a panacea for ischemic stroke. *N Engl J Med* 1997; 337: 1309–1310; discussion: 1313.
4. Committee of the ASITN E. Intraarterial thrombolysis: ready for prime time? *Am J Neuroradiol* 2001; 22: 55–58.
5. del Zoppo GJ, Poeck K, Pessin MS et al. Recombinant tissue plasminogen activator in acute thrombotic and embolic stroke. *Ann Neurol* 1992; 32: 78–86.
6. Zeumer H, Freitag HJ, Zanella F, Thie A, Arning C. Local intra-arterial fibrinolytic therapy in patients with stroke: urokinase versus recombinant tissue plasminogen activator (r-TPA). *Neuroradiology* 1993; 35: 159–162.
7. Gonner F, Remonda L, Mattle H et al. Local intra-arterial thrombolysis in acute ischemic stroke. *Stroke* 1998; 29: 1894–1900.
8. Rudolf J, Neveling M, Grond M, Schmulling S, Stenzel C, Heiss WD. Stroke following internal carotid artery occlusion – a contra-indication for intravenous thrombolysis? *Eur J Neurol* 1999; 6: 51–55.
9. Albers GW, Lansberg MG, Norbash AM et al. Yield of diffusion-weighted MRI for detection of potentially relevant findings in stroke patients. *Neurology* 2000; 54: 1562–1567.
10. Toni D, Fiorelli M, De Michele M et al. Clinical and prognostic correlates of stroke subtype misdiagnosis within 12 hours from onset. *Stroke* 1995; 26: 1837–1840.
11. Toni D, Del Duca R, Fiorelli M et al. Pure motor hemiparesis and sensorimotor stroke. Accuracy of very early clinical diagnosis of lacunar strokes. *Stroke* 1994; 25: 92–96.
12. Madden KP, Karanjia PN, Adams HP, Clarke WR. Accuracy of initial stroke subtype diagnosis in the TOAST study. Trial of ORG 10172 in Acute Stroke Treatment. *Neurology* 1995; 45: 1975–1979.
13. Toni D, Iweins F, von Kummer R et al. Identification of lacunar infarcts before thrombolysis in the ECASS I study. *Neurology* 2000; 54: 684–688.
14. Marler JR, Tilley BC, Lu M et al. Early stroke treatment associated with better outcome: the NINDS rt-PA stroke study. *Neurology* 2000; 55: 1649–1655.
15. Report of the Quality Standards Subcommittee of the American Academy of Neurology. Practice advisory: thrombolytic therapy for acute ischemic stroke – summary statement. *Neurology* 1996; 47: 835–839.
16. Adams HP, Brott TG, Furlan AJ et al. Guidelines for Thrombolytic Therapy for Acute Stroke: a Supplement to the Guidelines for the Management of Patients with Acute Ischemic Stroke. A statement for healthcare professionals from a Special Writing Group of the Stroke Council, American Heart Association. *Stroke* 1996; 27: 1711–1718.
17. Norris JW, Buchan A, Cote R et al. Canadian guidelines for intravenous thrombolytic treatment in acute stroke. A consensus statement of the Canadian Stroke Consortium. *Can J Neurol Sci* 1998; 25: 257–259.
18. Chapman KM, Woolfenden AR, Graeb D et al. Intravenous tissue plasminogen activator for acute ischemic stroke : a Canadian Hospital's experience. *Stroke* 2000; 31: 2920–2924.
19. Wang DZ, Rose JA, Honings DS, Garwacki DJ, Milbrandt JC. Treating acute stroke patients with intravenous tPA. The OSF stroke network experience. *Stroke* 2000; 31: 77–81.
20. Chiu D, Krieger D, Villar-Cordova C et al. Intravenous tissue plasminogen activator for acute ischemic stroke: feasibility, safety, and efficacy in the first year of clinical practice. *Stroke* 1998; 29: 18–22.

21 Siu YC, Wong TW, Lau CC. Candidates for thrombolytic treatment in acute ischaemic stroke – where are our patients in Hong Kong? *J Accid Emerg Med* 1999; 16: 412–417.

22 Lacy CR, Suh DC, Bueno M, Kostis JB. Delay in presentation and evaluation for acute stroke : stroke time registry for outcomes knowledge and epidemiology (S.T.R.O.K.E.). *Stroke* 2001; 32: 63–69.

23 Morris DL, Rosamond WD, Hinn AR, Gorton RA. Time delays in accessing stroke care in the emergency department. *Acad Emerg Med* 1999; 6: 218–223.

24 Hacke W, Kaste M, Fieschi C et al. Intravenous thrombolysis with recombinant tissue plasminogen activator for acute hemispheric stroke. The European Cooperative Acute Stroke Study (ECASS). *J Am Med Assoc* 1995; 274: 1017–1025.

25 Hacke W, Kaste M, Fieschi C et al. Randomised double-blind placebo-controlled trial of thrombolytic therapy with intravenous alteplase in acute ischaemic stroke (ECASS II). Second European-Australasian Acute Stroke Study Investigators. *Lancet* 1998; 352: 1245–1251.

26 Clark WM, Wissman S, Albers GW, Jhamandas JH, Madden KP, Hamilton S. Recombinant tissue-type plasminogen activator (Alteplase) for ischemic stroke 3 to 5 hours after symptom onset. The ATLANTIS Study: a randomized controlled trial. Alteplase Thrombolysis for Acute Noninterventional Therapy in Ischemic Stroke. *J Am Med Assoc* 1999; 282: 2019–2026.

27 del Zoppo GJ, Higashida RT, Furlan AJ, Pessin MS, Rowley HA, Gent M. PROACT: a phase II randomized trial of recombinant pro-urokinase by direct arterial delivery in acute middle cerebral artery stroke. PROACT Investigators. Prolyse in Acute Cerebral Thromboembolism. *Stroke* 1998; 29: 4–11.

28 Furlan A, Higashida R, Wechsler L et al. Intra-arterial prourokinase for acute ischemic stroke. The PROACT II study: a randomized controlled trial. Prolyse in Acute Cerebral Thromboembolism. *J Am Med Assoc* 1999; 282: 2003–2011.

29 Wardlaw JM, del Zoppo G, Yamaguchi T. Thrombolysis for acute ischaemic stroke. *Cochrane Database Syst Rev* 2000; 2.

30 Sulter G, Steen C, De Keyser J. Use of the Barthel index and modified Rankin scale in acute stroke trials. *Stroke* 1999; 30: 1538–1541.

31 Albers GW. Expanding the window for thrombolytic therapy in acute stroke. The potential role of acute MRI for patient selection. *Stroke* 1999; 30: 2230–2233.

32 Astrup J, Siesjo BK, Symon L. Thresholds in cerebral ischemia – the ischemic penumbra. *Stroke* 1981; 12: 723–725.

33 Hakim AM. The cerebral ischemic penumbra. *Can J Neurol Sci* 1987; 14: 557–559.

34 Hossmann KA. Viability thresholds and the penumbra of focal ischemia. *Ann Neurol* 1994; 36: 557–565.

35 Heiss WD, Graf R. The ischemic penumbra. *Curr Opin Neurol* 1994; 7: 11–19.

36 Hakim AM. Ischemic penumbra: the therapeutic window. *Neurology* 1998; 51: S44–S46.

37 Heiss WD. Ischemic penumbra: evidence from functional imaging in man. *J Cereb Blood Flow Metab* 2000; 20: 1276–1293.

38 Fisher M, Garcia JH. Evolving stroke and the ischemic penumbra. *Neurology* 1996; 47: 884–888.

39 Sharp FR, Lu A, Tang Y, Millhorn DE. Multiple molecular penumbras after focal cerebral ischemia. *J Cereb Blood Flow Metab* 2000; 20: 1011–1032.

40 Touzani O, Roussel S, MacKenzie ET. The ischaemic penumbra. *Curr Opin Neurol* 2001; 14: 83–88.

41 Xie Y, Mies G, Hossmann KA. Ischemic threshold of brain protein synthesis after unilateral carotid artery occlusion in gerbils. *Stroke* 1989; 20: 620–626.

42 Mies G, Ishimaru S, Xie Y, Seo K, Hossmann KA. Ischemic thresholds of cerebral protein synthesis and energy state following middle cerebral artery occlusion in rat. *J Cereb Blood Flow Metab* 1991; 11: 753–761.

43 Paschen W, Mies G, Hossmann KA. Threshold relationship between cerebral blood flow, glucose utilization, and energy metabolites during development of stroke in gerbils. *Exp Neurol* 1992; 117: 325–333.

44 Naritomi H, Sasaki M, Kanashiro M, Kitani M, Sawada T. Flow thresholds for cerebral energy disturbance and Na$^+$ pump failure as studied by in vivo ^{31}P and ^{23}Na nuclear magnetic resonance spectroscopy. *J Cereb Blood Flow Metab* 1988; 8: 16–23.

45 Hata R, Maeda K, Hermann D, Mies G, Hossmann KA. Dynamics of regional brain metabolism and gene expression after middle cerebral artery occlusion in mice. *J Cereb Blood Flow Metab* 2000; 20: 306–315.

46 Hata R, Maeda K, Hermann D, Mies G, Hossmann KA. Evolution of brain infarction after transient focal cerebral ischemia in mice. *J Cereb Blood Flow Metab* 2000; 20: 937–946.

47 Hossmann KA. The hypoxic brain. Insights from ischemia research. *Adv Exp Med Biol* 1999; 474: 155–169.

48 Hanson SK, Grotta JC, Rhoades H et al. Value of single-photon emission-computed tomography in acute stroke therapeutic trials. *Stroke* 1993; 24: 1322–1329.

49 Umemura A, Suzuka T, Yamada K. Quantitative measurement of cerebral blood flow by (99m)Tc-HMPAO SPECT in acute ischaemic stroke: usefulness in determining therapeutic options. *J Neurol Neurosurg Psychiatry* 2000; 69: 472–478.

50 Shimosegawa E, Hatazawa J, Inugami A et al. Cerebral infarction within six hours of onset: prediction of completed infarction with technetium-99m-HMPAO SPECT. *J Nucl Med* 1994; 35: 1097–1103.

51 Hughes RL, Yonas H, Gur D, Latchaw R. Cerebral blood flow determination within the first 8 hours of cerebral infarction using stable xenon-enhanced computed tomography. *Stroke* 1989; 20: 754–760.

52 Firlik AD, Rubin G, Yonas H, Wechsler LR. Relation between cerebral blood flow and neurologic deficit resolution in acute ischemic stroke. *Neurology* 1998; 51: 177–182.

53 Kaufmann AM, Firlik AD, Fukui MB, Wechsler LR, Jungries CA, Yonas H. Ischemic core and penumbra in human stroke. *Stroke* 1999; 30: 93–99.

54 Rubin G, Firlik AD, Levy EI, Pindzola RR, Yonas H. Relationship between cerebral blood flow and clinical outcome in acute stroke. *Cerebrovasc Dis* 2000; 10: 298–306.

55 Axel L. Cerebral blood flow determination by rapid-sequence computed tomography: theoretical analysis. *Radiology* 1980; 137: 679–686.

56 Rother J, Guckel F, Neff W, Schwartz A, Hennerici M. Assessment of regional cerebral blood volume in acute human stroke by use of single-slice dynamic susceptibility contrast-enhanced magnetic resonance imaging. *Stroke* 1996; 27: 1088–1093.

57 Koenig M, Klotz E, Luka B, Venderink DJ, Spittler JF, Heuser L. Perfusion CT of the brain: diagnostic approach for early detection of ischemic stroke. *Radiology* 1998; 209: 85–93.

58 Hunter GJ, Hamberg LM, Ponzo JA et al. Assessment of cerebral perfusion and arterial anatomy in hyperacute stroke with three-dimensional functional CT: early clinical results. *Am J Neuroradiol* 1998; 19: 29–37.

59 Aksoy FG, Lev MH. Dynamic contrast-enhanced brain perfusion imaging: technique and clinical applications. *Semin Ultrasound CT MR* 2000; 21: 462–477.

60 Koenig M, Kraus M, Theek C, Klotz E, Gehlen W, Heuser L. Quantitative assessment of the ischemic brain by means of perfusion-related parameters derived from perfusion CT. *Stroke* 2001; 32: 431–437.

61 Ackerman RH, Correia JA, Alpert NM et al. Positron imaging in ischemic stroke disease using compounds labeled with oxygen 15. Initial results of clinicophysiologic correlations. *Arch Neurol* 1981; 38: 537–543.

62 Lenzi GL, Frackowiak RS, Jones T. Cerebral oxygen metabolism and blood flow in human cerebral ischemic infarction. *J Cereb Blood Flow Metab* 1982; 2: 321–335.

63 Frackowiak RS, Lenzi GL, Jones T, Heather JD. Quantitative measurement of regional cerebral blood flow and oxygen metabolism in man using ^{15}O and positron emission tomography: theory, procedure, and normal values. *J Comput Assist Tomogr* 1980; 4: 727–736.

64 Wise RJ, Bernardi S, Frackowiak RS, Jones T, Legg NJ, Lenzi GL. Measurement of regional cerebral blood flow, oxygen extraction ratio and oxygen utilization in stroke patients using positron emission tomography. *Exp Brain Res* 1982; 182–186.

65 Hakim AM, Pokrupa RP, Villanueva J et al. The effect of spontaneous reperfusion on metabolic function in early human cerebral infarcts. *Ann Neurol* 1987; 21: 279–289.

66 Heiss WD, Graf R, Wienhard K et al. Dynamic penumbra demonstrated by sequential multi-tracer PET after middle cerebral artery occlusion in cats. *J Cereb Blood Flow Metab* 1994; 14: 892–902.

67 Marchal G, Beaudouin V, Rioux P et al. Prolonged persistence of substantial volumes of potentially viable brain tissue after stroke: a correlative PET-CT study with voxel-based data analysis. *Stroke* 1996; 27: 599–606.

68 Marchal G, Rioux P, Serrati C et al. Value of acute-stage positron emission tomography in predicting neurological outcome after ischemic stroke: further assessment. *Stroke* 1995; 26: 524–525.

69 Marchal G, Benali K, Iglesias S, Viader F, Derlon JM, Baron JC. Voxel-based mapping of irreversible ischaemic damage with PET in acute stroke. *Brain* 1999; 122: 2387–2400.

70 Furlan M, Marchal G, Viader F, Derlon JM, Baron JC. Spontaneous neurological recovery after stroke and the fate of the ischemic penumbra. *Ann Neurol* 1996; 40: 216–226.

71 Read SJ, Hirano T, Abbott DF et al. Identifying hypoxic tissue after acute ischemic stroke using PET and ^{18}F-fluoromisonidazole. *Neurology* 1998; 51: 1617–1621.

72 Read SJ, Hirano T, Abbott DF et al. The fate of hypoxic tissue on ^{18}F-fluoromisonidazole positron emission tomography after ischemic stroke. *Ann Neurol* 2000; 48: 228–235.

73 Sette G, Baron JC, Young AR et al. In vivo mapping of brain benzodiazepine receptor changes by positron emission tomography after focal ischemia in the anesthetized baboon. *Stroke* 1993; 24: 2046–2057; discussion 2057–2058.

74 Heiss WD, Graf R, Fujita T et al. Early detection of irreversibly damaged ischemic tissue by flumazenil positron emission tomography in cats. *Stroke* 1997; 28: 2045–2051; discussion 2051–2052.

75 Heiss WD, Kracht L, Grond M et al. Early [(11)C]Flumazenil/H(2)O positron emission tomography predicts irreversible ischemic cortical damage in stroke patients receiving acute thrombolytic therapy. *Stroke* 2000; 31: 366–369.

76 Heiss WD, Kracht LW, Thiel A, Grond M, Pawlik G. Penumbral probability thresholds of cortical flumazenil binding and blood flow predicting tissue outcome in patients with cerebral ischaemia. *Brain* 2001; 124: 20–29.

77 Le Bihan D, Breton E, Lallemand D, Grenier P, Cabanis E, Laval-Jeantet M. MR imaging of intravoxel incoherent motions: application to diffusion and perfusion in neurologic disorders. *Radiology* 1986; 161: 401–407.

78 Le Bihan D. Molecular diffusion, tissue microdynamics and microstructure. *NMR Biomed* 1995; 8: 375–386.

79 Moseley ME, Cohen Y, Mintorovitch J et al. Early detection of regional cerebral ischemia in cats: comparison of diffusion- and T_2-weighted MRI and spectroscopy. *Magn Reson Med* 1990; 14: 330–346.

80 Moseley ME, de Crespigny AJ, Roberts TP, Kozniewska E, Kucharczyk J. Early detection of regional cerebral ischemia using high-speed MRI. *Stroke* 1993; 24: 160–165.

81 Warach S, Chien D, Li W, Ronthal M, Edelman RR. Fast magnetic resonance diffusion-weighted imaging of acute human stroke. *Neurology* 1992; 42: 1717–1723.

82 Baird AE, Warach S. Magnetic resonance imaging of acute stroke. *J Cereb Blood Flow Metab* 1998; 18: 583–609.

83 Calamante F, Thomas DL, Pell GS, Wiersma J, Turner R. Measuring cerebral blood flow using magnetic resonance imaging techniques. *J Cereb Blood Flow Metab* 1999; 19: 701–735.

84 Darby DG, Barber PA, Gerraty RP et al. Pathophysiological topography of acute ischemia by combined diffusion-weighted and perfusion MRI. *Stroke* 1999; 30: 2043–2052.

85 Neumann-Haefelin T, Moseley ME, Albers GW. New magnetic resonance imaging methods for cerebrovascular disease: emerging clinical applications. *Ann Neurol* 2000; 47: 559–570.

86 Simonsen CZ, Ostergaard L, Smith DF, Vestergaard-Poulsen P, Gyldensted C. Comparison of gradient- and spin-echo imaging: CBF, CBV, and MTT measurements by bolus tracking. *J Magn Reson Imaging* 2000; 12: 411–416.

87 Ostergaard L, Weisskoff RM, Chesler DA, Gyldensted C, Rosen BR. High resolution measurement of cerebral blood flow using intravascular tracer bolus passages. Part I: Mathematical approach and statistical analysis. *Magn Reson Med* 1996; 36: 715–725.

88 Ostergaard L, Sorensen AG, Kwong KK, Weisskoff RM, Gyldensted C, Rosen BR. High resolution measurement of cerebral blood flow using intravascular tracer bolus passages. Part II: Experimental comparison and preliminary results. *Magn Reson Med* 1996; 36: 726–736.

89 Smith AM, Grandin CB, Duprez T, Mataigne F, Cosnard G. Whole brain quantitative CBF, CBV, and MTT measurements using MRI bolus tracking: implementation and application to data acquired from hyperacute stroke patients. *J Magn Reson Imaging* 2000; 12: 400–410.

90 Rempp KA, Brix G, Wenz F, Becker CR, Guckel F, Lorenz WJ. Quantification of regional cerebral blood flow and volume with dynamic susceptibility contrast-enhanced MR imaging. *Radiology* 1994; 193: 637–641.

91 Vonken EJ, van Osch MJ, Bakker CJ, Viergever MA. Measurement of cerebral perfusion with dual-echo multi-slice quantitative dynamic susceptibility contrast MRI. *J Magn Reson Imaging* 1999; 10: 109–117.

92 Sorensen AG, Copen WA, Ostergaard L et al. Hyperacute stroke: simultaneous measurement of relative cerebral blood volume, relative cerebral blood flow, and mean tissue transit time. *Radiology* 1999; 210: 519–527.

93 Calamante F, Gadian DG, Connelly A. Delay and dispersion effects in dynamic susceptibility contrast MRI: simulations using singular value decomposition. *Magn Reson Med* 2000; 44: 466–473.

94 Zaharchuk G, Yamada M, Sasamata M, Jenkins BG, Moskowitz MA, Rosen BR. Is all perfusion-weighted magnetic resonance imaging for stroke equal? The temporal evolution of multiple hemodynamic parameters after focal ischemia in rats correlated with evidence of infarction. *J Cereb Blood Flow Metab* 2000; 20: 1341–1351.

95 Baird AE, Benfield A, Schlaug G et al. Enlargement of human cerebral ischemic lesion volumes measured by diffusion-weighted magnetic resonance imaging. *Ann Neurol* 1997; 41: 581–589.

96 Sorensen AG, Buonanno FS, Gonzalez RG et al. Hyperacute stroke: evaluation with combined multi-section diffusion- weighted and hemodynamically weighted echo-planar MR imaging. *Radiology* 1996; 199: 391–401.

97 Back T, Hoehn-Berlage M, Kohno K, Hossmann KA. Diffusion nuclear magnetic resonance imaging in experimental stroke. Correlation with cerebral metabolites. *Stroke* 1994; 25: 494–500.

98 Kohno K, Hoehn-Berlage M, Mies G, Back T, Hossmann KA. Relationship between diffusion-weighted MR images, cerebral blood flow, and energy state in experimental brain infarction. *Magn Reson Imaging* 1995; 13: 73–80.

99 Hoehn-Berlage M, Norris DG, Kohno K, Mies G, Leibfritz D, Hossmann KA. Evolution of regional changes in apparent diffusion coefficient during focal ischemia of rat brain: the relationship of quantitative diffusion NMR imaging to reduction in cerebral blood flow and metabolic disturbances. *J Cereb Blood Flow Metab* 1995; 15: 1002–1011.

100 Mintorovitch J, Moseley ME, Chileuitt L, Shimizu H, Cohen Y, Weinstein PR. Comparison of diffusion- and T_2-weighted MRI for the early detection of cerebral ischemia and reperfusion in rats. *Magn Reson Med* 1991; 18: 39–50.

101 Rother J, de Crespigny AJ, D'Arceuil H, Iwai K, Moseley ME. Recovery of apparent diffusion coefficient after ischemia-induced spreading depression relates to cerebral perfusion gradient. *Stroke* 1996; 27: 980–986; discussion 986–987.

102 Li F, Han SS, Tatlisumak T et al. Reversal of acute apparent diffusion coefficient abnormalities and delayed neuronal death following transient focal cerebral ischemia in rats. *Ann Neurol* 1999; 46: 333–342.

103 Li F, Silva MD, Sotak CH, Fisher M. Temporal evolution of ischemic injury evaluated with diffusion-, perfusion-, and T_2-weighted MRI. *Neurology* 2000; 54: 689–696.

104 Li F, Liu KF, Silva MD et al. Transient and permanent resolution of ischemic lesions on diffusion-weighted imaging after brief periods of focal ischemia in rats : correlation with histopathology. *Stroke* 2000; 31: 946–954.

105 Marks MP, de Crespigny A, Lentz D, Enzmann DR, Albers GW, Moseley ME. Acute and chronic stroke: navigated spin-echo diffusion-weighted MR imaging. *Radiology* 1996; 199: 403–408.

106 Neumann-Haefelin T, Wittsack HJ, Wenserski F et al. Diffusion- and perfusion-weighted MRI in a patient with a prolonged reversible ischaemic neurological deficit. *Neuroradiology* 2000; 42: 444–447.

107 Lecouvet FE, Duprez TP, Raymackers JM, Peeters A, Cosnard G. Resolution of early diffusion-weighted and FLAIR MRI abnormalities in a patient with TIA. *Neurology* 1999; 52: 1085–1087.

108 Krueger K, Kugel H, Grond M, Thiel A, Maintz D, Lackner K. Late resolution of diffusion-weighted MRI changes in a patient with prolonged reversible ischemic neurological deficit after thrombolytic therapy. *Stroke* 2000; 31: 2715–2718.

109 Uno M, Harada M, Okada T, Nagahiro S. Diffusion-weighted and perfusion-weighted magnetic resonance imaging to monitor acute intra-arterial thrombolysis. *J Stroke Cerebrovasc Dis* 2000; 9: 113–120.

110 Kidwell CS, Alger JR et al. Diffusion MRI in patients with transient ischemic attacks . *Stroke* 1999; 30: 1174–1180.

111 Kidwell CS, Saver JL, Mattiello J et al. Thrombolytic reversal of acute human cerebral ischemic injury shown by diffusion/perfusion magnetic resonance imaging. *Ann Neurol* 2000; 47: 462–469.

112 Kidwell CS, Saver JL, Mattiello J et al. Late secondary injury in patients undergoing vessel recanalization with intra-arterial thrombolysis: visualization with MRI, frequency, and clinical correlates. *Stroke* 2001; 32: S317.

113 Kidwell CS, Saver JL, Mattiello J et al. A diffusion–perfusion MRI signature predicting hemorrhagic transformation following intra-arterial thrombolysis. *Stroke* 2001; 32: S318.

114 Kidwell CS, Alger JR, Saver JL et al. MR signatures of infarction vs. salvageable penumbra in acute human stroke: a preliminary model. *Stroke* 2000; 31: S275.

115 Tong DC, Adami A, Moseley ME, Marks MP. Relationship between apparent diffusion coefficient and subsequent hemorrhagic transformation following acute ischemic stroke. *Stroke* 2000; 31: 2378–2384.

116 Neumann-Haefelin T, Wittsack HJ, Wenserski F et al. Diffusion- and perfusion-weighted MRI. The DWI/PWI mismatch region in acute stroke. *Stroke* 1999; 30: 1591–1597.

117 Schlaug G, Benfield A, Baird AE et al. The ischemic penumbra: operationally defined by diffusion and perfusion MRI. *Neurology* 1999; 53: 1528–1537.

118 Thijs VN, Adam A, Neuman-Haeflin T et al. Relationship between the severity of MR perfusion deficit and DWI lesion evolution. *Neurology* 2001; 57: 1205–1211.

119 Schwamm LH, Koroshetz WJ, Sorensen AG et al. Time course of lesion development in patients with acute stroke: serial diffusion- and hemodynamic-weighted magnetic resonance imaging. *Stroke* 1998; 29: 2268–2276.

120 Beaulieu C, de Crespigny A, Tong DC, Moseley ME, Albers GW, Marks MP. Longitudinal magnetic resonance imaging study of perfusion and diffusion in stroke: evolution of lesion volume and correlation with clinical outcome. *Ann Neurol* 1999; 46: 568–578.

121 Barber PA, Darby DG, Desmond PM et al. Prediction of stroke outcome with echoplanar perfusion- and diffusion-weighted MRI. *Neurology* 1998; 51: 418–426.

122 Karonen JO, Liu Y, Vanninen RL et al. Combined perfusion- and diffusion-weighted MR imaging in acute ischemic stroke during the 1st week: a longitudinal study. *Radiology* 2000; 217: 886–894.

123 Warach S, Pettigrew LC, Dashe JF et al. Effect of citicoline on ischemic lesions as measured by diffusion-weighted magnetic resonance imaging. Citicoline 010 Investigators. *Ann Neurol* 2000; 48: 713–722.

124 Darby DG, Barber PA, Parsons MW et al. Outcome of MRI-delineated perfusion without diffusion weighted lesions in acute stroke. *Stroke* 2000; 31: S287.

125 Rordorf G, Koroshetz WJ, Copen WA et al. Regional ischemia and ischemic injury in patients with acute middle cerebral artery stroke as defined by early diffusion-weighted and perfusion-weighted MRI. *Stroke* 1998; 29: 939–943.

126 Barber PA, Davis SM, Darby et al. Absent middle cerebral artery flow predicts the presence and evolution of the ischemic penumbra. *Neurology* 1999; 52: 1125–1132.

127 Staroselskaya IA, Baird AE, Linfante I et al. Relationship between magnetic resonance arterial patency and perfusion–diffusion mismatch in acute ischemic stroke and its potential clinical use. *Arch Neurol* 2001; 58: 1069–1074

128 Lees KR. Advances in neuroprotection trials. *Eur Neurol* 2001; 45: 6–10.

129 DeGraba TJ, Pettigrew LC. Why do neuroprotective drugs work in animals but not humans? *Neurol Clin* 2000; 18: 475–493.

130 Muir KW, Grosset DG. Neuroprotection for acute stroke: making clinical trials work. *Stroke* 1999; 30: 180–182.

131 Suarez JI, Sunshine JL, Tarr R et al. Predictors of clinical improvement, angiographic recanalization, and intracranial hemorrhage after intra-arterial thrombolysis for acute ischemic stroke. *Stroke* 1999; 30: 2094–2100.

132 Fieschi C, Argentino C, Lenzi GL, Sacchetti ML, Toni D, Bozzao L. Clinical and instrumental evaluation of patients with ischemic stroke within the first six hours. *J Neurol Sci* 1989; 91: 311–321.

133 Bozzao L, Fantozzi LM, Bastianello S et al. Ischaemic supratentorial stroke: angiographic findings in patients examined in the very early phase. *J Neurol* 1989; 236: 340–342.

134 Barber PA, Darby DG, Yang Q et al. Reperfusion attenuates infarct growth and improves stroke outcome: a combined PI/DWI study. *Stroke* 2000; 31: S275: 59.

135 Marks MP, Tong DC, Beaulieu C, Albers GW, de Crespigny A, Moseley ME. Evaluation of early reperfusion and i.v. tPA therapy using diffusion- and perfusion-weighted MRI. *Neurology* 1999; 52: 1792–1798.

136 Lansberg MG, Tong DC, Norbash AM, Yenari MA, Moseley ME. Intra-arterial rtPA treatment of stroke assessed by diffusion- and perfusion-weighted MRI. *Stroke* 1999; 30: 678–680.

137 Jansen O, Schellinger P, Fiebach J, Hacke W, Sartor K. Early recanalisation in acute ischaemic stroke saves tissue at risk defined by MRI [letter]. *Lancet* 1999; 353: 2036–2037.

138 Schellinger PD, Jansen O, Fiebach JB et al. Feasibility and practicality of MR imaging of stroke in the management of hyperacute cerebral ischemia. *Am J Neuroradiol* 2000; 21: 1184–1189.

139 Parsons MW, Barber PA, Darby DG, Tress BM, Donnan GA, Davis SM. Hyperacute stroke diffusion- and perfusion-weighted MRI distinguishes t-PA responders. *Stroke* 2001; 32: S324: 181.

140 Temple R. Are surrogate markers adequate to assess cardiovascular disease drugs? *J Am Med Assoc* 1999; 282: 790–795.

141 van Everdingen KJ, van der Grond J, Kappelle LJ, Ramos LM, Mali WP. Diffusion-weighted magnetic resonance imaging in acute stroke. *Stroke* 1998; 29: 1783–1790.

142 Warach S, Dashe JF, Edelman RR. Clinical outcome in ischemic stroke predicted by early diffusion-weighted and perfusion magnetic resonance imaging: a preliminary analysis. *J Cereb Blood Flow Metab* 1996; 16: 53–59.

143 Lovblad KO, Baird AE, Schlaug G et al. Ischemic lesion volumes in acute stroke by diffusion-weighted magnetic resonance imaging correlate with clinical outcome. *Ann Neurol* 1997; 42: 164–170.

144 Baird AE, Lovblad KO, Dashe JF et al. Clinical correlations of diffusion and perfusion lesion volumes in acute ischemic stroke. *Cerebrovasc Dis* 2000; 10: 441–448.

145 Tong DC, Yenari MA, Albers GW, O'Brien M, Marks MP, Moseley ME. Correlation of perfusion- and diffusion-weighted MRI with NIHSS score in acute (6.5 hour) ischemic stroke. *Neurology* 1998; 50: 864–870.

146 Thijs VN, Lansberg MG, Beaulieu C, Marks MP, Moseley ME, Albers GW. Is early ischemic lesion volume on diffusion-weighted imaging an independent predictor of stroke outcome? : a multivariable analysis. *Stroke* 2000; 31: 2597–2602.

147 Albers GW, Lansberg MG, O'Brien MW et al. Evolution of cerebral infarct volume assessed by diffusion-weighted MRI: implications for acute stroke trials. *Neurology* 1999; 52: A453.

148 Saver JL, Johnston KC, Homer D et al. Infarct volume as a surrogate or auxiliary outcome measure in ischemic stroke clinical trials. The RANTTAS Investigators. *Stroke* 1999; 30: 293–298.

MRI as a tool in stroke drug development

Steven Warach

National Institute of Neurological Disorders and Stroke, Bethesda, MD, USA

The disappointingly slow progress in developing effective therapies for ischemic stroke, along with the clinical development of diffusion and perfusion MRI, has led to a re-evaluation of the strategies for the design of stroke clinical trials. Rapid, early MRI has been proposed and begun to be used in stroke trials as a means of optimizing patient selection and as a direct measure of the effect of treatments on cerebral infarction, as the marker of therapeutic response.

The need for a more rationale approach to clinical development of stroke therapeutics

The first and only success in developing an approved therapy culminated in the pivotal trials of intravenous recombinant tissue plasminogen activator (t-PA),[1] reported in 1995 and leading to regulatory approval in 1996. The key insight of the designers of these trials was optimizing the sample with regard to time to treatment, requiring patients to be treated within three hours from onset of symptoms. They recognized that very early stroke treatment would be more effective and that the earliest cases are most likely to still have the causative arterial occlusions, which may spontaneously lyse at later times. Thus, patients were included across the broad range of clinical features, and selection of patients by imaging confirmation of the diagnosis or pathologic features most amenable to the treatment was not necessary to prove the efficacy of intravenous t-PA for the less than 3 hours' time window. In the subsequent 6 years, many unsuccessful clinical trials for acute stroke have been reported and drug development for many once promising agents has been abandoned. In particular, trials of intravenous t-PA initiated up to 6 hours from symptom onset have failed to demonstrate efficacy in a sample of acute stroke patients selected without imaging confirmation of the diagnosis.[2-4]

Except for the trials of intravenous rt-PA in the treatment of ischemic stroke within the first 3 hours,[1] this traditional approach has lead to no approved therapies for stroke and a great degree of pessimism with regard to thrombolysis beyond 3 hours and to the general concept of neuroprotection in stroke. To demonstrate efficacy in a clinical trial with a treatment time window beyond 3 hours, other features of trial design need to be optimized, and proof of pharmacological activity in Phase 2 is needed before lengthy, expensive, labour intensive and potentially risky Phase III clinical trials are undertaken. The requirement of proof of concept Phase 2 studies will prevent the wastefulness of Phase 3 trials that are doomed to futility before they begin. Image-guided Phase 2 studies may answer the question of target biological activity in fewer than 200 patients, the sample size typical for Phase II trials. Trends toward benefit using clinical scales at Phase 2 have been notoriously poor predictors of clinical outcomes in Phase 3 trials on much larger samples.

Table 17.1. Uses of MRI (DWI, PWI, MRA) as a selection tool in stroke trials

Positive radiological diagnosis of ischemic stroke
Select by location appropriate to the therapeutic mechanism
Select by size
For reperfusion therapies select by presence of perfusion defect or by diffusion–perfusion mismatch
For neuroprotective drugs select by diffusion–perfusion mismatch or reperfusion depending on drug mechanism
Exclude if confounding subacute or chronic lesions

Patient selection (Table 17.1)

It would be unthinkable for clinical trials in cardiology or oncology to enrol patients by bedside clinical impression alone, without objective evidence from diagnostic testing confirming the pathology before inclusion of a patient. Yet this has been the traditional standard by which clinical trials for ischemic stroke have been conducted, because until recently there had been no practical alternative. Rapid MRI diffusion, perfusion, angiography and gradient echo imaging provides that alternative. In using MRI as a selection criterion, the goal would be a sample selection based upon a positive imaging diagnosis of a pathology rationally linked to the drug's mechanisms of action. Requiring a positive diagnosis of acute ischemic injury by DWI and PWI would ideally assure that no patients with diagnoses mimicking stroke are included in the sample, a desirable objective unachievable in trials using bedside impression and non-hemorrhagic CT as the basis of inclusion. The goal of image-based patient selection is to narrow the range of patient characteristics, leading to a more homogeneous sample, reducing within group variance, and increasing the statistical power (lowering sample size requirement) of the experimental design to demonstrate efficacy.

The principle of optimal patient selection by imaging confirmation of the relevant pathology was first demonstrated by the results of the intra-arterial pro-urokinase stroke study, PROACT II.[5]

Prior attempts to prove the efficacy of thrombolysis initiated between 3 and 6 hours from onset without a positive diagnosis of arterial occlusion or perfusion defect have not been successful.[2–4] However, in PROACT II[5] 180 patients were selected based on evidence of arterial occlusions at the M1 or M2 levels of the middle cerebral artery by conventional arteriography, and a significant clinical benefit was observed when thrombolysis was initiated up to 6 hours from symptom onset. The results of that trial suggested that a more prolonged study duration, increased expense and potential delay in treatment to complete a screening test may be justified by the greater chance of demonstrating clinical benefit by using a pathologically homogeneous and rational selection of patients.

A recent report of a pilot clinical trial of intravenous rt-PA between 3 and 6 hours from onset demonstrated in a subgroup of 16 patients with diffusion-perfusion mismatch a significant degree of recanalization, reperfusion and tissue salvage as well as a clinical benefit relative to untreated historical controls.[6] That sample size is an order of magnitude smaller than was required to show clinical benefits in the rt-PA trials, which did not select a homogeneous sample of patients on the basis of imaging pathology, and supports the concept that selection of an optimal sample may lead to smaller sample size requirements even for clinical endpoints.

Optimal patient selection would be based on a positive imaging evidence of the ischemic pathology that the therapy has been developed to treat. The simplest use as an inclusion criterion would include the presence of a lesion on DWI to increase the diagnostic certainty of ischemic stroke. For reperfusion therapies, the optimal target of therapy would be patients with evidence of an arterial occlusion or hypoperfusion with the greatest territory at risk for infarction: the diffusion–perfusion mismatch.[6–8] For neuroprotective drugs acting only in cortical areas of ischemic penumbra optimal selection of patients would be acute lesions involving the cerebral cortex. For some neuroprotective drugs the diffusion–perfusion mismatch may be the optimal target, for other agents that would protect against reperfusion injury or would not achieve sufficient concentration in oligemic tissue, the optimal target would be patients in whom reperfusion has occurred. Patients might also be excluded from the trial at screening if subacute or chronic lesions are found that may confound measurements of lesion volumes or clinical severity as outcome variables. Because of a relative large error of measurement associated with small lesions,[9] lesions larger than a minimum volume, e.g. 5 cm^3, may be desirable. Furthermore, an upper limit of lesion volume at enrolment would permit an opportunity for lesion growth and may better differentiate the effect on lesion size of an effective treatment from placebo. Selection of patients by DWI is also optimally suited for using change in lesion volume as a direct measure of the neuroprotective effect of the drug.

Proof of pharmacological principle using MRI as a marker of response to therapy: replicating the preclinical experiment in patients (Table 17.2)

Before an experimental stroke therapy is brought from the laboratory to clinical trial, it is necessary to demonstrate that the treatment causes reduction in lesion volume in experimental models. The fundamental premise of drug discovery and development in acute stroke is that treatments that reduce lesion size are those most likely to lead to clinical benefit. In clinical trial programmes that depend solely on clinical endpoints as indices of benefit, drugs may be brought to Phase 3 testing without the requirement of evidence that the drug will have the therapeutic effect observed in the experimental model. In practice, this traditional approach to stroke trials has been unsuccessful and often misleading.

Four major factors are hypothesized to predict tissue response and clinical efficacy in stroke trials: time to treatment, the salvageable tissue-at-risk, the relevance of the patient sample to the treatment and the intrinsic effectiveness of the therapeutic strategy. Time is an important factor,[10] but it is not the only important factor hypothesized to affect response to therapy. The amount of ischemically

Table 17.2. MRI as outcome measure

Necessary but not sufficient evidence of protective effect.
Protective effect may be attenuation of expected lesion growth or partial DWI lesion reversal
Clinical benefit unlikely if no protective effect on lesion volume (go/no go decision at phase 2).
Smaller sample size requirements than for typical clinical endpoints (~50–100 per arm)
May be confirmatory evidence supporting positive clinical endpoint trial for regulatory approval.

threatened and clinically symptomatic but potentially salvageable tissue-at-risk at the initiation of therapy is another factor that is likely to predict clinical response. The ideal sample in a clinical trial should also be treatment-congruent. A treatment-congruent sample is a sample composed of patients most likely to respond to therapy, patients who have the pathology that the therapy is intended to treat, e.g. an arterial occlusion for a thrombolytic trial, and who have other features predictive of a measurable response to therapy. The ideal treatment-congruent sample will also have no features predictive of serious adverse events. The fourth major factor is the intrinsic effectiveness of a therapeutic approach. Observations in experimental models suggest that reperfusion or neuroprotection by endogenous, pharmacological, or physical mechanisms reduce infarct volume, that reperfusion has a greater benefit on infarct reduction than neuroprotection, and that the effect of a combination of reperfusion and neuroprotection is yet greater. The relative effectiveness of a therapy depends not only on its pharmacological properties, but also on choices made in trial design, such as the dosing and method of administration.

Figure 17.1 illustrates the hypothesized relationship of these factors to efficacy in stroke trials using lesion growth on MRI as the marker of therapeutic response. The clinical trial optimized on all features would have the most robust response. When the trial is completely optimized on these factors, the pretreatment lesion on DWI is partially reversible. As the factors are progressively less optimized, the lesions are more likely to grow relative to the

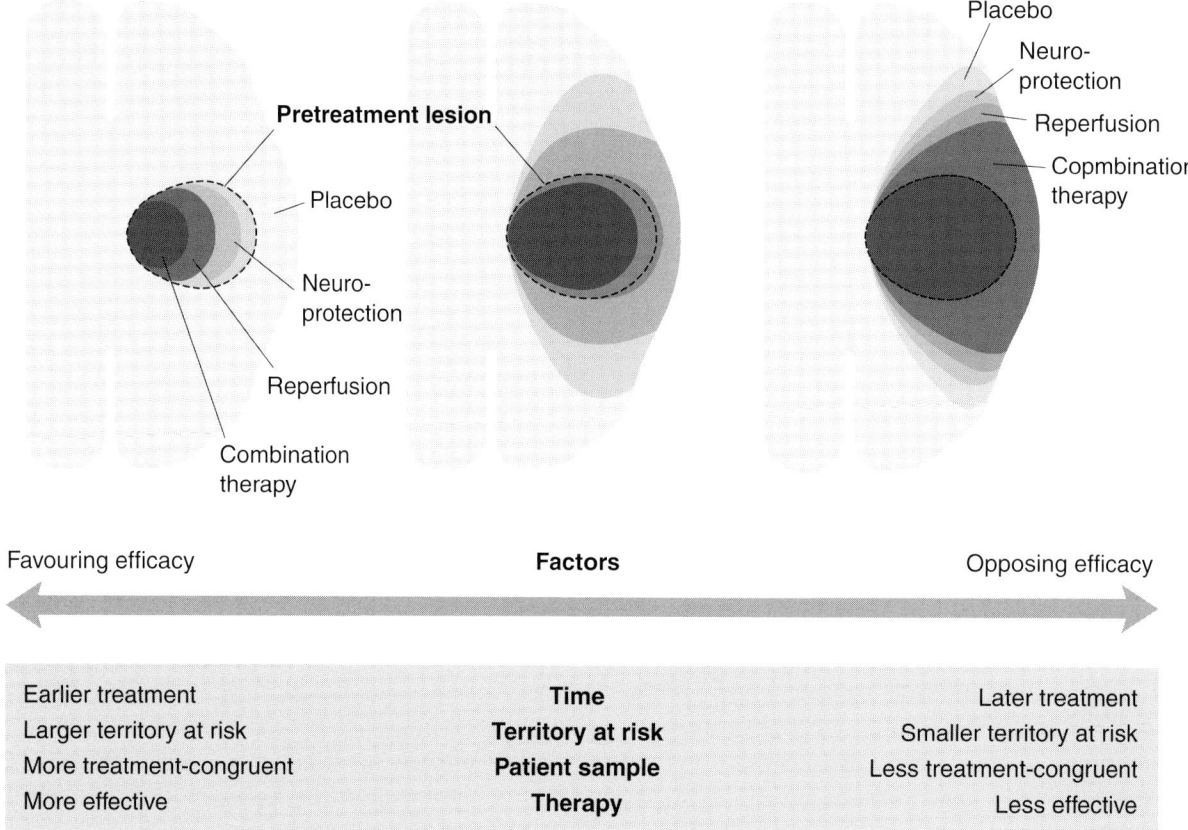

Fig. 17.1. Model of lesion responses in stroke clinical trials: a multifactorial continuum. The figure illustrates the principles hypothesized to affect tissue outcome in clinical trials, and the likelihood of demonstrating efficacy on either infarct volume or clinical variables. The three slices depict three points along the hypothetical continuum of tissue response in stroke trials according to the major factors (centre column) that are hypothesized to affect efficacy. The dashed ovals outline the pretreatment volume of tissue injury on DWI. The solid grey regions depict the final infarct volume as a function of treatment. The change in lesion volume from pretreatment volume is the MRI marker of therapeutic response. The untreated (placebo) patient will have an amount of lesion growth that is independent of factors affecting efficacy. Reperfusion therapy will have a greater lesion effect than neuroprotective therapy, and the combination of reperfusion and neuroprotection will be best. Trials optimized for efficacy have the features in the left column; trial characteristics that oppose efficacy for each factor are listed in the column on the right. The relative value along each of these dimensions in a clinical trial will interact to determine efficacy on infarct volume as well as clinical outcome. The factors are discussed in the text.

pretreatment volume and the differences among the types of treatment will progressively decrease to nil. Optimized on one feature, differences in trial efficacy will depend on the value of the other factors. A less effective therapy studied under optimized conditions may show greater efficacy in trials than a truly more effective one, if the latter is studied without optimizing the design along the other dimensions. For example, a later treatment window may nonetheless lead to a positive trial result if the trial design is optimized for efficacy on the other factors, despite lack of efficacy at those times on an indiscriminately selected sample.

As discussed above, optimizing sample selection may lead to smaller sample sizes, but the greatest advantage for increased power of MRI is the measurement of the pretreatment lesion against which to compare the final lesion. Such an approach to within subject variance must, by basic statistical principles, be more powerful than analysis of only the final lesion volume. The question of whether a treatment causes reduction of lesion volume may be answerable in the study of 100 to 200 patients in Phase 2, whereas five to ten times as many patients are typically tested in Phase 3 studies in order to evaluate the treatment with clinical endpoints. Thus, a Phase 2 MRI endpoint trial to replicate the preclinical experiment in a patient population may be a rational and cost effective basis of deciding whether or not to proceed with Phase 3 testing. A positive lesion outcome study in late Phase 2 would be supportive of the decision to proceed with Phase 3 trials. The citicoline MRI trials demonstrated this principle and also substantiated the claim that sample size requirements for an effect on lesion volume may be on the order of 50 to 100 patients when pre–post-lesion difference is used as the outcome variable. In the first citicoline MRI trial,[11] no significant difference was found on pre–post-percentage change in lesion volume between active and placebo, but from that study it was estimated 58 patients per treatment arm would have been required to achieve significance. In the next citicoline MRI trial using a higher dose, a significant effect of treatment of pre–post-lesion volume change was observed in 71 placebo and 62 citicoline-treated patients, using the baseline NIHSS as a covariate in the analysis.[12] By contrast, in that trial there were no differences in the final infarct size when pretreatment lesion volume assessment was not used, despite a sample size five times as great (337 placebo and 336 citicoline treated).

The first citicoline MRI trial[11] also confirmed observations from single centre natural history observations that the lesion volumes were significantly correlated with scores on clinical scales, and that the clinical severity (by baseline NIHSS) and the severity of the hemodynamic abnormality (volume of abnormality of PWI) were independent predictors of lesion growth, suggesting their value as covariates of lesion growth in subsequent trials.

Reducing the disabling sensory, motor and cognitive deficits associated with cerebral infarction is the clinical goal of acute stroke therapeutics, therefore reduction of infarct volume is the biological objective. A relative reduction in infarct volume in animal models is the necessary and sufficient evidence required to advance a drug into clinical trials. Replicating these preclinical observations in a clinical population is a logical step in clinical drug development, but has often been neglected. Treatments that do not lead to a smaller infarct in patients relative to an untreated cohort are unlikely to show a clinical benefit. Performing a dose escalation safety study, followed by large clinical endpoint trials at the maximum tolerated dose in the absence of evidence that the drug has the target biological effect in patients that it had in the animal models, has been tried and failed for treatments beyond the 3-hour time window. Pilot proof-of-principle studies toward defining the optimal sample on a biologically meaningful outcome variable are an important step.

Surrogate endpoint in Phase III trials

Ordinarily a drug must have a beneficial effect on a clinical endpoint or on a validated surrogate endpoint to demonstrate effectiveness and lead to registration. Current regulations governing the United States Food and Drug Administration state that a drug that has the potential to address unmet medical needs for serious and life-threatening conditions, such as stroke, may be approved if it has an effect on a surrogate endpoint that is reasonably likely to predict clinical benefit. Such surrogate endpoints are considered to be not validated because, while suggestive of clinical benefit, their relationship to clinical outcomes is not proven. The internationally accepted regulatory standards of the International Conference on Harmonization also state that surrogate endpoints may be used as primary endpoints when the surrogate is reasonably likely to predict clinical outcome.

Changes in volume of ischemic brain injury using diffusion-weighted (DWI) and T_2-weighted (T_2WI) MRI has been proposed as a surrogate marker of clinical outcome in stroke trials. Much of the thought on the use of biomarkers as measures of drug activity and potential surrogates have come from fields, such as oncology or cardiology, where death or a comparably objective and reliable assessment is the relevant clinical endpoint. For these disease categories, the biomarker does not fully capture the pathology underlying the disease as well as the clinical endpoint does. Principles of the use of biomarkers and potential surrogates are different for brain disorders in which disability defined by imperfect clinical rating scales rather than death is the relevant clinical variable, and in which the biomarker, macroscopic brain lesion, more fully captures the pathology than the clinical scales. Stroke is a special case among brain diseases because: it is a single event that is not progressive beyond the initial hours and days, there is a high rate of spontaneous clinical recovery (implying that clinical improvement is less reflective of drug effect), it requires rapid diagnosis under emergency conditions (the diagnostic certainty is less), a single discrete lesion fully captures the pathology (the clinical manifestations result from the size and location of the ischemic damage). For stroke the true clinical endpoint, disability, is difficult to measure, and only approximated by clinical scales. Furthermore, experts do not agree on how to measure outcome using clinical scales, and the criterion of 'complete recovery' used in many trials may include patients with significant disability. For these reasons, lesion volume as a biomarker is likely to be more helpful for stroke than in cancer and cardiac disorders.

MRI measurements of lesion volume acutely and chronically have proven to be a marker of clinical severity measured by stroke scales[13–16] and changes in lesion volume over time are associated with change in clinical severity.[11] The two citicoline DWI stroke trials both measured DWI within 24 hours of onset and T_2WI at Week 12. Volume measurements were performed in a central laboratory by a single reader blinded to clinical information and treatment assignment. Both protocols defined clinical improvement a priori as an improvement on NIHSS of 7 or more points. Exploratory analyses in the first trial (010; $n=81$) led to planned confirmatory analyses in the second trial (018; $n=133$). In both trials, the association of volume change to clinical improvement was highly significant ($P<0.0001$), and patients who improved had decreased volume change relative to those who did not ($P<0.01$). The

Table 17.3. Requirements of a validated surrogate for DWI and PWI

To fully establish diffusion and perfusion MRI as a validated surrogate in stroke trials several conditions need to be satisfied (the first four have been met, sufficient to meet the regulatory requirement for surrogate use of 'reasonably likely to predict outcome' on clinical variables):

1. DWI and PWI as biologic markers of the disease process in ischemic stroke.
2. The tests are sensitive and specific for the diagnosis of stroke in patients.
3. Lesion volumes correlate with clinical function as measured by clinical rating scales, predict outcome, and covary over time with clinical severity and clinical changes.
4. Rational covariates affecting lesion volumes outcomes identified.
5. Utility in identifying effective treatments in trials proven.

positive predictive value of a reduction in lesion volume predicting clinical improvement was 66% for the 010 trial and 76% for the 018 trial; the negative predictive values were 73% and 52%, respectively. The sensitivity of lesion volume decrease for detection of clinical improvement was 74% for the 010 trial and 70% for the 018 trial; the specificities were 64% and 60%, respectively. These results confirm that the change in lesion volume is a marker of clinical improvement in patients in these trials. Results on this marker in these and other trials have been consistent with results on clinical measures. Based upon the results of these trials, the regulatory standard is met: there is sufficient evidence to recommend MRI volume change as a surrogate endpoint that is reasonably likely to predict clinical outcome in stroke trials.

Although surrogates not yet validated may be used if reasonably likely to predict the outcome, eventual validation is a goal. The factors required for validation of MRI as a surrogate marker are summarized in Table 17.3. The first four of these requirements have been met. Confirmation of the

Table 17.4. Concordance of MRI and clinical results in clinical trials

Trials	Clinical benefit	MR surrogate benefit	MR natural history
i.v. t-PA (0–3 h)	+		+
i.v. t-PA (3–6 h)	– (+ secondary)	?	+
i.a. t-lysis	+	?	+
Citicoline	– (+ secondary)	+	
GAIN	–	–	
POST	–	–	

validity of many of these features of DWI and PWI in acute stroke has recently come from the first prospective multicentre stroke trial using MRI as an inclusion and primary outcome measure, the citicoline MRI stroke trial.[11]

The fifth criterion of validation, the concordance of effects on clinical outcomes and surrogate outcomes, continues to be evaluated in ongoing trials. Effective drugs should show benefit on both clinical and imaging outcome measures. To date several stroke trials have used MRI and the results seem concordant with the clinical endpoints. Table 17.4 summarizes these results. No randomized clinical trial with thrombolytic therapy using MRI has been reported, however for those therapies Table 17.4 lists results from natural history studies. The citicoline trials provide support for this wherein trends on clinical and effects on imaging outcomes measures have been observed.[11,12,17–19] Ineffective drugs will show benefit on neither clinical nor imaging outcome measures. The latter has been found for the GAIN and POST neuroprotective trials, which showed no effect on clinical or MRI surrogate outcomes.[20–23]

If the results on clinical endpoints and imaging endpoints were to be discordant, what are the possible explanations? If lesion volume shows a benefit but the clinical endpoint does not, the most likely explanation would be that the trial design or the choice of clinical endpoints is insensitive to the drug effect or that there is a toxicity affecting the measurement of clinical outcome that offsets the neuroprotective effect of the therapy. If clinical endpoint shows a benefit but lesion volume does not, this could either be that the imaging methods are insensitive to the drug effect or that the clinical benefit is not mediated by a direct effect on the evolving infarct. The latter possibility is not relevant to reperfusion or neuroprotective therapies, but may apply to classes of drugs that, for example, treat poststroke mood disorders or would lead to enhanced recovery through functional reorganization. This comparison is only meaningful if studies are optimally designed and equally powered to show effect on their respective outcome measures, i.e. the optimal sample size for imaging studies may be too small to show clinical effects.

Full validation must eventually be proven, but as we see from the regulatory standards it is not required in order to use lesion volume by MRI as a surrogate outcome in stroke trials. An imaging benefit may never stand alone as a surrogate, since there must also be evidence of clinical benefit. One could imagine a small but statistically significant volume reduction that would have a trivial or undetectable clinical effect. However, a benefit on the surrogate may be acceptable as an independent source of confirmatory data in support of benefit seen in clinical endpoint trials, but an application for registration of a stroke drug using MRI outcomes has not yet been submitted to regulatory agencies.

Concluding remarks

The pharmaceutical industry has taken the initiative, investigating this final step in validation. The results of several industry-sponsored drug trials using MRI as a surrogate will be known over the next several years, and those studies should provide the most

Table 17.5. Ongoing acute stroke trials using MRI (winter 2002)

Trial acronym	Intervention	Time window
Thrombolytic		
EPITHET	i.v. t-PA	3–6 h
DEFUSE	i.v. t-PA	3–6 h
DIAS	i.v. desmoteplase	3–9 h
MR SELECT	i.a. t-PA	6–12 h
ROSIE	i.v. abciximab/reteplase	3–24 h
Neuroprotective		
ARTIST MRI	i.v. AMPA antagonist	0–6 h
MR IMAGES	i.v. magnesium	0–12 h
SIS	i.v. sipatragine	0–12 h
COOL-AID I	hypothermia (i.v. catheter)	0–12 h

Table 17.6. Sample features of MRI-based stroke trials

1. MRI sequences:
   a. DWI: parenchymal injury
   b. PWI: hemodynamic abnormality
   c. MRA: arterial occlusion
   d. GRE: hemorrhage detection
   e. FLAIR: chronic and subacute lesions
2. Selection criteria:
   a. cortical DWI lesion > 5 cm^3
   b. diffusion-perfusion mismatch
   c. no pre-existing lesions in same vascular territory
3. Outcome variables:
   a. lesion volume change pre to post treatment
      i. absolute change
      ii. percentage change
      iii. proportion of patients reaching change criterion (e.g. volume decrease)
   b. final lesion volume on high resolution FLAIR at day 30 with baseline DWI volume of abnormality as a covariate
4. Data analysis
   a. Approach to non-normal distribution of lesion volumes
      i. transformed lesion volume (percentage change, log, cube root)
      ii. non-parametric statistical model
   b. covariance analysis on baseline variables:
      i. NIHSS
      ii. volume of hypoperfusion
      iii. initial lesion volume
      iv. others?
         1. age
         2. time to treatment

decisive information regarding the utility of MRI as a surrogate outcome measure in stroke trials. Several others are in progress (Table 17.5). There have been concerns raised in the past that the use of MRI in stroke clinical trials is impractical for technical and logistical reasons (e.g. scan duration and availability). The practical limitations have disappeared with the widespread availability of ultrafast echoplanar imaging with diffusion and perfusion capability on commercial MRI scanners. A highly motivated, well-coordinated centre can perform emergency diffusion and perfusion MRI with a latency to scan and scanning session duration approaching that of emergency head CT. There are now well over 100 centres worldwide that are capable and experienced in performing these types of acute MR exams in clinical trials. Key design issues with regard to the use of diffusion and perfusion MRI in stroke trials are proposed in Table 17.6. MRI-based recruitment into trials with time window of 6 hours have proven feasible, as has specifically selection based on lesion size, location, and the diffusion–perfusion mismatch. As the field of stroke clinical trials examines opportunities for improving trial design, positive imaging diagnoses in patient selection and use of imaging as treatment assessments is assuming an increasingly useful role. MRI is increasingly used as a selection tool and an outcome measure in stroke trials, reflecting recognition that direct pathophysiological imaging may provide a more rational approach to stroke therapeutics. Patient selection and outcomes based exclusively on clinical assessment and non-hemorrhagic CT scans may no longer be appropriate for all stroke trials.

REFERENCES

1 National Institute of Neurological Disorders and Stroke rt-PA Stroke Study Group. Tissue plasminogen activator for acute ischemic stroke. *N Engl J Med* 1995; 333(24): 1581–1587.

2 Hacke W, Kaste M, Fieschi C et al. Intravenous thrombolysis with recombinant tissue plasminogen activator for acute hemispheric stroke. The European Cooperative Acute Stroke Study (ECASS). *J Am Med Assoc* 1995; 274(13): 1017–1025.

3 Hacke W, Kaste M, Fieschi C et al. Randomised double-blind placebo-controlled trial of thrombolytic therapy with intravenous alteplase in acute ischaemic stroke (ECASS II). Second European–Australasian Acute Stroke Study Investigators. *Lancet* 1998; 352(9136): 1245–1251.

4 Clark WM, Wissman S, Albers GW, Jhamandas JH, Madden KP, Hamilton S. Recombinant tissue-type plasminogen activator (Alteplase) for ischemic stroke 3 to 5 hours after symptom onset. The ATLANTIS Study: a randomized controlled trial. Alteplase thrombolysis for acute noninterventional therapy in ischemic stroke. *J Am Med Assoc* 1999; 282(21): 2019–2026.

5 Furlan A, Higashida R, Wechsler L et al. Intra-arterial prourokinase for acute ischemic stroke. The PROACT II study: a randomized controlled trial. Prolyse in acute cerebral thromboembolism. *J Am Med Assoc* 1999; 282(21): 2003–2011.

6 Parsons MW, Barber PA, Chalk J et al. Diffusion- and perfusion-weighted MRI response to thrombolysis in stroke. *Ann Neurol* 2002; 51(1): 28–37.

7 Schellinger PD, Jansen O, Fiebach JB et al. Monitoring intravenous recombinant tissue plasminogen activator thrombolysis for acute ischemic stroke with diffusion and perfusion MRI. *Stroke* 2000; 31(6): 1318–1328.

8 Marks MP, Tong DC, Beaulieu C, Albers GW, de Crespigny A, Moseley ME. Evaluation of early reperfusion and i.v. tPA therapy using diffusion- and perfusion-weighted MRI. *Neurology* 1999; 52(9): 1792–1798.

9 Laubach HJ, Jakob PM, Lovblad KO et al. A phantom for diffusion-weighted imaging of acute stroke. *J Magn Reson Imaging* 1998; 8(6): 1349–1354.

10 Marler JR, Tilley BC, Lu M et al. Early stroke treatment associated with better outcome: the NINDS rt-PA stroke study. *Neurology* 2000; 55(11): 1649–1655.

11 Warach S, Pettigrew LC, Dashe JF et al. Effect of citicoline on ischemic lesions as measured by diffusion-weighted magnetic resonance imaging. Citicoline 010 Investigators. *Ann Neurol* 2000; 48(5): 713–722.

12 Warach S, Sabounjian LA. ECCO 2000 study of citicoline for treatment of acute ischemic stroke: Effects on infarct volumes measured by MRI. *Stroke* 2000; 31(1): 42.

13 Baird AE, Lovblad KO, Dashe JF et al. Clinical Correlations of diffusion and perfusion lesion volumes in acute ischemic stroke. *Cerebrovasc Dis* 2000; 10(6): 441–448.

14 Beaulieu C, de Crespigny A, Tong DC, Moseley ME, Albers GW, Marks MP. Longitudinal magnetic resonance imaging study of perfusion and diffusion in stroke: evolution of lesion volume and correlation with clinical outcome. *Ann Neurol* 1999; 46(4): 568–578.

15 Lovblad KO, Baird AE, Schlaug G et al. Ischemic lesion volumes in acute stroke by diffusion-weighted magnetic resonance imaging correlate with clinical outcome. *Ann Neurol* 1997; 42(2): 164–170.

16 van Everdingen KJ, van der Grond J, Kappelle LJ, Ramos LM, Mali WP. Diffusion-weighted magnetic resonance imaging in acute stroke. *Stroke* 1998; 29(9): 1783–1790.

17 Clark WM, Warach SJ, Pettigrew LC, Gammans RE, Sabounjian LA. A randomized dose-response trial of citicoline in acute ischemic stroke patients. Citicoline Stroke Study Group. *Neurology* 1997; 49(3): 671–678.

18 Clark WM, Williams BJ, Selzer KA, Zweifler RM, Sabounjian LA, Gammans RE. A randomized efficacy trial of citicoline in patients with acute ischemic stroke. *Stroke* 1999; 30(12): 2592–2597.

19 Clark WM, Wechsler LR, Sabounjian LA, Schwiderski UE. A phase III randomized efficacy trial of 2000 mg citicoline in acute ischemic stroke patients. *Neurology* 2001; 57(9): 1595–1602.

20 Lees KR, Asplund K, Carolei A et al. Glycine antagonist (gavestinel) in neuroprotection (GAIN International) in patients with acute stroke: a randomised controlled trial. GAIN International Investigators. *Lancet* 2000; 355(9219): 1949–1954.

21 Sacco RL, DeRosa JT, Haley EC Jr. et al. Glycine antagonist in neuroprotection for patients with acute stroke: GAIN Americas: a randomized controlled trial. *J Am Med Assoc* 2001; 285(13): 1719–1728.

22 Warach S, Kaste M, Fisher M. The effect of GV150526 on ischemic lesion volume: The GAIN Americas and GAIN International MRI Substudy. *Neurology* 2000; 54(Suppl 3): A87–A88.

23 Warach S, Hacke W, Hsu C et al. Effect of maxipost on ischemic lesions in patients with acute stroke: The POST-010 MRI Substudy. *Stroke* 2002; 33: 383.

Magnetic resonance spectroscopy in stroke

Dawn E. Saunders[1] and Martin M. Brown[2]

[1] Department of Neuroradiology, The National Hospital of Neurology and Neurosurgery, Queen Square, London, UK
[2] Stroke Medicine, Institute of Neurology, University College London, The National Hospital for Neurology and Neurosurgery, Queen Square, London UK

Magnetic resonance spectroscopy (MRS) is a non-invasive method that allows the in vivo investigation of biochemical changes in both animals and humans. The application of MRS to the study of stroke has made possible dynamic studies of intracellular metabolism in cerebral ischemia. The concentration of cerebral metabolites in the brain is very low (2–20 mM) compared to that of water (41.7 M of water or 83.4 M of protons). The evoked nuclear magnetic resonance (NMR) signal from the metabolite is therefore very much smaller than the signal from water used to generate an anatomical display in magnetic resonance imaging (MRI). Hence, the minimum voxel size required for MRS is larger and data acquisition times are longer than in MRI. MRS is more sensitive to local magnetic field inhomogeneities leading to difficulties in the quantitation of peak areas. MRS has therefore been limited to use as a research tool, until the last few years. Despite the relatively low signal-to-noise ratio of spectroscopy, improvements in magnet and gradient design, and the wider availability of magnets at higher field strength (1.5T), now enable good quality brain [^{1}H]-MRS spectra to be recorded on most modern clinical instruments.

The original spectroscopy work in animals and humans was carried out using phosphorus [^{31}P] MRS. However, not all metabolites contain phosphorus, and the MR application of this nucleus has been restricted to the study of energy and lipid metabolism. In the brain, [^{1}H]-MRS has two great advantages: the proton provides 15 times more sensitivity than [^{31}P]-MRS, and almost every compound in living tissue contains hydrogen. In theory, signals from ^{13}Carbon and ^{19}Fluorine can also be used to generate MRS but there has been little or no work in humans. The study of cerebral ischemia in humans is predominantly confined to [^{1}H]-MRS which is the subject of this chapter.

Until recently, data acquisition required the skills of an experienced spectroscopist to manually optimize the parameters for each scan and this could result in long examination times. The development of automated software programmes, e.g. the single voxel proton brain exam (PROBE, General Electric, Milwaukee, USA),[1] and their implementation on clinical systems has gone a long way to overcoming some of the problems of data collection. However, the low concentrations of visible metabolites requires the collection of data from a single voxel many times larger than that required for MR imaging. Appropriate coils and dedicated software are needed and for most purposes expert physics and spectroscopist backup is still required for the majority of applications. The patient will need to be able to tolerate the additional time in the scanner (20–30 minutes) required for MRS, if as is usually the case, conventional MRI is also performed. Quantification of metabolite concentrations requires off line analysis, but the spectra are usually displayed fairly rapidly allowing immediate reporting of major changes.

Chemical shift imaging (CSI) or multivoxel MR spectroscopic imaging is a more advanced form of spectroscopy that uses phase encoding to subdivide a large volume of interest into smaller acquisition voxels, thereby allowing the study of large and heterogeneous areas of brain. Single voxel MRS provides accurately quantifiable measures of metabolites within a region of interest. However, there is a limit to the number of single voxel measurements that can be made at a single MR examination, determined by the patient's tolerance, ranging in stroke patients from one to three examinations, and areas of partial ischemia or likely penumbra are not necessarily predictable from immediate MR images. CSI allows assessment of the extent and distribution of in vivo biochemical changes. Each voxel of a CSI map can be used to define all the biochemical changes that occur in stroke and the extent of the area examined allows the detection of metabolite concentration changes within, adjacent to and within the contralateral hemisphere in one acquisition. The disadvantages of CSI include greater sensitivity to motion, longer scan times and a large volume of data generated which may have to be manually analysed voxel by voxel. CSI is ideally suited to the study of stroke, particularly in the detection of the human penumbra. However, the complexity of image acquisition and data processing requires the availability of a dedicated spectroscopist and has limited the number of stroke studies carried out using CSI. Hence, CSI provides the promise of providing more clinically useful data than single voxel studies, but the technical demands of CSI have limited its application to stroke to date.

Basic requirements

The acquisition of a ^{1}H-MR spectrum requires the same basic equipment as that for a standard MR imaging system. The magnet must have a large enough bore to encompass a patient and be of sufficient strength (usually 1.0–1.5 T) to allow the collection of data with an adequate signal-to-noise ratio. The subject is placed within a radiofrequency coil and pulses of radiofrequency current generate a radiofrequency magnetic field which is experienced by the nuclei within the coil. Magnetic field gradients are required within the bore of the magnet to localize the signal to a well defined region (i.e. a voxel) in the same way as for imaging. Spatial localization techniques are not considered here and are more fully discussed in a review by Howe et al.[2] The signal is collected by a radio-receiver, amplified and passed to a dedicated computer which stores the signal, performs necessary calculations and displays either a spectrum or in the case of CSI, a metabolite map. The NMR pulse used for the majority of MRS experiments is the spin echo sequence.

Basic principles of MRS

Analogous to other spectroscopy methods, MR measures the effects of the transitions of nuclei between energy levels, which are induced by applying a pulse of radiofrequency (rf) radiation, corresponding to the required difference in the energy levels (Fig. 18.1). In MR, the energy difference is proportional to the magnetic field (B_0) and a constant specific to the nuclei of interest (e.g. protons), known as the gyromagnetic ratio, γ, and the radiofrequency required to cause a transition between two energy levels. This is known as the Larmor frequency. The MR equipment is described by either the magnetic field or the resonance frequency, $\omega_0 = \gamma B_0$, at that field. In vivo spectroscopy in humans is normally carried out at 1.5 T (64.2 MHz) and in animals can be carried out as high as 9.4 (400 MHz). A very few high field human systems at 2.0 and 3 T, and even one system at 7 T, are currently in use throughout the world.

In an NMR experiment, the nuclei of interest are excited at the Larmor frequency, causing the nuclei to adopt the higher energy level. At the end of the pulse of radiation the system relaxes back to thermal equilibrium at the lower energy level, by a process characterized by a longitudinal relaxation time (T_1). The resonant radiofrequency signal generated by this relaxation is known as the free induction decay. In addition to T_1 relaxation, the nuclei are relaxed due to the effects of the random variation of the magnetic fields of neighbouring nuclei, known as transverse relaxation, T_2. The signal decay described by T_2 relaxation is shorter than T_1 relaxation time. In a truly uniform magnetic field, the frequency of the signal emitted by relaxing nuclei would be identical to the exciting frequency, i.e. the

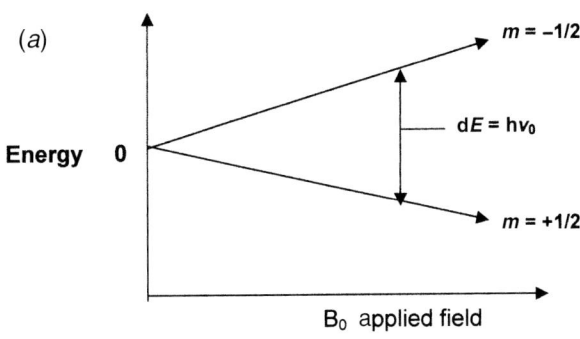

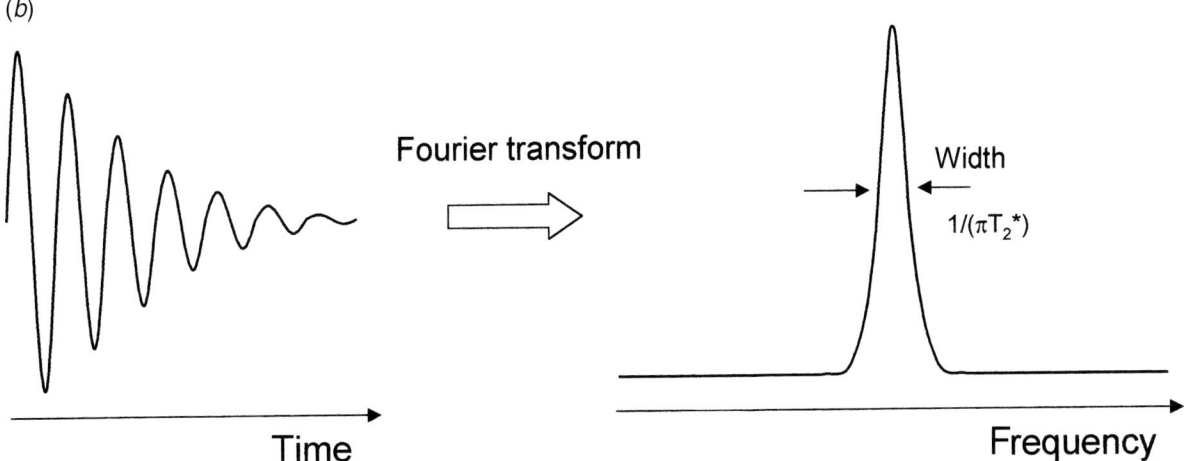

Fig. 18.1. (*a*) Diagram showing the energy level separation between the two spin states of a proton as a function of the magnetic field B_0. A higher field corresponds to a higher frequency v_0 and to a larger separation and resulting higher frequency.[40] (*b*) Correspondence between the NMR time domain signal and frequency spectrum. The signal decay rate (T_2^*) determines the spectral line width.

local frequency. However, electrons surrounding a nucleus shield it from the applied field, reducing the local field strength. The degree of reduction in the field strength depends on the strength of the chemical bonds surrounding the resonating nucleus and hence on the molecular compound containing the nucleus. The reduction in field strength results in a small change in the local resonant frequency, known as 'chemical shift'. MRS distinguishes the presence of different molecules (or different nuclei within a molecule) because of this sensitivity of the resonance frequency of magnetic nuclei to their local environment. The separation caused by chemical shift increases as the magnetic field increases. The sensitivity of a spectroscopic method is proportional to the difference between those nuclei at the higher energy level and those at the lower energy level (Fig. 18.1). MR sensitivity is low because the difference between the numbers of nuclei in these two energy states is only one per million at the field strengths currently being used clinically. As mentioned above, MRI overcomes this problem of sensitivity because water is highly concentrated in vivo (41.7 M) and the proton nucleus is 100% naturally abundant.

The various shifts in resonance associated with different metabolites in the brain result in a spectrum of resonant frequencies which is recorded during the MRS acquisition. In proton MRS, the signal contains the sum of all signals from ^1H containing nuclei that resonate close to the Larmor frequency. By Fourier transformation of the time-dependent signal the signals at different frequencies are separated and a spectrum is obtained (Fig. 18.1). The area under the peaks in the spectrum is proportional to the quantity of nuclei resonating at that frequency. In any real NMR experiment, the NMR signals decay much faster than T_2, at a rate denoted by T_2^*. This is the observed or effective T_2 relaxation and results from inhomogeneities of the static magnetic field. The larger the degree of inhomogeneity in the static magnetic field, the broader the line width of the spectral peak, and a method known as shimming is used to minimize the inhomogeneities of the magnetic field prior to the acquisition of a spectrum. The chemical shifts (δ) of a peak are expressed with respect to a reference line (v_0) and in parts per millions (ppm); $\delta = 10^6 (v-v_0)/v_0$ ppm. The large water peak is used as the reference peak in ^{1}H-MRS and by convention is assigned to be at 4.7 ppm. However, because the water peak is so much larger than that of the metabolites, it has to be suppressed and is not displayed in the spectrum or on CSI.

Water suppression techniques require an in-depth understanding of MR sequences and are beyond the scope of this chapter. The most commonly used technique is the chemical shift selective (CHESS) technique and readers requiring further information are referred to a comprehensive review of water suppression techniques.[3] The difference in the water concentration (41.7 M) compared to the metabolite concentration (2–20 mom), previously required suppression of the water signal to be of the order of 1000 to ensure visibility of the metabolite signal. These techniques required homogeneous and stable magnetic fields. Recent post processing techniques such as the HLSVD method remove the water without affecting the peaks of interest and have eliminated the need for such demanding water suppression techniques.[4]

Quantification of metabolites

To move MRS further into the clinical domain and allow the comparison of metabolite concentrations within and between institutions, automated methods of quantification need to be implemented to provide data analysis protocols for clinical studies. The concentration of detectable metabolites is directly proportional to the area under the peak of the spectra for that voxel. Early studies compared individual peak areas and peak area metabolite ratios were calculated from long echo time spectra. However, ratios can be misleading when metabolic concentrations of both the numerator and denominator peaks change in disease states. Although the majority of stroke studies have been carried out using metabolite ratios, some studies have used absolute quantification, of brain metabolites using the contralateral water as an internal standard.[5,6] In addition to the obvious advantages of absolute quantification this method allows the values to be corrected for the increased water concentration caused by cerebral edema associated with cerebral infarction.

The accuracy of the metabolite estimation depends on the accuracy of the fitting method. Various fitting routines have been incorporated in the frequency domain[7] (the conventional domain of MRS data analysis) (Fig. 18.2) and the time domain,[8,9] to overcome the problem of contributions to peak area estimates from the underlying baseline and adjacent peaks to improve the accuracy of metabolite quantification. Analysis in the time domain by the variable projection method (VARPRO) allows a smoother baseline to be obtained without subjective assumptions being made by the operator (Fig. 18.3). It has the advantage that initial data points of the frequency induction decay (FID) can be excluded from the analysis to avoid artefacts from receiver distortion and some of the contributions due to short T^2 components. The addition of prior knowledge such as peak positions, multiplet structures, and linewidths to the data analysis significantly improve the fit of the *myo*-inositol, creatine, choline, NAA and lactate peaks. 'Metabolite nulling' has been employed to simplify the spectrum and overcome the problems of the incorporation of the broad background signal into the peak area estimates of short echo proton spectroscopy (Fig. 18.4).[10]

The normal [^{1}H]-MRS spectrum (Fig. 18.2)

Histochemical and cell culture studies have shown that specific cell types or structures have metabolites that give rise to particular [^{1}H]-MRS peaks. A change in the signal intensity of the peaks may reflect loss or damage of the specific cell type or a change in the NMR visibility of the metabolite. The acquisition of long echo time data (TE = 270 ms, TR = 3 s) only allows the detection of *N*-acetylaspartate (NAA), total creatine (Cr/PCr) and choline (Cho) in the normal brain, plus lactate (Lac) in regions of

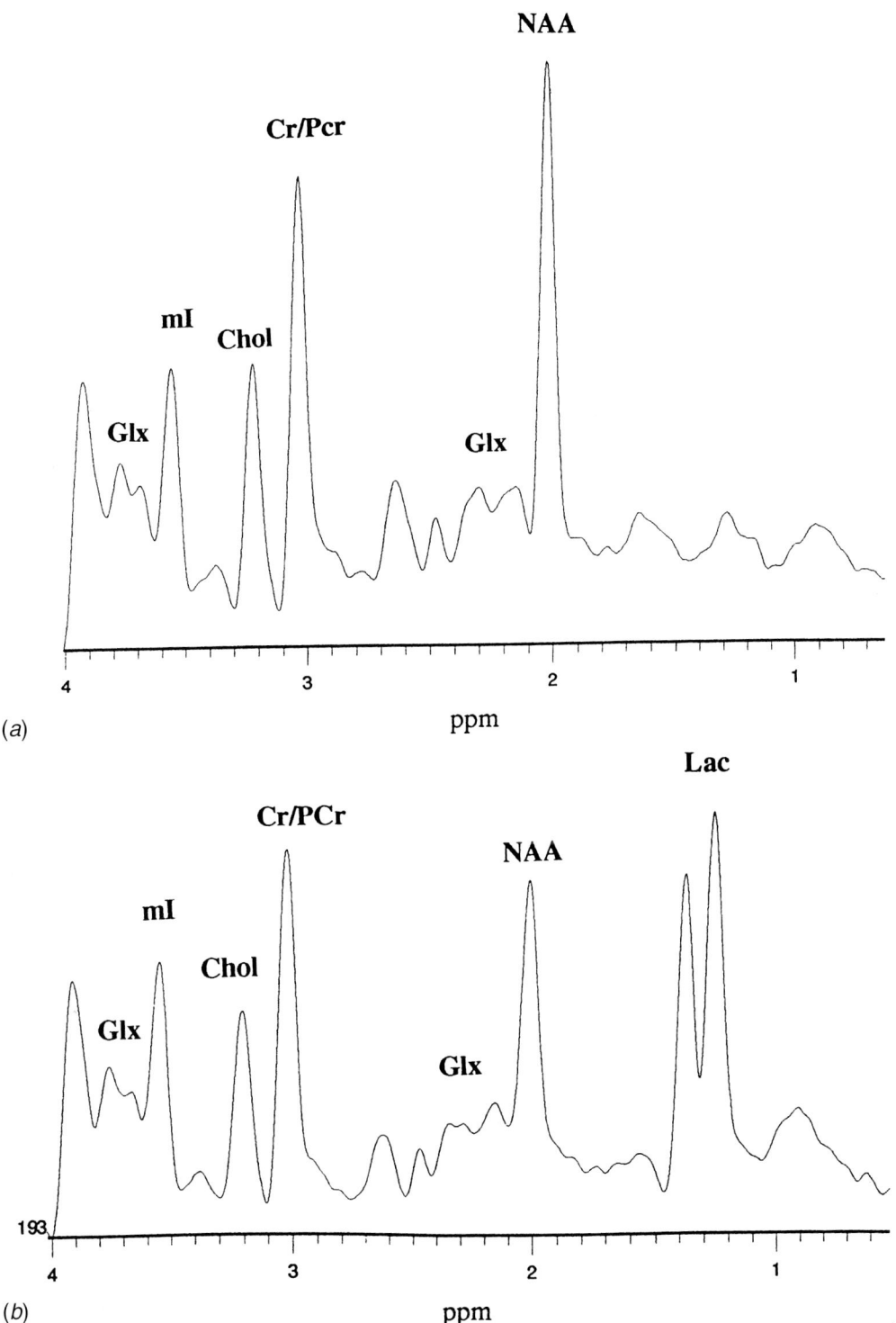

Fig. 18.2. Short echo time proton spectra (TE=30 ms, TR=2020 ms) obtained in the acute phase from the centre of an infarct (*b*) and the homologous region of the normal contralateral hemisphere (*a*). Resonance peaks are: glutamate and glutamine (Glx) at 3.8 and 2.1–2.45 parts per million (ppm), *myo*-inositol (mI) at 3.56 ppm, choline containing compounds (Chol) at 3.22 ppm, total creatine (Cr/PCr) methyl singlet at 3.03 ppm, *N*-acetyl aspartate (NAA) methyl singlet at 2.01 ppm, and lactate doublet (Lac) at 1.33 ppm. The concentration of NAA and Cr/PCr are reduced and lactate is elevated in the infarct core compared to the contralateral hemisphere.

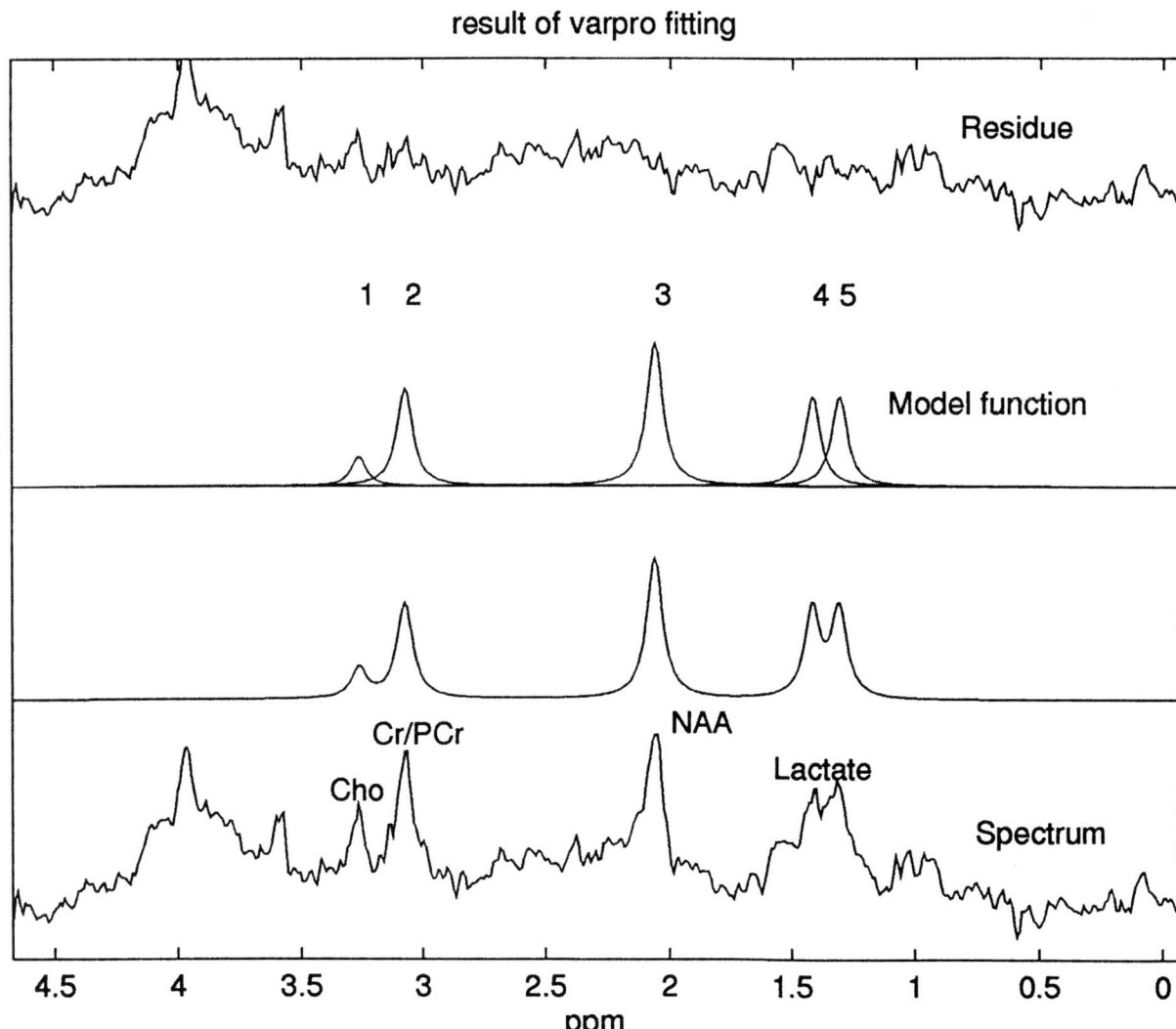

Fig. 18.3. Tracings show the variable projection (VARPRO) analysis of ^{1}H-MR spectrum (TR = 2020 ms, TE = 30 ms) from the infarct region of a stroke patient. The acquired spectrum is shown at the bottom with no line broadening. The model function is shown in the centre spectra as individual peaks (upper) and summation (lower). The residual spectrum is calculated from the difference between the model function and the acquired spectrum. This contains peaks from metabolites such as glutamate and glutamine and a broad baseline from as yet undetermined resonances. Reduction in the NAA peak and a large lactate doublet is seen in the infarct. Identification of the peaks is seen in the acquired (lower) spectrum. Cho = choline containing compounds, Cr/PCr = total creatine, NAA = N-acetyl aspartate.

ischemia. T_2 losses result in lower signal-to-noise ratios and increase the difficulty of absolute quantification, because the signal loss due to T_2 relaxation is not easily determined. The acquisition of short echo time data (TE = 30 ms, TR = 2 s) reduces the effects of signal loss due to T_2 relaxation, and therefore provides spectra with increased signal-to-noise ratios. Short echo time spectroscopy detects additional complex resonances from metabolites such as *myo*-inositol (mI), glutamate and glutamine (Glu). These are not seen at long echo times because the signals from these metabolites cancel due to phase modulation ('J-coupling'). Whilst providing more information, short echo time data

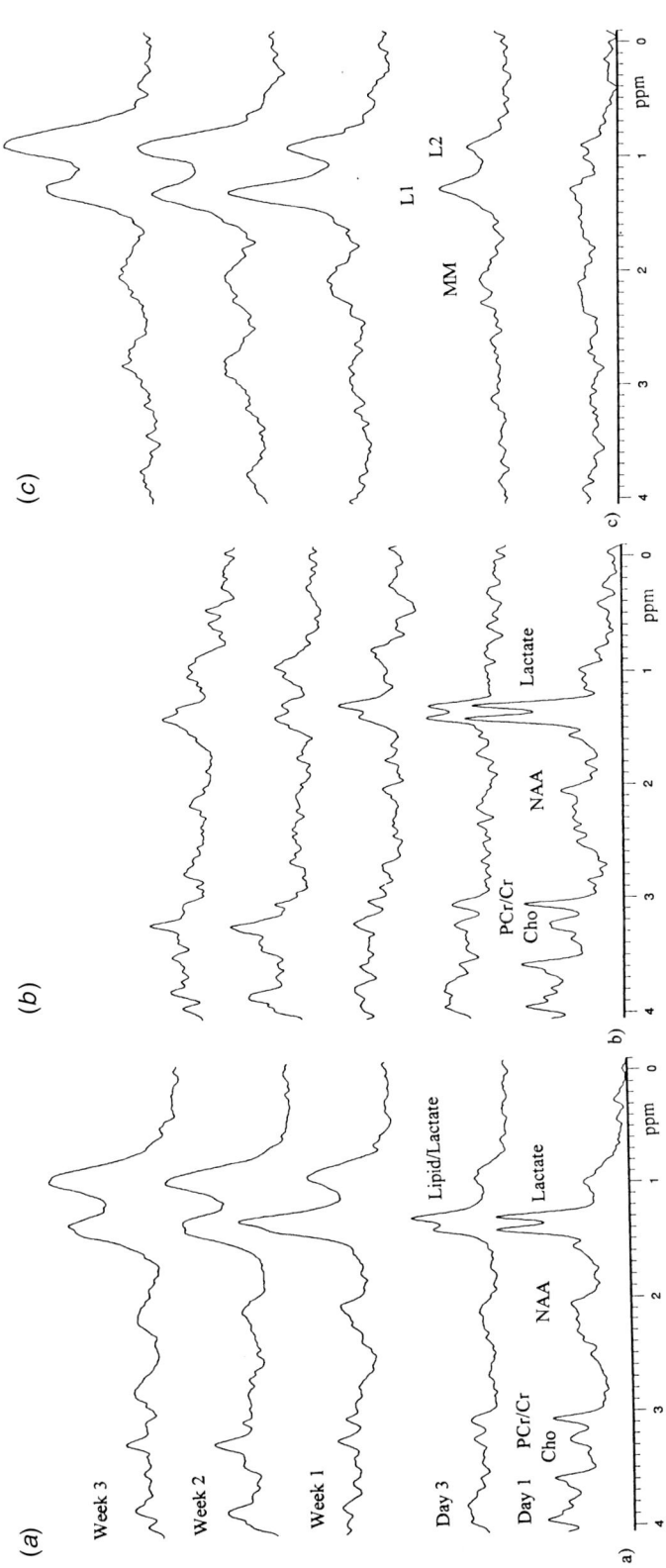

Fig. 18.4. Longitudinal data acquired from a 35-year-old patient 24 hours to 3 weeks after infarction. (*a*) The 'standard' spectra showing a large lipid peak developing under the lactate doublet within 3 days of stroke onset. (*b*) The 'difference' spectra or 'pure metabolite' spectrum obtained by subtracting the 'metabolite nulled' spectra from the 'standard' spectra. (*c*) The 'metabolite nulled' spectra acquired from the underlying lipids/macromolecules and showing a large peak at the position of the lactate doublet (1.33 ppm). Cr/PCr = total creatine, Cho = choline containing compounds, NAA = *N*-acetyl aspartate, MM = macromolecules, L1 and L2 = lipid-containing compounds.

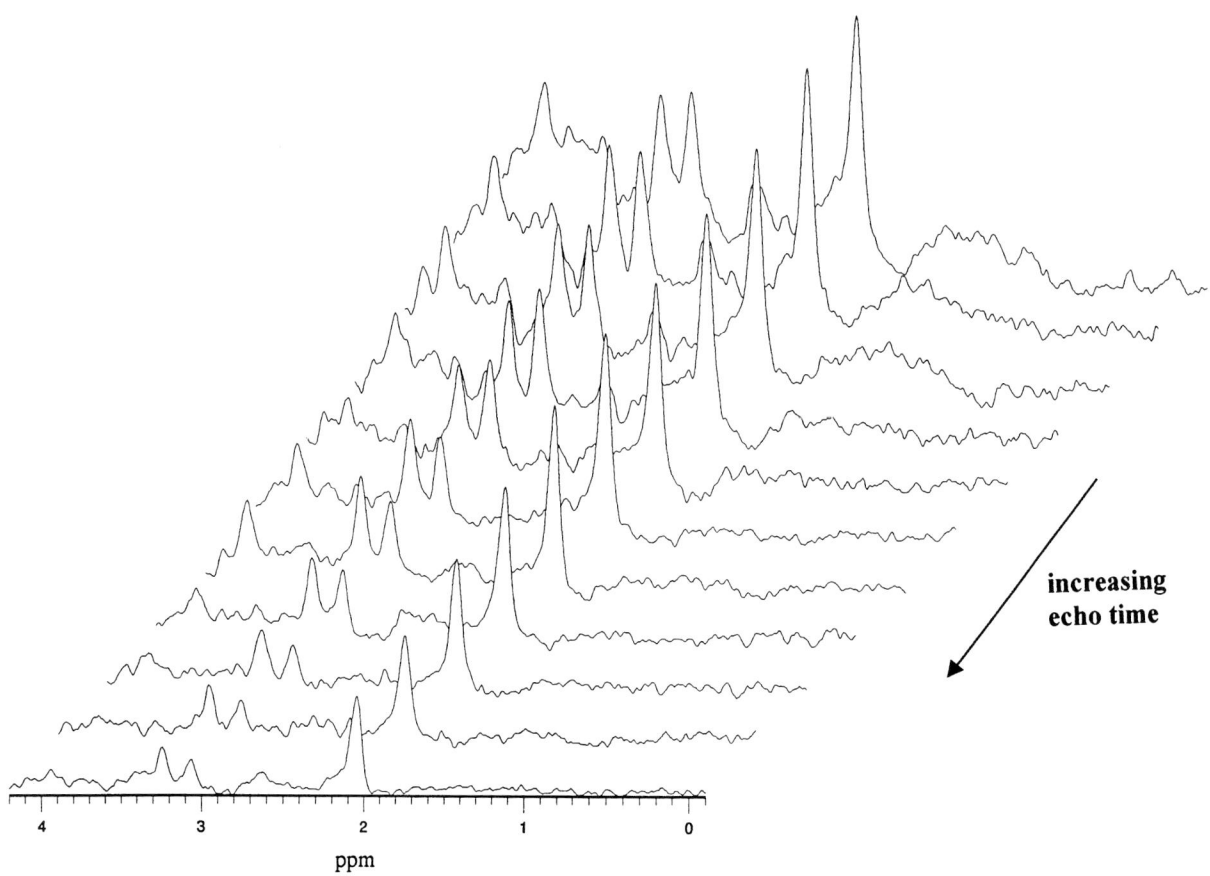

Fig. 18.5. In vivo ^{1}H-MR spectra acquired from the parietal white matter of a normal volunteer as a function of echo times at 30, 40, 50, 90, 120, 160, 220, 290, 360 and 408 ms and scaled together. The signal decreases as the echo time increases due to T_2 losses, and contributions from the baseline diminish as the echo time increases.

include a broad background signal consisting of low concentration metabolites, and macromolecules and lipids with short T_2 relaxation times, which increases the difficulty of accurate peak area estimation. Therefore, both the signal and the contribution from the baseline diminish as the echo time increases (Fig. 18.5).

N-acetyl aspartate (2.01 ppm)

The methyl resonance of NAA produces a large, sharp peak at 2.01 ppm. NAA is almost exclusively confined to neurons in the human brain, where it is found predominantly in axons and nerve processes.[11] It has been found in the oligodendrocyte type II astrocyte progenitor cell in rats,[12] but these cells represent only 2–3 % of the glial population in man.[13] The NAA peak therefore acts as a marker of healthy neurons. Reduction in the size of the NAA peak provides a useful indicator of neuronal disease or loss, including infarction after stroke. NAA was first identified in 1956, and there has been a large body of literature on its synthesis and distribution reviewed by Birken and Oldendorf[14] and Williams.[15] However, although NAA is very prominent in MRS, its function remains unknown.

In children, the interpretation of the NAA signal is complicated by increases in the concentration of NAA during development[16] when it is thought to have a role in supplying acetyl groups for myelin synthesis.[15] In adults, the concentration is known to vary in different areas in the brain. For example, the concentration of NAA is higher in grey than white matter, which is explained by the higher neuronal density in grey matter.[17] This can be overcome in the study of stroke patients by comparing spectra from an area of suspected abnormality with spectra from a homologous region of the contralateral normal hemisphere.[5]

Creatine (3.94 and 3.03 ppm)

Both creatine and phosphocreatine have signals at 3.94 ppm (methylene singlet) and 3.03 ppm (methyl singlet) which makes it impossible to distinguish between the two compounds and therefore total creatine (Cr/PCr) signals are measured by [^{1}H]-MRS. Other resonances seen at 3.00 ppm arise from the γ-amino butyric acid (GABA)[18] and cytosolic macromolecules, which become incorporated into the Cr/PCr peak.[19,20] Cr/PCr is found in both neurones and glial cells[13] and acts as a phosphate buffer transport system and energy buffer within the cell. Little information can be gleaned about phosphocreatine metabolism because the signal comes from the sum of creatine and phosphocreatine. The complete absence of creatine signal probably reflects necrotic tissue, but the interpretation of reduced total creatine levels is uncertain at present.

Choline (3.22 ppm)

The trimethylamine resonance of choline-containing compounds is present at 3.22 ppm. In normal brain, the Cho peak is thought to consist predominantly of glycerolphosphocholine and phosphocholine. Both compounds are involved in membrane synthesis and degradation.[21] Taurine and the N-CH$_2$ resonance of phosphoryletholamine will also contribute to the signal.[15] Reduction in the choline peak has been proposed as a marker of membrane damage.

Lipid/macromolecule resonances

Lipid peaks are detectable by short echo proton spectroscopy but are not seen at long echo times because they have short T$_2$ decay constants and so the signal is lost at longer repetition times. Lipid/macromolecule peaks have been assigned at 0.9, 1.3 and 1.45 ppm in normal appearing brain.[6,22] Increase in these resonances have been reported in stroke[6] and demyelination.[22,23] The 0.9 and 1.3 ppm resonances are assigned to the methylene and methyl groups of lipid, respectively.[24] Recent work in animal models has shown that contributions to these resonances also arise from mobile protons,[20] and correlate with the peaks found in humans.[10] The significance of these peaks is as yet unknown and may only represent increased MRS visibility of cell membrane lipids following cell breakdown. The assignment of these signals will, however, influence the interpretation of proton spectra obtained from the cerebral cortex.

[^{1}H]-MRS changes in cerebral ischemia

MRS in patients with stroke has largely been limited to the study of cerebral ischemia. The most striking changes in patients with acute cerebral infarction on MRS is the appearance of lactate with reduction in NAA and total Cr/PCr within the infarct compared to the contralateral hemisphere.[5] Large variations in the initial concentrations of Cho have been observed in the region of infarction.[5,25] These changes are described in detail below.

The presence of a significant quantity of blood in the brain disrupts the homogeneity of the magnetic field due to the presence of the iron from the hemoglobin molecule, and spectroscopy cannot be carried out in patients with large intracerebral hemorrhages. However, it is possible to sufficiently shim the magnetic field away from areas of hemorrhagic transformation or subarachnoid hemorrhage and acquire spectra of acceptable linewidths. Petechial hemorrhage may result in spectra with broader line widths due to field inhomogeneity, but the spectra may still be of acceptable quality.

Lactate (doublet at 1.33 ppm)

The detection of lactate on MRS, an end product of glycolysis, is a particularly useful measure of anaerobic metabolism. Lactate is not detected by MRS in normal brain. The concentration of lactate rises when the glycolytic rate exceeds the tissue's capacity to catabolize it or remove it from the bloodstream. The rise in brain lactate that results from the mismatch between glycolysis and oxygen supply has been demonstrated by numerous [^{1}H]-MRS experiments, making it an important hallmark for the detection of cerebral ischemia.[5,25,26]

The persistence of lactate for weeks or months after stroke onset is a common observation.[5,26] Removal of lactate depends on the permeability of the blood–brain barrier (BBB) and diffusion of the metabolite through the damaged tissue. A fall in lactate concentration has been shown to occur during a period of hyperemia.[26] Using [1–^{13}C]-labelled glucose, the metabolic activity of the lactate pool associated with a 32-day-old infarct has demonstrated that all the cerebral lactate arises from the glycolysis of serum glucose. This supports the hypothesis that elevated lactate is the product of ongoing lactate synthesis in the brain.[27] It is not possible to establish whether this originates from tissue which is still ischemic after stroke onset or comes from metabolically active macrophages, which have infiltrated the infarct. The presence of lactate beyond the time in which active phagocytosis occurs supports the theory of persistently ischemic tissue in some cases.[28]

Spectroscopic imaging studies have demonstrated that lactate is not confined to areas of infarction determined by T_2-weighted imaging and in one study was even found in the contralateral hemisphere.[29] In this study, the lactate levels in regions adjacent to infarcts as shown by T_2 changes were not significantly different from those found in the infarcted brain. It seems likely that this is the result of diffusion of lactate out of the infarct, but the extent to which there is local production of lactate in peri-infarct tissue remains uncertain.

NAA (2.01 ppm)

The concentration of NAA is almost invariably reduced within the core of cerebral infarction, when measured within 24 hours of onset. Longitudinal studies in humans have demonstrated a further decline in NAA concentration following the initial reductions in NAA detected in the first spectra after the onset of cerebral infarction (Fig. 18.6).[5,25,26] The continuing fall in NAA concentration over the course of the first week after stroke onset cannot be explained simply by an increase in edema because changes in the concentration of water within the infarct have been corrected for by using the contralateral water signal as the internal standard.[5] It has been suggested that NAA is actively degraded by enzymes within the injured neurones in the first few days or hours following infarction.[23] This remains a possibility but it seems unlikely that enzymes would remain active for up to 7–10 days within an ischemic neurone. The gradual decline in NAA concentration and the persistence of lactate within the region of infarction over a period of a number of days may suggest a period of ongoing ischemia[5] and has implications in the timing of therapeutic intervention. Alternatively, it may reflect breakdown of NAA, removal by phagocytosis or diffusion, or alteration in the physicochemical surrounding of the metabolite associated with cell dissolution so that it is no longer MRS visible.

Cr/PCr (3.94 and 3.03 ppm)

Initial reductions in Cr/PCr are identified following infarction and further reductions have been demonstrated up to 10 days following the time of onset.[5] The pathological correlate is thought to be gliosis of the tissue. The reduction in NAA in the infarct region is more marked than the reduction in Cr/PCr and this is thought to reflect the increased sensitivity of neurons to ischemia, compared to glial tissue.

Choline (3.22 ppm)

The choline peak has been shown to be increased, decreased and stay the same following cerebral infarction.[5,25,26] The changes in the choline peak are thought to reflect changes in the MR visibility of the choline containing compounds that make up the cell membrane. We have shown a fall and then a late rise, maximal 3 months after onset of stroke.[5] This may represent loss of membrane function, followed by late gliosis.

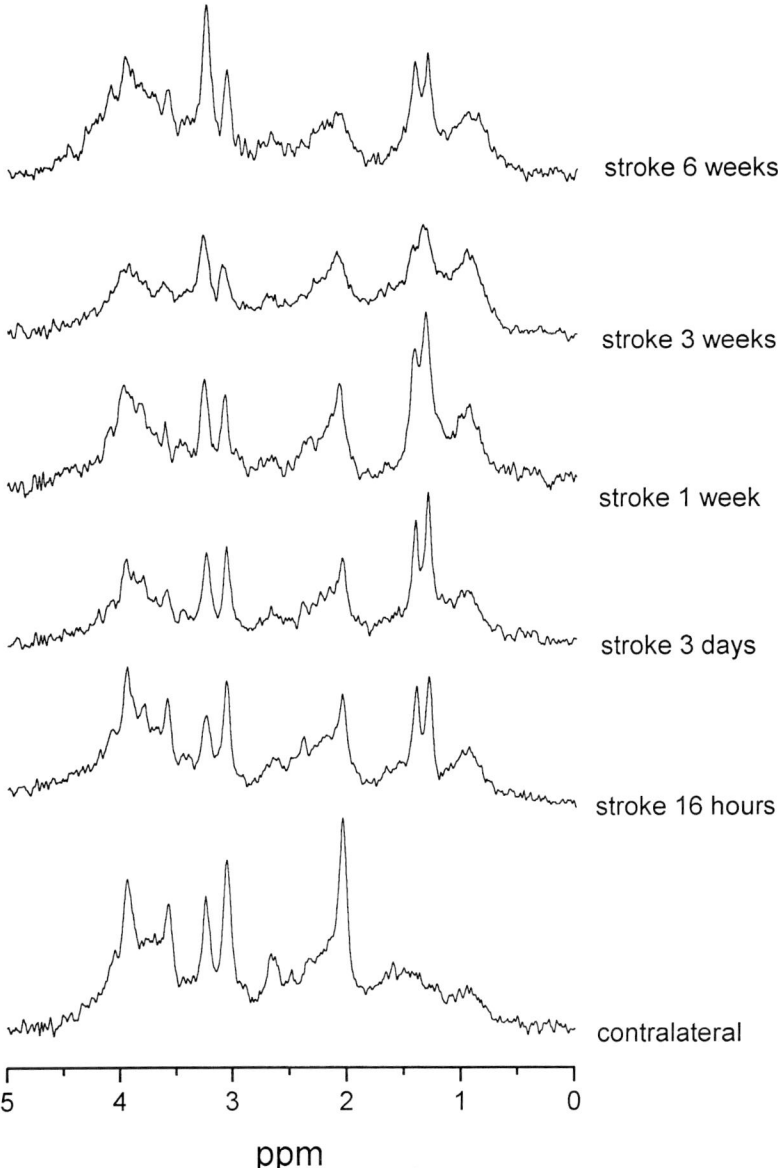

Fig. 18.6. A longitudinal study of MRS in a 32-year-old women from the core of a middle cerebral infarct. NAA and Cr/PCr continue to fall over 6 weeks following infarction. Lactate is visible within 16 hours and persists for 6 weeks. The lactate peak can be seen to increase further with some contribution from underlying lipids. Choline increases up to 6 weeks which reflects increased visibility of choline containing compounds within the membrane due to cell necrosis (see Fig. 18.2 for peak assignment).

Glutamate and other amino acids

It would be useful to be able to measure the concentration of excitotoxic amino acids, such as glutamate and glutamine, which are released in ischemia and may be responsible for neuronal injury in the penumbra. Glutamate and glutamine have strongly coupled spins and the chemical shift of 2.1–2.5 ppm at 1.5T overlaps with the NAA peak. Other amino acids, such as GABA, aspartate and alanine are also difficult to detect because of their low concentrations and/or overlap with more intense resonances from other compounds.[30] To date, there is very little work in cerebral ischemia on the detection of glutamate and glutamine in humans, reflecting the difficulty of spectral analysis. Higher strength fields may improve our ability to detect these neurotransmitters, which will be particularly relevant to the study of the ischemic penumbra.

Lipids/macromolecules

Signals from lipids pose particular problems in [^{1}H]-MRS by obscuring the resonances from the methyl group of lactate. It has been postulated that membrane lipids in the brain under normal conditions are not mobile enough to generate sharp spectral peaks in vivo. During ischemia, degradation of the membrane leads to the release of free fatty acids that produce well defined, but broad, resonances in the region of the lactate peak with resulting difficulties in the accurate quantification of lactate. The 'metabolite nulling' technique has been used to separate the lipid from the lactate signal.[6,10] The technique is based on the observation that lipids and macromolecule signals have short T_1 relaxation times (100–200 ms), whereas highly mobile metabolites have long T_1 relaxation times (1,200–2,000 ms). Using the inversion recovery technique, metabolite-nulled spectra are obtained that contain the signal from lipids and macromolecules with minimal contribution from the smaller highly mobile metabolites. The difference between a standard and metabolite-nulled short echo time spectrum yields a difference spectrum composed of narrow metabolite peaks with the lipids and macromolecule resonances removed thereby allowing the accurate quantitation of lactate and other metabolites. In addition, the metabolite-nulled spectra allow the separate evaluation of the changes in lipids and macromolecules (Fig. 18.4).

Reversible changes detected by [^{1}H]-MRS

The identification of the ischemic penumbra by [^{1}H]-MRS depends on the observation of the reversibility of metabolic changes within the region of infarction. Spectroscopy studies have reported a reversible reduction of NAA in acute multiple sclerosis lesions[22,23,31] and mitochondrial encephalopathy with lactic acidosis and stroke-like episodes (MELAS).[31] CSI studies in MELAS have observed high levels of lactate return to undetectable levels, in normal appearing regions of the brain separate from the areas of infarction. Although slight reductions in NAA were later observed, the presence of high lactate concentrations did not result in complete infarction.[29] In MELAS the primary defect is mitochondrial and, as NAA is synthesized in mitochondria, the results suggest that the reversibility of NAA reflects metabolic impairment of synthesis rather than ischemic damage to cells. Similarly, it has been suggested that, in the demyelinating lesions of multiple sclerosis, the function of the mitochondria is reversibly impaired during inflammation resulting in the reversible reduction of the production of NAA within the damaged neurone.[22] No convincing reports of reversible NAA within the core of cerebral infarction have been published. However, we have observed reversible falls in NAA concentration at the edge of infarcts in patients recovering from stroke in association with reciprocal change in lactate concentration (Fig. 18.7).[32] The interpretation of these changes is uncertain but they may represent recovery in the penumbra, stunned neurons, a toxic effect of lactate or the effects of neuronal disconnection.

Prediction of outcome

Selection and comparison of treatments for acute stroke would be facilitated by more accurate prediction of stroke outcome from early MR studies. In our studies, we have shown that infarct volume determined by T_2-weighted images is a fairly good predictor of outcome in patients with cortical infarction within the middle cerebral artery territory. Patients with large infarcts invariably did badly, while patients with small infarcts (<80 cm^3) all survived until the 3 months follow-up study.[33] However, some patients with small infarcts remained severely disabled, while others made a

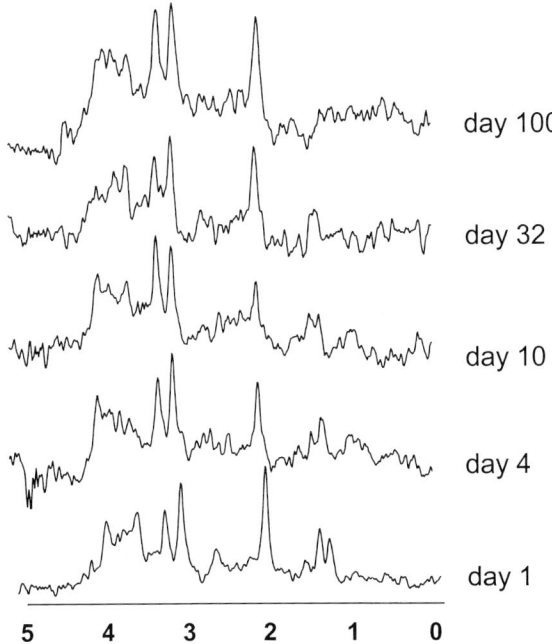

Fig. 18.7. Serial MRS recorded 6 hours after onset (day 1) to 3 months after onset (100 days) from identical voxels placed at the edge of a middle cerebral artery infarct. At onset, the patient had severe dysphasia and hemiparesis. His condition was similar at the day 4 and 10 examinations, but by day 32 he had improved considerably and by day 100 he was communicating well and was independently mobile. The spectra show a decline in the NAA peak associated with the presence of lactate up to day 10, followed by a recovery in NAA as the lactate disappears.

good recovery. The addition of the core NAA concentration to infarct volume allowed better prediction of patients' outcome, than either NAA concentration or infarct volume alone.[34] For example, in patients with infarcts smaller than 70 cm^3, low NAA (<7 mmol) in the initial scan predicted poor outcome (dead or dependent), while preserved NAA (>7 mmol) predicted independent recovery. In contrast, all patients with large infarct volumes (>70 cm^3) were dead or dependent at 3 months, irrespective of the initial NAA concentration. In another small number of serially studied patients, the best recovery was also seen in those patients with relatively preserved NAA, total creatine and choline peaks.[35]

The importance of lactate in the pathogenesis of cerebral infarction has been studied extensively. The degree and extent of tissue damage has been correlated with the content of lactic acid in animals,[36] and an increase in morbidity and mortality in hyperglycemic animals has been linked to excessive lactate production and the resulting acidosis.[37] The correlation of lactate with outcome in humans has been variable. Although, a single study has shown lactate to correlate with acute stroke severity and outcome,[25] other studies have failed to demonstrate a relationship between outcome and infarct lactate concentration.[34] In a study of 50 patients, large infarcts were associated with high lactate and reduced NAA but not the clinical stroke syndrome, timing of the scan, blood velocity measured by Doppler ultrasound, or amount of infarct swelling.[38] This work agreed with earlier work in a cat cerebral infarct model that demonstrated that animals with the largest and most prolonged reductions in cerebral blood flow developed the largest infarcts, but the amount of edema in the infarct varied between animals and was independent of the amount of lactate detected in the infarct.[37] The likely explanation for the discrepancy in the literature between the animal and many of the human studies is that completely occluded middle cerebral artery animal models may not have similar rates of lactate generation and clearance compared with human stroke, where there is often partial vessel occlusion and collateral flow.[39] Another very likely reason is the varying time points at which stroke patients are studied, often a day or more after onset. It is well known that lactate concentrations decrease after infarction at a variable rate over the subsequent few days and weeks.[5]

Understanding disability

There is often a poor correlation between the size of chronic cerebral infarction and persisting deficit. MRS has the potential to provide useful information to improve our understanding of the mechanisms underlying recovery and persistent

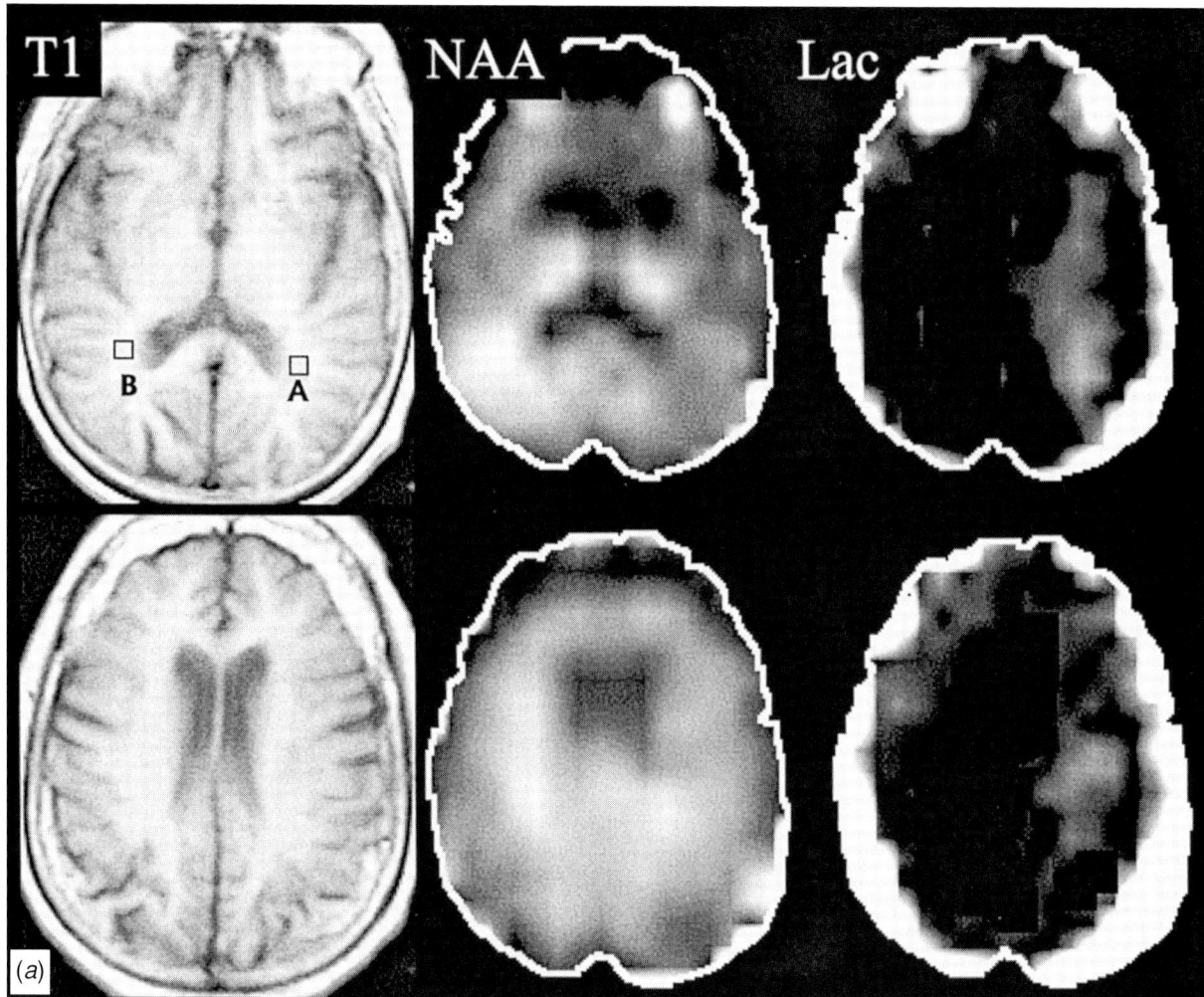

Fig. 18.8. Selected slices from multimodal imaging acquired from an 83-year-old woman who presented with global aphasia, right hemianopia and hemiparesis. T_1 images and chemical shift images (CSI) show the distribution of NAA and lactate at two levels (a). Single voxels have been selected from the CSI grid as marked on the T_1 images, at sites A in the infarct and B in the contralateral normal hemisphere, and the individual spectra displayed (b). T_2 images, apparent diffusion coefficient (ADC) maps and perfusion imaging were recorded on the same occasion (c). Follow-up T_2 images were obtained at 3 months following very little recovery (d). The sequences show that lactate was elevated in the initial CSI map in an area of the middle cerebral artery territory which was much larger than the areas of reduced NAA and abnormal T_2 signal. The single voxel MRS confirms elevated lactate and reduced NAA and creatine in the infarct compared to the contralateral hemisphere. The perfusion deficit is larger than the area of increased T_2 and restricted diffusion and corresponds more closely to the distribution of lactate on the CSI map. The final area of infarction at 3 months also corresponds better to the area of increased lactate and reduced perfusion. (Figure courtesy of Dr Peter Barker, Johns Hopkins University Hospital, Baltimore, Maryland, USA.)

disability. Measuring just the size of an infarct does not take into account variations in lesion location or shape. Recent work using a mask of the corticospinal tract and spectroscopy demonstrated that the maximal cross-sectional overlap of the corticospinal tracts and the infarct showed a more linear relationship to motor deficit and axonal injury, as measured by the loss of NAA from the internal capsule, than did the stroke volume.[40]

Magnetic resonance spectroscopy in stroke 247

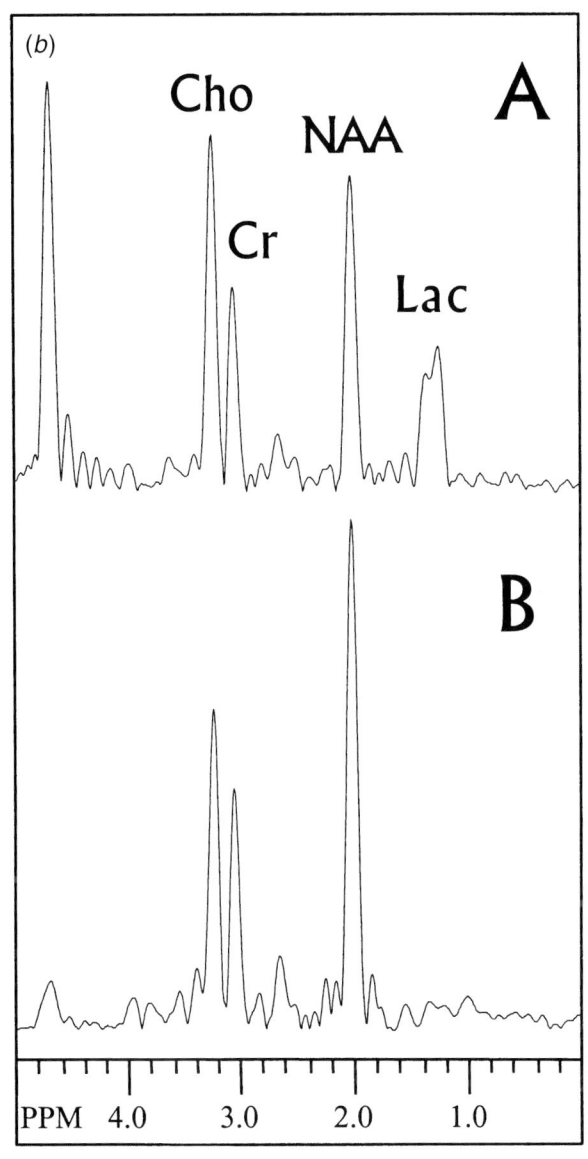

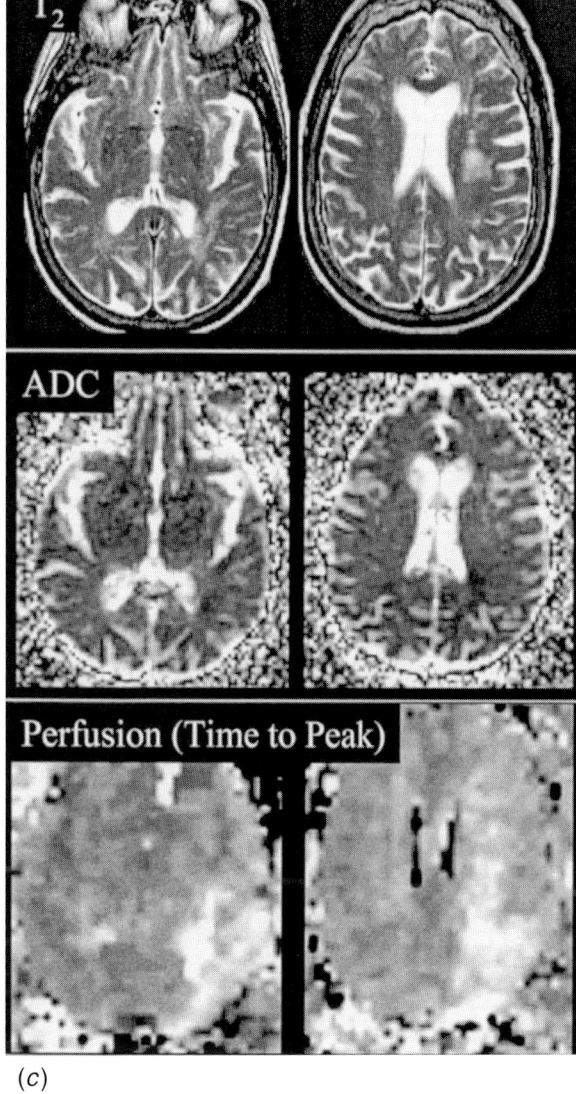

Fig. 18.8. (cont.)

Selection of patients for treatment

The addition of [^{1}H]- MRS to diffusion and perfusion imaging studies of acute stroke may well improve the utility of multimodal imaging (Fig. 18.8). An important role for new MR techniques is likely to be in the selection of patients for thrombolysis or new neuroprotective agents. In an elegant study of 19 patients in whom diffusion-weighted imaging was combined with single voxel [^{1}H]-MRS, a strong correlation was found between patients' clinical outcome and the acute (mean 11.1 hours) and subacute (mean 3.9 days) lactate/choline ratios. This was better than the correlation of outcome with NAA/choline ratios or infarct volume. The correlation with outcome improved further when the lactate/choline ratio was combined with the acute DWI lesion volume. The authors postulate that the lactate producing cells are a marker for tissue that will ultimately infarct in the absence of intervention.[39] Clearly, such changes might identify candidates for

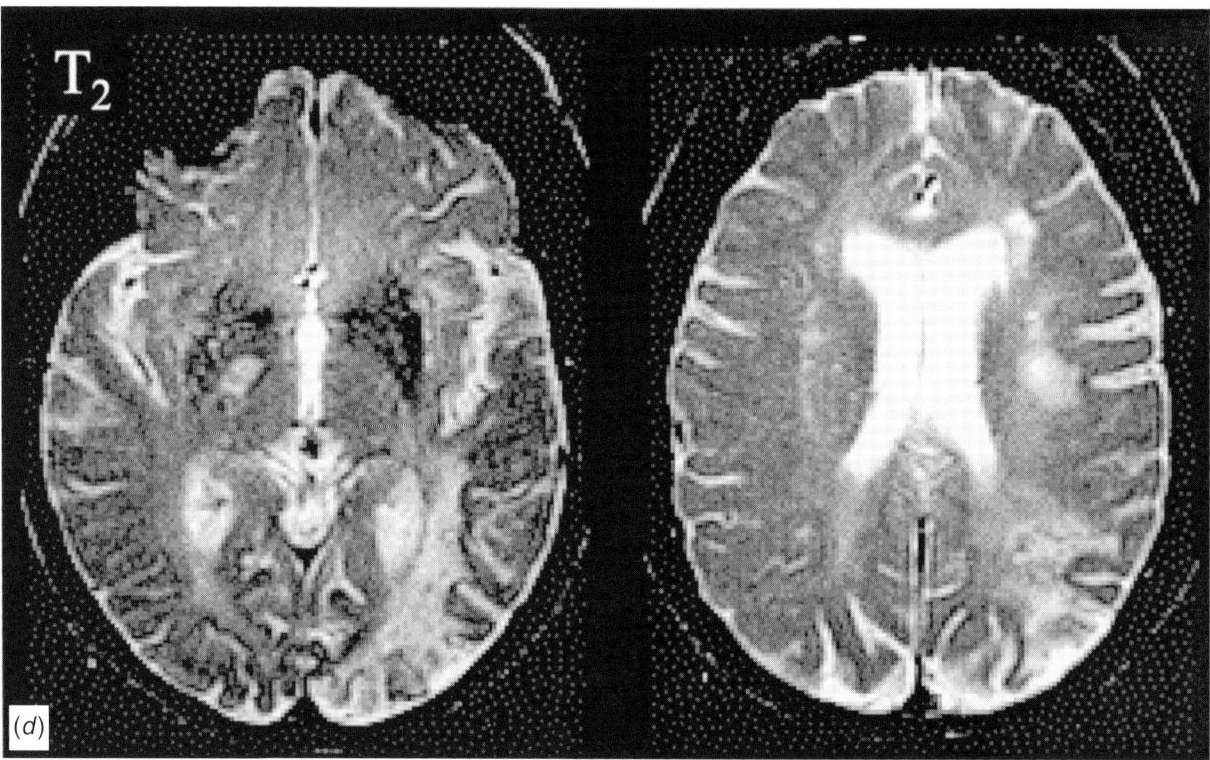

Fig. 18.8. (*cont.*)

thrombolysis or neuroprotective therapy. The effect of thrombolytic therapy on metabolic changes within regions of ischemia have been demonstrated in animals but there is little published work in man. In a study using a rat stroke model, an improvement of perfusion and a reduction of the area of elevated lactate was demonstrated only after short treatment delays.[41] Of particular interest to the treatment of humans, the authors demonstrated a critical value for the lactate/NAA ratio of 0.7 independent of the treatment delay above which metabolic recovery was not seen.

Conclusions

MR spectroscopy and multivoxel MR spectroscopic imaging have proven to be valuable tools in the study of cerebrovascular disease. Their role in the detection of potentially salvageable ischemic tissue suitable for treatment with thrombolytic and neuroprotective agents has not yet been fully realized in humans. The combined use of diffusion-weighted and perfusion imaging with [^{1}H]-MRS may have value in the diagnosis of acute stroke, especially when diffusion-weighted imaging is negative. The ability of multivoxel CSI to detect changes throughout the brain makes it the most suitable spectroscopic technique for the study of cerebral ischemia. Further development of CSI and data processing techniques are required to move the use of spectroscopy further into the clinical domain. It is likely that the development of high field strength single voxel MRS will provide interesting data from the analyses of additional metabolites in stroke.

ACKNOWLEDGEMENT

Franklyn Howe PhD kindly contributed to the description of the physics of MRS.

REFERENCES

1 Webb PG, Sailasuta N, Kohler SJ, Raidy T, Moats RA, Hurd R. Automated single voxel proton MRS: technical development and multisite variation. *Magn Res Med* 1994; 31, 365–373.

2 Howe FA, Maxwell RJ, Saunders DE, Brown MM, Griffiths JR: Proton spectroscopy *in vivo*. *Magn Reson Q* 1993, 9: 31–59.

3 Van Zijl PCM, Moonen CTW. Solvent suppression strategies for in vivo spectroscopy. *NMR Basic Princ Progr* 1992; 26: 67–108.

4 Pijnappel WWF, van den Boogaart A, de Beer R, van Ormondt. SVD based quantification of magnetic resonance signals. *J Magn Reson* 1992; 97: 122–134.

5 Saunders DE, Howe FA, van den Boogaart A, McLean MA, Griffiths JR, Brown MM. Continuing ischaemic damage following acute middle cerebral artery infarction in man demonstrated by short echo proton spectroscopy. *Stroke* 1995; 26: 1007–1013.

6 Saunders DE, Howe FA, van den Boogaart A, Griffiths JR, Brown MM. Discrimination of metabolite from lipid and macromolecule resonances in cerebral infarction using short echo proton spectroscopy. *J Magn Reson Imaging* 1997; 7: 1116–1121.

7 Provencher SW. Estimation of metabolite concentrations from localised in vivo proton NMR spectra. *Magn Reson Med* 1993; 30: 672–679.

8 de Beer R, van Ormondt D, Pijnappel WWF, van der Veen JWC. Quantitative analysis of magnetic resonance signals in the time domain. *Isr J Chem* 1988; 28: 249–261.

9 van der Veen JWC, de Beer R, Luyten PR, van Ormondt D. Accurate quantification of in vivo ^{31}P NMR signals using the variable projection method and prior knowledge. *Magn Reson Med* 1988; 6: 92–98.

10 Behar KL, Rothamn DL, Spencer DD, Petroff OAC. Analysis of macromolecule resonances in ^{1}H-NMR spectra in human brain. *Magn Reson Med* 1994; 32: 292–302.

11 Tallan HH, Moore S, Stein WH. *N*-acetyl-L-aspartic acid in the brain. *J Biochem* 1956; 219: 257–264.

12 Urenjak J, Williams SR, Gadian DG, Noble M. Proton magnetic resonance spectroscopy unambiguously identifies different neural cell types. *J Neurosci* 1993; 13: 981–989.

13 Wolswijk G, Munro PMG, Riddle PN, Noble M. Origin growth factor responses, and ultrastructure characteristics of an adult-specific glial progenitor-cell. *Ann NY Acad Sci* 1991; 633: 502–504.

14 Birken DL, Oldendorf WH. *N*-acetyl-L-aspartic acid: a literature review of a compound prominent in ^{1}H-NMR spectroscopic studies of the brain. *Neurosci Biobehav Rev* 1989; 13: 23–31.

15 Williams SR. In vivo proton spectroscopy. Experimental aspects and potentials. In: Rudin M, Seelig J. (eds). *NMR – Basic Principles and Progress: In Vivo Magnetic Resonance Spectroscopy*. Heidelberg: Springer, 1992; 55–72.

16 Kreis R, Ernst T, Ross BD. Development of the human brain: in vivo quantification of metabolite and water content with proton magnetic resonance spectroscopy. *Magn Res Med* 1993; 30: 424–427.

17 Kreis R, Ernst T, Ross BD. Absolute quantification of water and metabolites in the human brain. II Metabolite concentrations. *J Magn Reson* 1993; 102: 9–19.

18 Rothman DL, Petroff OAC, Behar KL, Mattson RH. Localised ^{1}H-NMR measurements of γ-amino butyric acid in human brains *in vivo*. *Proc Natl Acad Sci USA* 1993; 90: 5662–5666.

19 Behar KL, Ogino T. Characterisation of macromolecule resonances in the ^{1}H-NMR spectrum of rat brain. *Magn Reson Med* 1993; 30: 38–44.

20 Kauppinen RA, Kokko H, Williams SR. Detection of mobile proteins by proton magnetic resonance spectroscopy in the guinea pig brain *ex vivo* and their partial purification. *J Neurochem* 1992; 58: 967–974.

21 Miller BL. A review of chemical issues in ^{1}H-NMR spectroscopy; *N*-acetyl-L-aspartate, creatine and choline. *NMR Biomed* 1991; 4: 47–52.

22 Davie CA, Hawkins CP, Barker GJ, Tofts PS, Miller DH, McDonald WI. Serial proton magnetic resonance spectroscopy in acute multiple sclerosis lesions. *Brain* 1994; 117: 49–58.

23 Arnold DL, Matthews PM, Francis GS, O'Connor J, Antel JP. Proton magnetic resonance spectroscopic imaging for metabolic characterisation of demyelinating plaques. *Ann Neurol* 1992; 31: 235–241.

24 May GL, Wright LC, Holmes KT et al. Assignment of methylene proton magnetic resonances in NMR spectra of embryonic and transformed cells to plasma triglyceride. *J Biol Chem* 1986; 261: 3048–3053.

25 Graham GD, Blamire AM, Rothman DL et al. Early temporal variation of cerebral metabolites after human stroke. A proton magnetic resonance spectroscopy study. *Stroke* 1993; 24: 1891–1896.

26 Gideon P, Henrikson O, Sperling B et al. Early time course of *N*-acetyl aspartate, creatine and phosphocreatine, and compounds containing choline in the brain after acute stroke. A proton magnetic resonance study. *Stroke* 1992; 23: 1566–1572.

27 Rothman DL, Howseman AM, Graham GD et al. Localised proton NMR observation of (3-^{13}C)-lactate in stroke after (1-^{13}C)-glucose infusion. *Magn Reson Med* 1991; 21: 302–307.

28 Houkin K, Kwee IL, Nakada T. Persistent high lactate level as a sensitive MR spectroscopy of complete infarction. *Brain Pathol* 1994; 4: 23–36.

29 Gilliard JH, Barker PB, van Zijl PCM, Bryan RN, Oppenheimer SM. Proton MR spectroscopy in acute middle cerebral artery stroke. *Am J Neuroradiol* 1996; 17: 873–886.

30 Williams SR. Cerebral amino acids studied by nuclear magnetic resonance spectroscopy in vivo. *Progr Nucl Magn Reson Spectr* 1999; 34: 301–326.

31 De Stafano N, Matthews PM, Arnold DL. Reversible decreases in *N*-acetyl aspartate after acute brain injury. *Magn Reson Med* 1995; 34: 721–727.

32 Pereira AC. Magnetic resonance imaging and ^{1}H spectroscopy in stroke. MD Thesis, Cambridge 1999.

33 Saunders DE, Clifton A, Brown MM. The value of MR imaging in determining the prognosis of acute stroke. *Stroke* 1995; 26: 2272–2276.

34 Pereira AC, Saunders DE, Doyle VL et al. Measurement of initial *N*-acetyl aspartate concentration using MRS and initial infarct volume using MRI predicts outcome in patients with middle cerebral artery territory infarcts. *Stroke* 1999, 30: 1577–1582.

35 Ford CC, Griffey RH, Matwiywoff NA, Rosenberg GA. Multi-voxel ^{1}H-MRS of stroke. *Neurology* 1992; 42: 1408–1412.

36 Pulsinelli WA, Waldman S, Rawlinson D, Plum F. Moderate hyperglycaemia augments ischaemic brain damage: a neuropathologic study in the rat. *Neurology* 1982; 32: 1239–1246.

37 Siemkowicz E, Gjedde A. Post ischaemic coma in rats: effect of different pre-ischaemic blood glucose levels on cerebral metabolic recovery after ischaemia. *Acta Physiol Scand* 1980; 110: 225–232.

38 Wardlaw JM, Marshall I, Wild J, Dennis MS, Cannon J, Lewis SC. Studies of acute ischaemic stroke with proton magnetic resonance spectroscopy. Relation between time from onset, neurological deficit, metabolite abnormalities in the infarct, blood flow and clinical outcome. *Stroke* 1998; 29: 1618–1624.

39 Parsons MW, Barber PA, Darby DG et al. Combined ^{1}H-MR spectroscopy and diffusion-weighted MRI improves the prediction of stroke outcome. *Neurology* 2000; 55: 498–505.

40 Pineiro R, Pendlebury ST, Smith S et al. Relating MRI changes to motor deficit after ischaemic stroke by segmentation of functional motor pathways. *Stroke* 2000; 31: 672.

41 Franke C, Brinker G, Pillekamp F, Hoehn M. Probability of metabolic tissue recovery after thrombolytic treatment of experimental stroke: a magnetic resonance spectroscopic imaging study in rat brain. *J Cereb Blood Flow Metab* 2000; 20: 583–591.

Functional MRI and stroke

Amy Brodtmann, Leeanne Carey and David G. Darby

Department of Neurology, Royal Melbourne Hospital, Parkville and Brain Imaging Research Institute, Heidelberg, Victoria, Australia

Introduction

The role of functional magnetic resonance imaging (FMRI) in patients with stroke is still in evolution. Most of the MRI advances in stroke to date have focused on improved sensitivity for localizing infarcted tissue, or methods for earlier or more reliable imaging of the ischemic penumbra. This has largely been driven by the desire to better determine pathophysiology, and to improve the utility of thrombolysis and other new therapeutic interventions. However, FMRI cannot directly measure damaged brain tissue. It aims to detect healthy tissue by means of imaging changes in local cerebral blood flow, yoked to regional brain function. This correlative relationship is well defined in healthy brain, but is more complex in ischemic brain complicating the interpretation of FMRI in acute stroke. Hence, it seems unlikely that FMRI will have a role in hyperacute stroke (less than 6 hours) because of problems inherent in the duration of the study and choosing an appropriate activation paradigm in the hyperacute period. It is not surprising that most poststroke studies are in the subacute phase or in the chronic recovery period. In this chapter we will briefly describe the history of FMRI development, outline recent contributions to the understanding of stroke-related brain dysfunction and end with recommendations for future research in stroke using FMRI.

Technical background

Functional magnetic resonance imaging

The first report of the mapping of functional changes in regional human brain function using FMRI was by Belliveau et al.[1] They quantitated cerebral blood volume by measuring the area under the concentration–time curve of infused gadolinium during or without photic stimulation. By subtraction, they showed detectable increases in visual cortex perfusion during stimulation, and for the first time displayed regional neural correlates of perception in awake healthy humans. Subsequently, intrinsic non-invasive methods have usurped this original technique, based on work from the early 1990s.[2] The method, blood oxygenation level dependent (BOLD) contrast, is dependent on the relative regional decrease in tissue deoxyhemoglobin level that occurs near active brain tissue. Deoxyhemoglobin, but not oxyhemoglobin, is paramagnetic. Hence, tissues with a relative increase in deoxyhemoglobin will show more rapid local dephasing (shortened T_2^*) and increased susceptibility effects, leading to decreased MR imaging signal intensity on T_2^*-weighted images. Conversely, those with an increase in oxyhemoglobin will be associated with a relative increase in MR imaging signal intensity. Whilst increased neuronal activity is associated with a local increase in blood flow, only a small amount of the excess oxygen delivered to neurones is utilized, resulting in a relative *decrease* in deoxyhemoglobin. Hence, rapid acquisition of T_2^*-weighted images during an activation task will be associated with an increase in MR signal intensity reflecting neuronal activation. Echoplanar techniques have made very rapid imaging possible,[3,4] and resolution is improved by higher field strengths.[5–7] Changes in regional BOLD signal intensity localize changes in neural activity, and activation can be detected by comparing signal obtained during rest and active conditions. A relative increase in blood flow in a particular area of the brain indicates an increase in the synaptic activity associated with greater demand being placed on the region during the particular behavioural task. However, the system is complicated, as distant active neurones may inhibit imaged areas and it is not possible to differentiate whether the activation is excitatory or inhibitory in nature. In addition, both 'activations' and 'deactivations' occur, complicating the interpretation of correlative neuronal ensemble activity. The BOLD related changes actually occur in postcapillary venous vessels,[6,8,9] raising difficulties in the interpretation of regional activation and the anatomical correspondence to upstream neuronal activity. High reproducibility of human FMRI studies is imperative for clinical applications. This issue is being investigated as the technique develops.[10]

Arterial and capillary perfusion techniques have also been applied to functional imaging.[11–16] In principle, incident arterial water protons are spin labelled before they enter the region of interest. Subtracting a non-labelled baseline image from that with intrinsic contrast leads to an image of incident perfusion only. Time-delayed imaging allows arterial phase to capillary blush to be separately visualized. Cognitive paradigms can also be combined with such perfusion techniques to localize regional perfusion changes correlated with neuronal activity.[17,18] Each technique has strengths and limitations with BOLD being the most widely used technique currently. It is also possible to combine these sequences to visualize both precapillary and venous circulations.[13,15,16]

Trial design and paradigm selection

Imaging sequences are only one important aspect of FMRI. A whole new discipline has been spawned related to careful design of behavioural and cognitive paradigms.[19,20] Since FMRI is based on measurement of change, paradigm designs must ensure that both baseline and active behavioural states are controlled. Ideally, both states will be identical in terms of perception, response selection and cognitive processing except for the one difference of interest. For example, a study interested in the regional ensembles involved in colour processing might present baseline greyscale scenes and their equivalents in colour whilst keeping the overall luminance the same.[21] Retinotopy and multiple visual areas have been mapped by variations on this theme.[22,23] More complex paradigms might have multiple perceptual elements and response requirements that differ only in the elements to which the subject must selectively attend.[24,25] Yet more complex paradigms have been used to investigate the relationships between cooperating brain loci.[26–31]

Since the aim of FMRI is to compare two or more behavioural states, the paradigms and sequences must be coordinated in a logical manner so their differential effects can be appreciated.[32] A two-state paradigm might be presented in alternating blocks several times (e.g. ABABAB) so their images can be extracted and analysed separately. Blocked trial designs are simple and conceptually appealing and can accommodate more than two states (e.g. ABCABCABCA), so that cognitive processes can be 'loaded' and stepwise changes in activation appreciated. Blocked trial designs were partly designed to overcome the approximately 5–8 second lag in BOLD signal rising to a steady state after a cognitive state change.[33–36] However, experiments can also use a 'single trial design' where the cognitive state trials are presented in a balanced randomized order many times. The unique contribution of each brain region to the cognitive process can then be extracted by averaging techniques (sourced from evoked potential studies) without requiring stabilization of BOLD signal.[5,37]

Data analysis and statistics

At present there is no accepted standard method of analysing FMRI data. Typical experiments use multiple brain levels, time-points and repetitions leading to several thousand images being usual. Each image contains a variable number of pixels (picture elements) with image matrices varying between 64 and 256. Note that the term 'voxel' refers to the volume elements to which the pixels relate. Hundreds of megabytes of data are therefore generated. Statistical techniques to compare these range from simple averaging and magnitude subtraction, through non-parametric techniques (e.g. Kolmgorov–Smirnov d statistic) and correlational time or frequency domain analysis[38,39] to complicated modelling of systematic signal intensity change and statistical parametric maps (see Fig. 19.1, in colour plate section, for example).[28,40–44] Sophisticated computer programs have aided these analyses and are able to statistically minimize the confounds caused by incidental jaw or head movement, boundary susceptibility or other artefacts. It is no wonder that successful FMRI experimentation requires a multidisciplinary approach.

Mapping with FMRI

The majority of FMRI work to date has focused on academic studies clarifying brain–behaviour relationships. In particular, this has involved mapping or localizing normal cognitive functions such as language generation and laterality,[45–52] working memory,[53–55] visuospatial function[56–59] or sensorimotor processing of simple and complex hand movements.[60,61] Most early studies used healthy subjects for two several reasons. Firstly, normals provided a substrate from which to correlate and extend previous clinico-anatomical, neuroimaging and electrophysiological work. Secondly, patients with neurological illnesses were usually incapable of complying with paradigms that were often laborious and required movement-free cooperation for periods lasting several hours.

FRMI has made an extensive contribution to our understanding of the mechanisms underlying normal plasticity in the adult human brain. Studies examining plasticity in patients who have sustained perinatal injury[62] or insults during childhood (particularly work done on patients posthemispherectomy,)[63] has also contributed enormously. Findings from studies using FMRI in healthy subjects have clarified the regional reorganization underlying normal motor adaptation. For example, it has been found that novel tasks are associated with initial widespread activation, particularly involving prefrontal association cortex. With task repetition and established automaticity, the association cortices no longer participate leaving relatively small activation loci in the primary motor regions.[61,64] This suggests that cortical reorganization during the learning of novel motor tasks is a dynamic process with differing cortical bases dependent upon the stage of adaptation to the task. Further mechanisms of reorganization also occur. For example, recruitment of ipsilateral pathways or contralateral hemispheric cortex can occur during complex lateralized tasks, such as complicated motor movements.[64,65]

More recently, advances in paradigm design, scan duration, and computerized analysis techniques have allowed some acute patient populations to be studied, including those with stroke. Most of the studies in stroke patients performed to date have been replications of previous studies using positron emission tomography (PET),[66,67] event-related potentials, transcranial magnetic stimulation,[68] transcranial Doppler ultrasonography[69] and magnetoencephalography.[70] However, there have also been novel single case paradigms catering to individual patients that have provided new insights into the mechanisms and pathways underlying stroke recovery.[71] FMRI has several advantages in the investigation of stroke recovery. It is a non-invasive neuroimaging technique that provides images of high spatial (submillimetre) and relatively high temporal resolution. Serial investigation is possible and signal-to-noise ratio is adequate to permit single subject image analysis. Structural anatomical images can be readily obtained at the same session, thus facilitating interpretation of the functional neuroanatomy associated with recovery. However, in stroke, FMRI is most suited to the study of the activity of the remaining undamaged tissue, since infarcted or ischemic tissue perfusion will not display the normal autoregulatory changes with activity.[72–74]

Neural plasticity post-stroke

The neuronal mechanisms of recovery following stroke are still relatively poorly understood. Neural plasticity has been defined as 'short-term modulations of function and long term structural changes'.[75] These changes may occur at both cellular and systems levels in the brain. Pathophysiological studies suggest that the changes fall into two main groups: recovery of damaged or ischemic neural networks, and increased activation and recruitment of non-damaged areas.[76–79] Recruitment of new areas may be a function of a reduction in remote functional inhibition or may involve a reactivation of sites of dormant functionality, as is seen with utilization of ipsilateral corticospinal tracts in childhood recovery from hemispherectomy.[63] Cellular level changes, such as cortical reorganization via synaptic sprouting, and the formation of new cortical connections may also contribute to recovery. Findings of the functional neuroanatomy associated with stroke recovery, such as expansion of cortical representation of the damaged area of the cortex into adjacent areas, use of ipsilateral pathways in the intact hemisphere and activation of other cortical and subcortical regions distant to the lesion[62,66–68,78,80] are consistent with these earlier findings.

Factors contributing to the recovery of ischemic tissue include reperfusion, resolution of edema or local inflammation. Location and extent of infarction have also been indicated as important factors.[81] In addition, there are patient-specific factors which may alter recovery from brain damage. These include demographic factors, such as age, gender, ethnicity and education. Handedness is also a known determinant of patterns of motor cortex activation.

The right motor cortex is activated mostly during contralateral finger movements in both right- and left-handed subjects, but the left motor cortex is activated predominantly during ipsilateral movements in left-handed subjects. This phenomenon appears to be even more marked in right-handed subjects.[60] These factors are complex but will require due consideration if the true nature of brain plasticity is to be understood.

Imaging motor recovery

The majority of FMRI mapping studies in stroke patients have focused on the sites associated with recovery of motor function. Previous neuroimaging studies suggest that there are common patterns of reorganization across subjects, as well as individual differences.[66–68,80] To date, most patients with primary motor cortex infarction investigated with FMRI have been shown to activate an enlarged volume of contralesional primary sensorimotor cortex during movements of the paretic hand,[62,82–84] possibly via recruitment of the 10–15% of uncrossed corticospinal tracts present in humans.[85,86] Often this is also associated with peri-infarct activation in extant sensorimotor cortex in the infarcted hemisphere. The superior spatial resolution of FMRI studies over positron emission tomography allows more precise identification of the infarct borders as well as activation loci.[82,83,87] Additional sites of activation outside the primary motor cortex associated with movements of a paretic hand in the recovered brain are reported in the supplementary motor area, postcentral gyrus, and premotor areas. Anterior cingulate cortex activation has also been seen, and is presumed to be associated with increased attentional demands and concentration in motivated stroke patients performing effortful tasks. These areas of activation are similar to those reported in PET activation studies with a few exceptions. For example, activation of contralesional primary sensorimotor cortex is more commonly reported in FMRI than PET studies. The reasons for this require further investigation, but may be a function of individual vs. group analyses or better spatial resolution with MRI.

In studies to date, patients have typically been assessed at one point in time after marked recovery of hand function has been demonstrated clinically. There have been few longitudinal studies serially examining recovery of motor deficits after stroke.

Thus the nature and extent of change associated with recovery over time or with different levels of recovery is still relatively unknown. One recent FMRI study has investigated subjects who recovered well a few days post-stroke and at 3 to 6 months.[88] They found an evolution of early contralesional primary sensorimotor cortex activation followed by late ipsilesional activity, consistent with the findings of Silvestrini et al.[69] Few studies have directly compared mechanisms of recovery following cortical or subcortical infarction, although both stroke subtypes have been included in analyses.[83,87,88] Use of alternative motor paradigms, such as the study of imagined movements,[89–91] might also demonstrate differences in the functioning of the motor system relative to healthy volunteers and may be associated with recovery.

Recovery in post-stroke aphasia

Again, FMRI studies have usually attempted to replicate the results of earlier PET data.[92,93] However, FMRI studies have significant advantages allowing non-invasive radioisotope-free serial studies of recovering association cortex. Furthermore, sophisticated paradigms were developed for the original FMRI studies which involved healthy subjects performing a variety of lexical, semantic and verbal tasks that can be used in patients. The restricted and lateralized nature of language function has allowed assessment of prognosis dependent upon the early post-stroke sites of activation and extent of residual language activation in the non-dominant (unaffected) and dominant hemispheres. Differences between PET and FMRI results have been reported, raising important questions about what these techniques purport to measure.[94–97] For example, recent PET data has suggested that language recovery was facilitated when the right hemisphere contributed significantly to language recovery, but that restoration of left hemisphere language networks was associated with even better language outcome, particularly if the left temporal areas were preserved and could be integrated into the functional network.[92,95] These conclusions were based on 23 patients imaged sequentially at 2 and 8 weeks post-stroke, and compared with 11 controls.

The aphasic patients were a heterogeneous group, comprising 9 subcortical, 7 frontal and 7 temporal infarcts. These results have been challenged in part by similar though smaller FMRI studies. Cao et al.[87] correlated functional language recovery in 7 aphasic patients with FMRI at 5 months or more post-stroke with activation patterns. They found that restitution of left hemisphere networks was associated with improved recovery in language but inversely related to the extent of activation in the right hemisphere. Further support for the latter position comes from a single case report with serial FMRI studies at 2 and 4 weeks then 7 months post-stroke,[98] but this is refuted by another two case reports.[99]

The duration of continued post-stroke reorganization has been investigated in one study. Welch et al. examined whether patients continue to recover 12 months or more after infarction, and sought to delineate the expansion of cortical language networks at this time.[71] They found that brain activation associated with improvement on language tests could be exclusively in the right hemisphere out to 22 months post-stroke (involving right inferior parietal, superior temporal and anterior cingulate gyri), but that different cortical regions in both the right and left hemispheres were activated at 32 months (including bilateral inferior parietal and superior temporal, right inferior frontal and left anterior cingulate gyri). In addition, they performed tissue segmentation using T_1- and T_2-weighted MRI, and were able to delineate four heterogeneous zones in the patient's infarct at 22 months (6 at 35 months). Two zones of slightly elevated T_2 levels and decreased T_1 levels were felt to be capable of recovery, and brain reactivation was documented in these zones at 32 months. They concluded that the restored cortical activity in partially damaged tissue was in part associated with the patient's documented language improvement.

Other FMRI studies of stroke recovery

Little FMRI work has been done to date to examine recovery following damage to other brain areas or functions, however limited case studies have provided useful information. For example, in visual research, one study attempted to correlate FMRI activation, dynamic susceptibility imaging (as a measure of relative cerebral blood volume perfusion), and standard visual field mapping.[100] They found that FMRI alone could accurately map both functional and perfusion deficits. Another report compared two patients with contrasting visual perceptual deficits to determine that first- and second-order motion systems were mediated by regionally separate mechanisms.[101] Brandt et al. studied the extent of sensorimotor control achieved for each hemisphere (separately or together) 5–7 days following the development of homonymous hemianopia secondary to infarction.[102]

Mechanisms of neglect and executive dysfunction, or recovery of these, have not been systematically examined. Judging by abstracts and presentations, it is a popular subject of research, but little has made its way into the literature. Novel case reports and small case series have examined language and calculation within the parietal lobe,[103] parietal and cingulate processes in central pain,[104] and the mechanisms of sensory recovery following stroke.[105] Much remains to be done.

Future directions

Further FMRI-based investigations in stroke need to focus on specific questions in specific patient subgroups. It is to be hoped that delineation of early postinfarction patterns of functional activation may predict extent of recovery, provide direction for the development of rehabilitative and therapeutic strategies, and supplement other functional evaluative techniques including neuropsychology. At present, FMRI remains in an early mapping stage without standardized protocols for specific clinical or anatomical stroke syndromes. This will require an understanding of the mechanisms underlying the considerable interpatient variability observed in patterns of recovery following hemispheric stroke (e.g. ipsilateral hemispheric activation, vs. restoration of activation to the contralateral, damaged hemisphere in novel and peri-infarct sites). Studies differentiating patient stroke subtype, or cortical vs. subcortical location are required, as are studies of differences between anterior and posterior circulation infarcts and their patterns of activation. Patient factors also need to be considered including handedness, age, race, and gender. Handedness associated hemispheric asymmetries in particular has not been explicitly addressed in previous FMRI stroke studies, and may be found to account for some of the variability in recovery patterns. Age related effects on cerebral blood flow are well documented in other neuroimaging literature, but normative data for each decade does not yet exist in FMRI,[106] with most of the mapping activation studies performed on healthy young controls. Gender differences in language activation patterns exist, which may also contribute to observed interhemispheric asymmetries.[107–109] Current FMRI work looking at sex differences in language processing is raising as many questions as it answers, and appears to be increasing the degree of controversy in the field.[110,111] Racial differences have not yet been studied.

More work could also be done in the early post-stroke period and longitudinally, to establish whether acute mechanisms of recovery differ from those seen months to years later. Some of the recent FMRI studies in post-stroke aphasia have in part attempted to address this question. However, differences in activation sites between patients making a good recovery in the first few days compared to those improving over weeks to months have not been evaluated. Nor have attempts yet been made to correlate the timing of recovery and of the FMRI study on the patient with the site and size of infarct, factors which are known to impact on prognosis. Comparison of patterns of reorganization observed in those who show good vs. poor behavioural recovery also requires further investigation, as does the effect of rehabilitative training on cerebral reorganization.

Future integrative research correlating perfusion–diffusion characteristics and site of FMRI activation might shed light on factors predictive of recovery.[71] Combined MRI techniques can provide not only the anatomical site of the infarct, but also the state of the surrounding ischemic penumbra, cerebral blood flow, and functional activation. This information could be used to improve understanding of the pathophysiological mechanisms of stroke. Correlative study designs using dual measures of functional activation in normal subjects, could be relatively easily translated into patient-based studies following stroke.[37,112–114]

Overall, the field of FMRI is in its infancy in applying these new techniques to the unique dysfunctions characteristic of stroke, and in the prediction of recovery. Its singular advantages are balanced by the complicated nature of the studies, and the need for a well integrated team of neurologists, neuroradiologists, neuroscientists, allied health professionals, MRI technicians, physicists and specialised information technologists and statisticians, to name the bare minimum, with access to an MRI scanner complete with the information technology to perform this work. Therefore, it is difficult to predict the future of this discipline in the post-stroke area. Hopefully, interesting and useful practical insights into the mechanisms underlying brain plasticity will ensue, and also possibly into the pathophysiology of acute stroke. However, this will only occur with the interaction of multidisciplinary FMRI teams, working in concert to best contribute to these studies.

REFERENCES

1 Belliveau JW, Kennedy DN, Jr, McKinstry RC et al. Functional mapping of the human visual cortex by magnetic resonance imaging. *Science* 1991; 254: 716–719.
2 Ogawa S, Lee TM, Kay AR, Tank DW. Brain magnetic resonance imaging with contrast dependent on blood oxygenation. *Proc Natl Acad Sci USA* 1990; 87: 9868–9872.
3 Kwong KK. Functional magnetic resonance imaging with echo planar imaging. *Magn Reson Q* 1995; 11: 1–20.
4 Stehling MK, Turner R, Mansfield P. Echo-planar imaging: magnetic resonance imaging in a fraction of a second. *Science* 1991; 254: 43–50.
5 Le Bihan D. Functional MRI of the brain principles, applications and limitations. *J Neuroradiol* 1996; 23: 1–5.
6 Menon RS, Ogawa S, Hu X, Strupp JP, Anderson P, Ugurbil K. BOLD based functional MRI at 4 Tesla includes a capillary bed contribution: echo-planar imaging correlates with previous optical imaging using intrinsic signals. *Magn Reson Med* 1995; 33: 453–459.
7 Ugurbil K, Garwood M, Ellermann J et al. Imaging at high magnetic fields: initial experiences at 4 T. *Magn Reson Q* 1993; 9: 259–277.
8 Ogawa S, Menon RS, Tank DW et al. Functional brain mapping by blood oxygenation level-dependent contrast magnetic resonance imaging. A comparison of signal characteristics with a biophysical model. *Biophys J* 1993; 64: 803–812.
9 Ogawa S, Menon RS, Kim SG, Ugurbil K. On the characteristics of functional magnetic resonance imaging of the brain. *Annu Rev Biophys Biomol Struct* 1998; 27: 447–474.
10 Moser E, Teichtmeister C, Diemling M. Reproducibility and postprocessing of gradient-echo functional MRI to improve localization of brain activity in the human visual cortex. *Magn Reson Imaging* 1996; 14: 567–579.
11 Edelman RR, Siewert B, Darby DG et al. Qualitative mapping of cerebral blood flow and functional localization with echo-planar MR imaging and signal targeting with alternating radio frequency. *Radiology* 1994; 192: 513–520.
12 Kim SG, Tsekos NV. Perfusion imaging by a flow-sensitive alternating inversion recovery (FAIR) technique: application to functional brain imaging. *Magn Reson Med* 1997; 37: 425–435.
13 Kim SG, Tsekos NV, Ashe J. Multi-slice perfusion-based functional MRI using the FAIR technique: comparison of CBF and BOLD effects. *NMR Biomed* 1997; 10: 191–196.
14 Kim SG, Ugurbil K. Comparison of blood oxygenation and cerebral blood flow effects in fMRI: estimation of relative oxygen consumption change. *Magn Reson Med* 1997; 38: 59–65.
15 Li TQ, Kastrup A, Takahashi AM, Moseley ME. Functional MRI of human brain during breath holding by BOLD and FAIR techniques. *Neuroimage* 1999; 9: 243–249.
16 Zaini MR, Strother SC, Anderson JR et al. Comparison of matched BOLD and FAIR 4.0T-fMRI with [15O]water PET brain volumes. *Med Phys* 1999; 26: 1559–1567.
17 Darby DG, Nobre AC, Thangaraj V, Edelman R, Mesulam MM, Warach S. Cortical activation in the human brain during lateral saccades using EPISTAR functional magnetic resonance imaging. *Neuroimage* 1996; 3: 53–62.

18. Nobre AC, Darby DG, Edelman R, Mesulam MM, Warach S. Cortical activation during spatial attention tasks in the human brain shown by EPISTAR magnetic resonance imaging (abstract). In *Society for Neuroscience* 1994; 434.
19. Bandettini PA, Wong EC. Magnetic resonance imaging of human brain function. Principles, practicalities, and possibilities. *Neurosurg Clin N Am* 1997; 8: 345–371.
20. Nadeau SE, Crosson B. A guide to the functional imaging of cognitive processes. *Neuropsychol, Neuropsychiatry, Behav Neurol* 1995; 8: 143–162.
21. Sakai K, Watanabe E, Onodera Y et al. Functional mapping of the human colour centre with echo-planar magnetic resonance imaging. *Proc R Soc Lond B Biol Sci* 1995; 261: 89–98.
22. Sereno MI, Dale AM, Reppas JB et al. Borders of multiple visual areas in humans revealed by functional magnetic resonance imaging. *Science* 1995; 268: 889–893.
23. Tootell RB, Reppas JB, Kwong KK et al. Functional analysis of human MT and related visual cortical areas using magnetic resonance imaging. *J Neurosci* 1995; 15: 3215–3230.
24. O'Craven KM, Rosen BR, Kwong KK, Treisman A, Savoy RL. Voluntary attention modulates fMRI activity in human MT-MST. *Neuron* 1997; 18: 591–598.
25. Engel SA, Rumelhart DE, Wandell BA et al. fMRI of human visual cortex. *Nature* 1994; 369: 525.
26. Courtney SM, Ungerleider LG, Keil K, Haxby JV. Object and spatial visual working memory activate separate neural systems in human cortex. *Cereb Cortex* 1996; 6: 39–49.
27. Courtney SM, Ungerleider LG, Keil K, Haxby JV. Transient and sustained activity in a distributed neural system for human working memory. *Nature* 1997; 386: 608–611.
28. Friston KJ, Frith CD, Frackowiak RS, Turner R. Characterizing dynamic brain responses with fMRI: a multivariate approach. *Neuroimage* 1995; 2: 166–172.
29. Friston KJ, Frith CD, Liddle PF, Frackowiak RS. Functional connectivity: the principal-component analysis of large (PET) data sets. *J Cereb Blood Flow Metab* 1993; 13: 5–14.
30. Friston KJ, Price CJ, Fletcher P, Moore C, Frackowiak RS, Dolan RJ. The trouble with cognitive subtraction. *Neuroimage* 1996; 4: 97–104.
31. Friston KJ, Zarahn E, Josephs O, Henson RN, Dale AM. Stochastic designs in event-related fMRI. *Neuroimage* 1999; 10: 607–619.
32. Bandettini PA, Wong EC, Hinks RS, Tikofsky RS, Hyde JS. Time course EPI of human brain function during task activation. *Magn Reson Med* 1992; 25: 390–397.
33. Duyn JH, Moonen CT, van Yperen GH, de Boer RW, Luyten PR. Inflow versus deoxyhemoglobin effects in BOLD functional MRI using gradient echoes at 1.5 T. *NMR Biomed* 1994; 7: 83–88.
34. Kennan RP, Scanley BE, Innis RB, Gore JC. Physiological basis for BOLD MR signal changes due to neuronal stimulation: separation of blood volume and magnetic susceptibility effects. *Magn Reson Med* 1998; 40: 840–846.
35. Rees G, Howseman A, Josephs O et al. Characterizing the relationship between BOLD contrast and regional cerebral blood flow measurements by varying the stimulus presentation rate. *Neuroimage* 1997; 6: 270–278.
36. Schwarzbauer C, Heinke W. Investigating the dependence of BOLD contrast on oxidative metabolism. *Magn Reson Med* 1999; 41: 537–543.
37. McCarthy G, Puce A, Luby M, Belger A, Allison T. Magnetic resonance imaging studies of functional brain activation: analysis and interpretation. *Electroencephalogr Clin Neurophysiol* 1996; 47: 15–31.
38. McCarthy G, Adrignolo A, Spicer M, Luby M, Gore JC, Alison T. Localized brain activation with visual stimulus motion studied by functional magnetic resonance imaging in humans. *Hum Brain Mapp* 1995; 2: 234–243.
39. Bandettini PA, Jesmanowicz A, Wong EC, Hyde JS. Processing strategies for time-course data sets in functional MRI of the human brain. *Magn Reson Med* 1993; 30: 161–173.
40. Aguirre GK, Zarahn E, D'Esposito M. Empirical analyses of BOLD fMRI statistics. II. Spatially smoothed data collected under null-hypothesis and experimental conditions. *Neuroimage* 1997; 5: 199–212.
41. Friston KJ, Josephs O, Rees G, Turner R. Nonlinear event-related responses in fMRI. *Magn Reson Med* 1998; 39: 41–52.
42. Friston KJ, Josephs O, Zarahn E, Holmes AP, Rouquette S, Poline J. To smooth or not to smooth? Bias and efficiency in fMRI time-series analysis. *Neuroimage* 2000; 12: 196–208.
43. Zarahn E, Aguirre GK, D'Esposito M. Empirical analyses of BOLD fMRI statistics. I. Spatially unsmoothed data collected under null-hypothesis conditions. *Neuroimage* 1997; 5: 179–197.

44 Friston KJ, Holmes AP, Price CJ, Buchel C, Worsley KJ. Multisubject fMRI studies and conjunction analyses. *Neuroimage* 1999; 10: 385–396.

45 Binder JR. Neuroanatomy of language processing studied with functional MRI. *Clin Neurosci* 1997; 4: 87–94.

46 Binder JR, Rao SM, Hammeke TA et al. Lateralized human brain language systems demonstrated by task subtraction functional magnetic resonance imaging. *Arch Neurol* 1995; 52: 593–601.

47 Cuenod CA, Bookheimer SY, Hertz-Pannier L, Zeffiro TA, Theodore WH, Le Bihan D. Functional MRI during word generation, using conventional equipment: a potential tool for language localization in the clinical environment. *Neurology* 1995; 45: 1821–1827.

48 Frackowiak RS. Functional mapping of verbal memory and language. *Trends Neurosci* 1994; 17: 109–115.

49 Habib M, Demonet JF, Frackowiak R. [Cognitive neuroanatomy of language: contribution of functional cerebral imaging]. *Rev Neurol* (Paris) 1996; 152: 249–260.

50 Hinke RM, Hu X, Stillman AE et al. Functional magnetic resonance imaging of Broca's area during internal speech. *Neuroreport* 1993; 4: 675–678.

51 McCarthy G, Blamire AM, Rothman DL, Gruetter R, Shulman RG. Echo-planar magnetic resonance imaging studies of frontal cortex activation during word generation in humans. *Proc Natl Acad Sci USA* 1993; 90: 4952–4956.

52 Rueckert L, Appollonio I, Grafman J et al. Magnetic resonance imaging functional activation of left frontal cortex during covert word production. *J Neuroimaging* 1994; 4: 67–70.

53 Belger A, Puce A, Krystal JH, Gore JC, Goldman-Rakic P, McCarthy G. Dissociation of mnemonic and perceptual processes during spatial and nonspatial working memory using fMRI. *Hum Brain Mapp* 1998; 6: 14–32.

54 Cohen JD, Forman SD, Braver TS, Casey BJ, Servan-Schreiber D, Noll DC. Activation of prefrontal cortex in a non-spatial working memory task with functional MRI. *Hum Brain Mapp* 1994; 1: 293–304.

55 McCarthy G, Puce A, Constable RT, Krystal JH, Gore JC, Goldman-Rakic P. Activation of human prefrontal cortex during spatial and nonspatial working memory tasks measured by functional MRI. *Cereb Cortex* 1996; 6: 600–611.

56 Gauthier I, Skudlarski P, Gore JC, Anderson AW. Expertise for cars and birds recruits brain areas involved in face recognition. *Nat Neurosci* 2000; 3: 191–197.

57 Grinvald A, Slovin H, Vanzetta I. Non-invasive visualization of cortical columns by fMRI. *Nat Neurosci* 2000; 3: 105–107.

58 Puce A, Allison T, Asgari M, Gore JC, McCarthy G. Differential sensitivity of human visual cortex to faces, letterstrings, and textures: a functional magnetic resonance imaging study. *J Neurosci* 1996; 16: 5205–5215.

59 Puce A, Allison T, Gore JC, McCarthy G. Face-sensitive regions in human extrastriate cortex studied by functional MRI. *J Neurophysiol* 1995; 74: 1192–1199.

60 Kim SG, Ashe J, Hendrich K et al. Functional magnetic resonance imaging of motor cortex: hemispheric asymmetry and handedness. *Science* 1993; 261: 615–617.

61 Rao SM, Binder JR, Bandettini PA et al. Functional magnetic resonance imaging of complex human movements. *Neurology* 1993; 43: 2311–2318.

62 Cao Y, Vikingstad EM, Huttenlocher PR, Towle VL, Levin DN. Functional magnetic resonance studies of the reorganization of the human hand sensorimotor area after unilateral brain injury in the perinatal period. *Proc Natl Acad Sci USA* 1994; 91: 9612–9616.

63 Holloway V, Gadian DG, Vargha-Khadem F, Porter DA, Boyd SG, Connelly A. The reorganization of sensorimotor function in children after hemispherectomy. A functional MRI and somatosensory evoked potential study. *Brain* 2000; 123: 2432–2444.

64 Karni A, Meyer G, Jezzard P, Adams MM, Turner R, Ungerleider LG. Functional MRI evidence for adult motor cortex plasticity during motor skill learning. *Nature* 1995; 377: 155–158.

65 Just MA, Carpenter PA, Keller TA, Eddy WF, Thulborn KR. Brain activation modulated by sentence comprehension. *Science* 1996; 274: 114–116.

66 Chollet F, DiPiero V, Wise RJ, Brooks DJ, Dolan RJ, Frackowiak RS. The functional anatomy of motor recovery after stroke in humans: a study with positron emission tomography. *Ann Neurol* 1991; 29: 63–71.

67 Weiller C, Chollet F, Friston KJ, Wise RJ, Frackowiak RS. Functional reorganization of the brain in recovery from striatocapsular infarction in man. *Ann Neurol* 1992; 31: 463–472.

68 Liepert J, Bauder H, Wolfgang HR, Miltner WH, Taub E, Weiller C. Treatment-induced cortical reorganization after stroke in humans. *Stroke* 2000; 31: 1210–1216.

69 Silvestrini M, Cupini LM, Placidi F, Diomedi M, Bernardi G. Bilateral hemispheric activation in the early recovery of motor function after stroke. *Stroke* 1998; 29: 1305–1310.

70 Rossini PM, Tecchio F, Pizzella V et al. On the reorganization of sensory hand areas after mono-hemispheric lesion: a functional (MEG)/anatomical (MRI) integrative study. *Brain Res* 1998; 782: 153–166.

71 Welch KM, Cao Y, Nagesh V. Magnetic resonance assessment of acute and chronic stroke. *Prog Cardiovasc Dis* 2000; 43: 113–134.

72 Heiss WD, Huber M, Fink GR et al. Progressive derangement of periinfarct viable tissue in ischemic stroke. *J Cereb Blood Flow Metab* 1992; 12: 193–203.

73 Wise RJ, Bernardi S, Frackowiak RS, Legg NJ, Jones T. Serial observations on the pathophysiology of acute stroke. The transition from ischaemia to infarction as reflected in regional oxygen extraction. *Brain* 1983; 106: 197–222.

74 Wise RJ, Rhodes CG, Gibbs JM et al. Disturbance of oxidative metabolism of glucose in recent human cerebral infarcts. *Ann Neurol* 1983; 14: 627–637.

75 Dobkin DH. Plasticity in motor and neural networks. In: Dobkin DH, ed. *Neuroscientific Foundations in Rehabilitation*. Philadelphia: FA Davis Co; 1996. p. 4.

76 Feeney DM, Baron JC. Diaschisis. *Stroke* 1986; 17: 817–830.

77 Merrill EG, Wall PD. Plasticity of connections in the adult nervous system. In: Cotman CW, ed. *Neuronal Plasticity*. New York: Raven Press; 1978: 97–111.

78 Nudo RJ, Wise BM, SiFuentes F, Milliken GW. Neural substrates for the effects of rehabilitative training on motor recovery after ischemic infarct. *Science* 1996; 272: 1791–1794.

79 Stroemer RP, Kent TA, Hulsebosch CE. Enhanced neocortical neural sprouting, synaptogenesis, and behavioral recovery with D-amphetamine therapy after neocortical infarction in rats. *Stroke* 1998; 29: 2381–2393; discussion 93–95.

80 Weiller C, Ramsay SC, Wise RJ, Friston KJ, Frackowiak RS. Individual patterns of functional reorganization in the human cerebral cortex after capsular infarction. *Ann Neurol* 1993; 33: 181–189.

81 Weiller C. Imaging recovery from stroke. *Exp Brain Res* 1998; 123: 13–17.

82 Cramer SC. Stroke recovery. Lessons from functional MR imaging and other methods of human brain mapping. *Phys Med Rehab Clin N Am* 1999; 10: 875–886.

83 Cramer SC, Nelles G, Benson RR et al. A functional MRI study of subjects recovered from hemiparetic stroke. *Stroke* 1997; 28: 2518–2527.

84 Cramer SC, Moore CI, Finklestein SP, Rosen BR. A pilot study of somatotopic mapping after cortical infarct. *Stroke* 2000; 31: 668–671.

85 Glees P, Cole J. Ipsilateral representation in the cerebral cortex: its significance in relation to motor function. *Lancet* 1952; 1: 1191–1192.

86 Nyberg-Hansen R, Rinvik E. Some comments on the pyramidal tract, with special reference to its individual variations in man. *Acta Neurol Scand* 1963; 39: 1–30.

87 Cao Y, D'Olhaberriague L, Vikingstad EM, Levine SR, Welch KM. Pilot study of functional MRI to assess cerebral activation of motor function after poststroke hemiparesis. *Stroke* 1998; 29: 112–122.

88 Marshall RS, Perera GM, Lazar RM, Krakauer JW, Constantine RC, DeLaPaz RL. Evolution of cortical activation during recovery from corticospinal tract infarction. *Stroke* 2000; 31: 656–661.

89 Crammond DJ. Motor imagery: never in your wildest dream. *Trends Neurosci* 1997; 20: 54–57.

90 Sirigu A, Cohen L, Duhamel JR et al. Congruent unilateral impairments for real and imagined hand movements. *Neuroreport* 1995; 6: 997–1001.

91 Sirigu A, Duhamel JR, Cohen L, Pillon B, Dubois B, Agid Y. The mental representation of hand movements after parietal cortex damage. *Science* 1996; 273: 1564–1568.

92 Heiss WD, Kessler J, Thiel A, Ghaemi M, Karbe H. Differential capacity of left and right hemispheric areas for compensation of poststroke aphasia. *Ann Neurol* 1999; 45: 430–438.

93 Musso M, Weiller C, Kiebel S, Muller SP, Bulau P, Rijntjes M. Training-induced brain plasticity in aphasia. *Brain* 1999; 122: 1781–1790.

94 Devlin JT, Russell RP, Davis MH et al. Susceptibility-induced loss of signal: comparing PET and fMRI on a semantic task. *Neuroimage* 2000; 11: 589–600.

95 Karbe H, Thiel A, Weber-Luxenburger G, Herholz K, Kessler J, Heiss WD. Brain plasticity in poststroke aphasia: what is the contribution of the right hemisphere? *Brain Lang* 1998; 64: 215–230.

96 Small SL, Noll DC, Perfetti CA, Hlustik P, Wellington R, Schneider W. Localizing the lexicon for reading aloud: replication of a PET study using fMRI. *Neuroreport* 1996; 7: 961–965.

97 Veltman DJ, Friston KJ, Sanders G, Price CJ. Regionally specific sensitivity differences in fMRI and PET: where do they come from? *Neuroimage* 2000; 11: 575–588.

98 Miura K, Nakamura Y, Miura F et al. Functional magnetic resonance imaging to word generation task in a patient with Broca's aphasia. *J Neurol* 1999; 246: 939–942.

99 Thulborn KR, Carpenter PA, Just MA. Plasticity of language-related brain function during recovery from stroke. *Stroke* 1999; 30: 749–754.

100 Sorensen AG, Wray SH, Weisskoff RM et al. Functional MR of brain activity and perfusion in patients with chronic cortical stroke. *Am J Neuroradiol* 1995; 16: 1753–1762.

101 Vaina LM, Cowey A, Kennedy D. Perception of first- and second-order motion: separable neurological mechanisms? *Hum Brain Mapp* 1999; 7: 67–77.

102 Brandt T, Bucher SF, Seelos KC, Dieterich M. Bilateral functional MRI activation of the basal ganglia and middle temporal/medial superior temporal motion-sensitive areas: optokinetic stimulation in homonymous hemianopia. *Arch Neurol* 1998; 55: 1126–1131.

103 Cohen L, Dehaene S, Chochon F, Lehericy S, Naccache L. Language and calculation within the parietal lobe: a combined cognitive, anatomical and fMRI study. *Neuropsychologia* 2000; 38: 1426–1440.

104 Peyron R, Garcia-Larrea L, Gregoire MC et al. Parietal and cingulate processes in central pain. A combined positron emission tomography (PET) and functional magnetic resonance imaging (fMRI) study of an unusual case. *Pain* 2000; 84: 77–87.

105 Carey LM, Abbott DF, Puce A, Jackson GD, Syngeniotis A, Donnan GA. Reemergence of activation with post-stroke somatosensory recovery. (in press) 2001.

106 Martin AJ, Friston KJ, Colebatch JG, Frackowiak RS. Decreases in regional cerebral blood flow with normal aging. *J Cereb Blood Flow Metab* 1991; 11: 684–689.

107 Harasty J, Double KL, Halliday GM, Kril JJ, McRitchie DA. Language-associated cortical regions are proportionally larger in the female brain. *Arch Neurol* 1997; 54: 171–176.

108 Healey JM, Waldstein S, Goodglass H. Sex differences in the lateralization of language discrimination vs language production. *Neuropsychologia* 1985; 23: 777–789.

109 Inglis J, Ruckman M, Lawson JS, MacLean AW, Monga TN. Sex differences in the cognitive effects of unilateral brain damage. *Cortex* 1982; 18: 257–275.

110 Frost JA, Binder JR, Springer JA et al. Language processing is strongly left lateralized in both sexes. Evidence from functional MRI. *Brain* 1999; 122: 199–208.

111 Harasty J. Language processing in both sexes: evidence from brain studies. *Brain* 2000; 123: 404–406.

112 Macdonell RA, Jackson GD, Curatolo JM et al. Motor cortex localization using functional MRI and transcranial magnetic stimulation. *Neurology* 1999; 53: 1462–1467.

113 Puce A, Allison T, McCarthy G. Electrophysiological studies of human face perception. III: Effects of top-down processing on face-specific potentials. *Cereb Cortex* 1999; 9: 445–458.

114 Puce A, Constable RT, Luby ML et al. Functional magnetic resonance imaging of sensory and motor cortex: comparison with electrophysiological localization. *J Neurosurg* 1995; 83: 262–270.

Index

Numbers in italics indicate *tables* or *figures*, *cp* denotes colour plate.

N-acetyl aspartate (NAA)
  levels in cerebral ischemia *237, 238*, 242, *cp*
  levels in normal brain *237*, 240–1
  in outcome prediction 185, 245
  reversible changes 244, *245*
age and stroke therapy 9
ancrod 113
aneurysms, detection of 95–6
animal stroke models
  DWI studies 114, *cp*
    neuroprotective therapy 116–17, *cp*
    reperfusion injury 114–15
  DWI–PWI combined studies
    diffusion–perfusion mismatch 115
    mechanical reperfusion 117
    neuroprotective therapy 118
    thrombolytic therapy 117–18
  PWI studies 115, 117, 168
  use in preclinical evaluation of therapies 113–14, 116
aortic embolisms 6
apparent diffusion coefficient (ADC)
  anisotropic 59
  effects of ischemia on 114, 198–9
  effects of reperfusion on 114–15, 210
  maps *57, 60*, 122
  trace ADC 61
arterial hemorrhagic infarcts 79
arterial obstruction, detection by CT 32, 36
arterial spin labelling (ASL) 62–3, 148, 161–74
  clinical applications in stroke 168–71
  labelling strategies
    continuous 162–3, *163–4*
    pulsed 163
    to overcome transit delays 171–2
  motion artefact reduction 164–6
  multislice imaging 166–7
  perfusion mapping in animal models 168
  principle 161–2
  quantification of perfusion 164
  subtraction method 162, *163*
  validation 168
aspirin 1

blood
  appearance in MR images 85
  see also cerebral blood flow (CBF) evaluation; cerebral blood volume (CBV) evaluation
blood oxygen level dependent (BOLD) imaging 202, 251–2
blood pressure
  management in intracerebral hemorrhage 50–1
  and stroke risk 8
blood–brain barrier 148
brain imaging in stroke
  goals 208
  importance 15
  modalities compared *176*
  patient factors 15
  see also specific imaging modalities
brain tissue swelling, detection by CT 32–5, 36
brain tumors, differentiation from infarcts 79, 81

cardiac-origin embolism 6, 182
carotid artery, imaging by MRA 89–93, *94*
carotid endarterectomy 7, 89
CE 3DMRA *see* contrast-enhanced MRA (CE-MRA)
cerebral blood flow (CBF) evaluation
  acute stroke 48–9
  chronic cerebral ischemia 49–50
  CT-based 47–54
  intracerebral hemorrhage 50–1
  PET-based 24
  PWI-based 62, *63*, 152–4
  subarachnoid hemorrhage 51
  vasospasm 51
cerebral blood volume (CBV) evaluation
  PET-based 24–5
  PWI-based 62, 150–2
cerebral glucose metabolism, measurement by PET 25
cerebral oxygen metabolism, measurement by PET 25
cerebral perfusion pressure (CPP) 154–5
cerebral venous thrombosis 4
cerebritis, differentiation from infarcts 81, 83
cerebrovascular reserve, characterization with ASL 169, *170*, 171
Cerestat 116

Ceretec 22
cervical vascular lesions 7
chemical shift imaging (CSI) 185–6, 233, 234
choline measurement by MRS
  cerebral ischemia *237*, 242
  normal brain *237*, 241
circle of Willis, evaluation by MRA 93–7
citicoline trials 183, 227
computed tomographic angiography (CTA) 18–19, 52, 90–1, 94, 95
computed tomographic perfusion imaging (CTP) 19, 51–2, 196, *197*
computed tomography (CT)
  CBF evaluation 47–54
  in pregnancy 16
  principle 16
  radiation exposure 16
  sequence of changes after stroke 16
  in TIA 136
computed tomography (CT) in acute stroke 31–45
  advantages 15, *16*
  compared with other imaging modalities *176*
  detection capability
    arterial obstruction 32
    brain tissue swelling 32
    intracranial hemorrhage 31–2
    ischemic brain edema 32–5
    stroke location and extent 122, 125
  diagnostic accuracy 35
    arterial obstruction 36, *37*
    brain tissue swelling 36
    intracranial hemorrhage 36
  diagnostic impact 36–7
    intracranial hemorrhage 37
    ischemic brain edema 37–9, *40*
  impact on patient outcome 40–3
  limitations 16–18
  therapeutic impact 39–40
contrast-enhanced MRA (CE-MRA) 59
  advantages 76, 88
  compared with time of flight 89
  contrast agent dosage and timing 88
  drawbacks 88
  technical considerations 88–9
contrast-enhanced T_1-weighted sequences 70–1, 73, *74*, 76

creatine measurement by MRS *237*, 241, 242
CSI *see* chemical shift imaging (CSI)
CT *see* computed tomography (CT)
CTA *see* computed tomographic angiography (CTA)
cytotoxic edema 69, 114

dark blood techniques 85–6
deoxyhemoglobin 105, 147–8
diffusion tensor imaging (DTI) 59, 61
diffusion–perfusion (DWI/PWI) mismatch 115, 180–1, 197, *200*, 212
diffusion-weighted MR imaging (DWI) 121–33
  clinical representations of results 121–2
  compared with other imaging modalities *176*
  diagnosis of acute and chronic ischemia 177–9
  factors influencing lesion evolution 211–12
  false negatives 123
  infarct pathogenesis studies 182–3
  ischemic penumbra 196–9, 209–11
  motion artefacts 61
  multiple infarcts 126–7, *128, 129, 130*
  in patient selection for therapy 183–5, 200, 224–5
  prognostic value 179–80
  and stroke extent 125–6
  and stroke location 122–4
  surrogate endpoint in drug trials 183, 214, 227–9
  technical aspects 59–61, 121
  therapeutic impact 127–8, *130, 131, 132*
  thrombolytic therapy monitoring 212–13
  TIA studies 137–42
  typical examination 60–1
  in a typical stroke protocol *56*
  see also animal stroke models: DWI studies
digital subtraction angiography 6
drug development *see* stroke drug development

ECASS *see* European Cooperative Acute Stroke Studies (ECASS I and II)
echoplanar magnetic resonance imaging (EPI) 21
  techniques summarized *177*
  see also specific techniques
elliptico-centric phase-encoding 89
embolism, in stroke pathogenesis 7
encephalitis, differentiation from infarct 81–3
endothelin antagonist 118
EPISTAR 63
European Cooperative Acute Stroke Studies (ECASS I and II) 31, *36*, 40–3, 208
exametazime 22
extracranial stenoses 89–91

flow-driven adiabatic inversion 163–4
fluid-attenuated inversion recovery (FLAIR) imaging 57–8, 70, 76, *77*
flumenazil 209
^{18}F-fluoromisonidazole (FMISO) 193, 209
FOCI pulses 167
functional magnetic resonance imaging (FMRI) 251–61

data analysis 253
future directions 256–7
mapping of normal functions 253
paradigm selection 252
stroke recovery studies 253–4, *cp*
  language recovery 255–6
  motor recovery 254–5
  other studies 256
technical background 251–2
trial design 252

gadolinium
  magnetic susceptibility effect 149
  relaxivity effect 148, 149
  T1/T2 shortening 57, 58, 148
  use in MRA 59, 88
  use in PWI 62, 148–9
gamma variate curves *62, 63*
glutamate/glutamine detection by MRS 243–4
gradient echo sequences in PWI 149
gyromagnetic ratio 234

heat shock protein 70 (HSP 70) *194*, 195
hemodynamic stroke 7–8
hemoglobin degradation 103
hemorrhagic infarction 4, 77–9, *80–1*
Herpes simplex encephalitis 81–3
hypertension 8
hypoxia inducible factor 1 (HIF-1) *194*, 195

intracranial hemorrhage (ICH)
  blood pressure management 50–1
  detection by CT 31–2, 36, 37
  etiology 103, 104
  local pathological processes 109
  MRI
    hyperacute stage 104–8
    acute stage 103–4
    subacute and chronic stages 104
    etiological information 104
    signal characteristics summarized 104
  sensitivities of MRI and CT 103
  subarachnoid hemorrhage *see* subarachnoid hemorrhage (SAH)
  surgery for 108–9
  Xe CT 50–1
intracranial stenoses 7, 93–4
intracranial veins, imaging by MRA 97
ischemic brain edema, detection by CT 32–5, 36, 37–9, *40*
ischemic core
  and DWI lesions 210, 211
  molecular definition 194
  operational definitions *197*
  variability between patients 209
ischemic penumbra 191–206
  biochemical definition 208
  current concept *212*
  DWI of 196–9, 209–11
  DWI/PWI mismatch 115, 180–5, 197, *200*, 212
  flow thresholds 192
  functional definition 191
  identification by PET 208–9
  importance 191
  molecular zones 194–5

MRS of 185–6, 200–1, *cp*
operational definitions 195, *197*
  CT perfusion 196
  DWI/PWI *197*
  PET 195–6
  SPECT 196
  Xe-CT 196
PWI of 199, 211
time-relatedness 192–3
trials of prediction of response to therapy 184–5
ischemic stroke diagnosis 9–10
  acute stroke 4–5
  approach summarized *6*
  assessment of stroke risk factors 8
  importance in patient management 9–10
  stroke mechanism
    embolism 7
    hemodynamic stroke 7–8
    migrainous 8
    thrombosis 7
  stroke severity 9
  vascular lesions 5–6
ischemic stroke management
  acute stroke 4, 5
  aortic lesions 6–7
  cardiac-origin embolism 6
  cervical vascular lesions 7
  hemodynamic stroke 8
  individualized 8, 9
  intracranial stenoses 7
  migrainous stroke 8

k-space sampling 97–8

lactate measurement by MRS 185, *186*, 200–6, *cp*
  in cerebral ischemia 241–2
  levels and stroke outcome 245
lacunar infarcts 3, 79, 182, 183
language recovery poststroke, FMRI studies 255–6
Larmor frequency 234
lightbulb sign 178, *179*
lipid measurement by MRS *239*, 241, 244
longitudinal relaxation time (T_1) 55, 148

magnetic resonance angiography (MRA) 85–101
  clinical applications 76
  carotid and vertebral arteries 89–93, *94*
  circle of Willis 93–7
  contrast-enhanced *see* contrast-enhanced MRA (CE-MRA)
  penumbral patterns 180–1
  phase-contrast 58–9, *75, 76, 78*, 86–8
  principles 85
  time of flight 58, 59, 76, 85–6, *87*, 89, *91*
  in a typical stroke protocol *56*
  work in progress 97–8
magnetic resonance imaging (MRI)
  advantages in stroke 19
  appearances of ischemic infarction 70–6
  compared with other imaging modalities *176*
  integrated stroke protocols 55, *56*
  limitations in stroke 19–20

practical application in acute stroke 5
sensitivity to early ischemia 20
T_1-weighted *see* T_1-weighted MRI
T_2-weighted *see* T_2-weighted MRI
see also intracranial hemorrhage (ICH): MRI; *specific MRI modalities*
magnetic resonance spectroscopy (MRS) 233–50
　chemical shift imaging 185–6, 233, 234
　clinical utility 185–6, *cp*
　data collection 233
　equipment 234
　ischemic penumbra 185–6, 200–1, *cp*
　long and short echo time data 236, 238, 240
　normal spectrum 64, *65*, 237
　　N-acetyl aspartate 240–1
　　choline 241
　　creatine 241
　　lipids/macromolecules 241
　nuclei applied 233
　outcome prediction 244–5, 247
　peaks in cerebral ischemia 241
　　N-acetyl aspartate 242
　　choline 242
　　creatine 242
　　glutamate/glutamine 243–4
　　lactate 241–2
　　lipids/macromolecules *239*, 244
　principles 63–4, 234–6
　quantification of metabolites 236, *237*, *238*, *239*
　reversible changes in metabolites 244
　selection of patients for treatment 247–8
　TIAs 137
　in understanding disability 245–6
　water suppression techniques 236
magnetic resonance venography (MRV) 79, *80*–1
magnetization transfer 167
magnetization transfer contrast (MTC) 76
mean transit time (MTT) 61, 152, 154
MELAS 244
methemoglobin, shortening effects of 57, 58
migrainous stroke 8
motor recovery poststroke, FMRI studies 254–5
moyamoya disease 95
MRA *see* magnetic resonance angiography (MRA)
MRI *see* magnetic resonance imaging (MRI)
MRS *see* magnetic resonance spectroscopy (MRS)
multiple sclerosis 244
multivoxel MRS *see* chemical shift imaging (CSI)

neural plasticity poststroke 254
Neurolite 22
neuroprotective drugs, MRI studies in animals 116–17, 118, *cp*
neurospectroscopy *see* magnetic resonance spectroscopy (MRS)
NINDS trial 4, *36*, 207

oxyhemoglobin 105

parallel imaging in MRA 98
parenchymal hemorrhage detection
　CT 31–2
　MRI 78
perfusion 61, 147
perfusion-based FMRI 252
perfusion-weighted MR imaging (PWI) 147–59, *cp*
　clinical utility 155–6, *158*, 179
　compared with other imaging modalities *176*
　contrast agents
　　endogenous 147–8, *see also* arterial spin labelling (ASL)
　　exogenous 61–2, 148–9
　　reasons for rapid bolus injection 152
　factors influencing lesion evolution 211–12
　image interpretation 154–6
　image postprocessing computations
　　deconvolution 154
　　mean transit time 152, 154
　　rCBF 152–4
　　rCBV 150–2
　infarct pathogenesis studies 182
　of ischemic penumbra 199, 211
　in patient selection for therapy 155, 183–5, *224*
　prognostic value 179–80
　pulse sequences 149–50
　raw images 150, *151*
　sample imaging parameters 150
　surrogate endpoint in drug trials 183, 214, 227–9
　thrombolytic therapy monitoring 212–13
　in a typical stroke protocol *56*
　see also animal stroke models: PWI studies; diffusion–perfusion (DWI/PWI) mismatch
phase contrast MRA 58–9, *75*, *76*, *78*, 86–8
phosphocreatine (PCr) measurement by MRS *237*, 241, 242
positron emission tomography (PET)
　advantages in stroke *24*
　compared with other imaging modalities *176*
　image acquisition 23–4
　ischemic penumbra *192*, 195–6, *197*, 208–9
　language recovery studies 255
　limitations in stroke *24*, 25
　measurements
　　CBF 24
　　CBV 24–5
　　cerebral glucose metabolism 25
　　cerebral oxygen metabolism 25
pregnancy, CT in 16
PROACT II trial *36*, 113, 224
proton density weighted images 58
proton magnetic resonance spectroscopy *see* magnetic resonance spectroscopy (MRS)
proUrokinase
　evaluation in rats 117–18
　see also PROACT II trial
pulsed magnetic field gradient technique 59–60
PWI *see* perfusion-weighted MR imaging (PWI)

randomized stroke trials, design problems 1–2
reperfusion injury, DWI studies in animal models 114–15
RS-87476 116
rt-PA (tissue plasminogen activator) *see* thrombolytic therapy

short tau inversion recovery (STIR) imaging 57–8
single photon emission computed tomography (SPECT)
　advantages in stroke *21*, 22–3, 177, *cps*
　compared with other imaging modalities *176*
　image acquisition 21–2
　ischemic penumbra studies *192*, 196, *197*
　limitations *21*, 23, 177, *cp*
　qualitative 22
　radiolabelled tracers 22
　semiquantitative 22
spin echo sequences in PWI 149
spin-lattice relaxation time (T1) 55, 148
spiral imaging in MRA 97
spreading depression *194*, 195
steady-state free precession (SSFP) techniques 97
Stejskal–Tanner (ST) technique 59–60
STIR (short tau inversion recovery) imaging 57–8
stroke
　determination of prognosis 9
　diagnosis
　　cerebral venous thrombosis 4
　　hemorrhagic stroke 4
　　importance in patient management 9–10
　　initial step 3
　　ischemic stroke *see* ischemic stroke diagnosis
　multiple possible causes 8–9
　new therapies 2
　pathology of ischemic infarction 69
　risk factors 8
　subtype classifications 2–3
　term 1
　see also ischemic stroke management
stroke drug development 223–31
　factors affecting clinical efficacy 225–6
　rational approach 17
　stroke trials
　　design issues, MRI-based trials *230*
　　ongoing *230*
　　positive trials to date 113, *see also specific trials*
　traditional approach 223, *224*
　use of animal models *see* animal stroke models
　use of MRI
　　marker of therapeutic response 225–7
　　outcome measure *225*
　　patient selection 224–5
　　phase II trials 227
　　surrogate marker in phase III trials 183, 214, 227–9
stroke MRI protocols 55, *56*
Stroke Therapy Ancrod Trial (STAT) 113

subarachnoid hemorrhage (SAH)
    CT 32, 108
    MRI 20, 70, 108
    Xe CT 51
surrogate endpoints 183, 214, 227–9

T_1-weighted MRI 55, 57–8, 70–6, 148
T_2-shine-through effect 122
T_2-weighted MRI 57, 58, 69–70, 70–5
    see also fluid-attenuated inversion recovery (FLAIR) imaging
T_2^* 4, 62, 235
^{105}technetium ethyl cysteinate dimer 22
^{105}technetium hexamethylpropyleneamine oxime (105Tc-HMPAO) 22
thrombolytic therapy
    clinical trials 4, 40–3, 184, 207–9, 224
        future 214–9
    monitoring by DWI/PWI 212–13
        in animals 117–18
    MRS studies of ischemic regions 248
    patient selection
        by DWI/PWI 155–6, 183–5, 200, 224–5
        limitations of CT 17–18
        limitations of standard MRI 20
    response related to baseline CT, ECASS findings 40–3

thrombosis in stroke pathogenesis 7
TIAs see transient ischemic attacks (TIAs)
time of flight (TOF) MRA 58, 59, 76, 85–6, 87, 89, 91
tissue plasminogen activator (rt-PA) see thrombolytic therapy
TOAST stroke classification system 2, 3
TOF MRA see time of flight (TOF) MRA
transcranial Doppler (TCD) 51, 93–4
transient ischemic attacks (TIAs)
    definitions
        conventional 135, 142
        new (tissue-based) 143
        research 143
        time-based 142–3
    diffusion MRI studies 137–42
        clinical utility 141–2
        pathophysiological insights 141
        prognostic value 142
    standard MRI studies 136
    tissue patterns on MRI 135
transverse relaxation time (T_2) 58

validation of MRI as a surrogate marker 228–9
variable projection method (VARPRO) 236, 238

vascular malformation, evaluation by MRA 96–7
vasogenic edema 69
vasospasm 51
velocity-encoding sensitivity (VENC) 86–7
venous infarcts 79
vertebral artery dissections 92, 93
Virchow–Robin spaces 79, 81
visual recovery poststroke, FMRI studies 256
voxels 253

water suppression techniques (MRS) 236

X-ray angiography (XRA) 85, 89, 98
xenon enhanced CT (Xe CT)
    advantages 47–8
    clinical applications 48
        acute stroke 48–9, cps
        chronic cerebral ischemia 49–50
        intracerebral hemorrhage 50–1
        subarachnoid hemorrhage 51
        vasospasm 51
    ischemic penumbra studies 192, 196, 197
    principle 47
    technical problems 48

ZD9379 117